RECENT ADVANCES IN PHARMACOLOGY

THIRD EDITION

by

J. M. ROBSON

M.D., D.Sc., F.R.S.E.

Professor of Pharmacology, University of London,
Guy's Hospital Medical School

and

R. S. STACEY

M.A., M.D.

Professor of Pharmacology and Therapeutics, University
of London, St. Thomas's Hospital Medical School

With 68 Illustrations

J. & A. CHURCHILL LTD

104 Gloucester Place, London, W.1

1962

First Edition (Robson & Keele) 1950
Reprinted   1951
Second Edition (Robson & Keele) 1956
Third Edition (Robson & Stacey) 1962

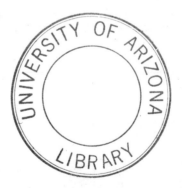
Printed in Great Britain

PREFACE

We have called this the third edition of *Recent Advances in Pharmacology* as there have been two previous editions. In fact, it is a completely new book, necessitated by the rapid progress in the subject. This has also made it impossible for two authors to present a reasonably up-to-date account of all subjects to be covered and we have been fortunate in enlisting the co-operation of a number of experts in various fields who have, occasionally with some prompting, quite rapidly prepared their manuscripts.

The chapters they have written are indicated in the Table of Contents. In addition, in Chapter 2, the section on the Clinical Use of Psychotropic Drugs was contributed by Dr. C. M. B. Pare and that on Experimental Methods in Psychopharmacology by Dr. Hannah Steinberg. We are sorry not to have had the collaboration on this occasion of Professor Keele who has been occupied in producing the new edition of Samson Wright's *Applied Physiology*. Indicative of a trend in the subject is the fact that some of our co-authors are clinicians actively engaged in the study of human pharmacology.

As in the past, we have tried to present pharmacology as a science covering all aspects of the action of drugs, from the study of their basic mechanism of action to their use in the treatment of disease and this has been our aim in selecting the topics discussed and the approach to them. We are well aware that there has perforce had to be selection and that we may have left out aspects of the subject even more important than those we have chosen. In at least some cases, e.g. the significance of membranes and the chemotherapy of virus infections, to choose but two examples, we thought that the time was not yet ripe for a fruitful discussion.

We offer our thanks to those authors who have kindly allowed us to reproduce figures and photographs and to the Editors of the Journals in which these were published. We are grateful to Miss Tredgold of the Department of Medical Illustration at Guy's for her help and advice in the preparation of a number of figures, to Dr. W. Hewitt of the Department of Anatomy at St. Thomas's who greatly helped in disentangling many problems of anatomical nomenclature encountered in the preparation of Chapter 1 and we should like to express our appreciation of the untiring help which Mrs. S. Robson has given to the collection of the literature and of the constant helpful co-operation of Mr. J. A. Rivers of Messrs. J. & A. Churchill Ltd.

J. M. ROBSON
R. S. STACEY

CONTRIBUTORS

W. J. H. BUTTERFIELD, O.B.E., M.A., M.D., F.R.C.P.
Professor of Experimental Medicine, Guy's Hospital Medical School, London.

L. G. GOODWIN, M.B., B.S., B.Pharm., B.Sc.
Head, The Wellcome Laboratories of Tropical Medicine, London.

R. F. MAHLER, B.Sc., M.B., Ch.B., M.R.C.P.
Senior Lecturer in Experimental Medicine, Guy's Hospital Medical School, London.

M. D. MILNE, B.Sc., M.D., F.R.C.P.
Professor of Medicine, Westminster Hospital Medical School, London.

C. M. B. PARE, M.D., M.R.C.P., D.P.M.
Physician, Department of Psychological Medicine, St. Bartholomew's Hospital, London.

M. SCHACHTER, M.D., C.M., M.Sc.
Reader in Physiology, University College, London.

HANNAH STEINBERG, B.A., Ph.D.
Lecturer in Pharmacology, University College, London.

J. R. VANE, B.Sc., D.Phil.
Reader in Pharmacology, Institute of Basic Medical Sciences, Royal College of Surgeons, London.

CONTENTS

ACKNOWLEDGEMENTS

Permission to reproduce a number of the illustrations in this book has kindly been given by publishers and by the editors of journals. Their names are listed below:

Charles C. Thomas, Fig. 20; The McGraw - Hill Book Co., Fig. 29; The Editors of *American Journal of Medical Science*, Fig. 49; *Annales de l'Institut Pasteur*, Figs. 56 and 57; *A.M.A. Archives of Internal Medicine*, Figs. 41 and 47; *Biochemical Pharmacology*, Fig. 7; *British Medical Journal*, Figs. 43, 45, 51, 52 and 54; *British Journal of Pharmacology*, Figs. 59, 63 and 64; *Deutsche Medizinische Wochenschrift*, Fig. 8; *Diabetes*, Fig. 30; *Journal of the American Medical Association*, Fig. 46; *Journal of Anatomy*, Plate I; *Journal of Pharmacology and Experimental Therapeutics*, Figs. 3, 5 and 7; *The Lancet*, Figs. 44, 48 and 51; *Science*, Fig. 4; *Toxicology and Applied Pharmacology*, Fig. 42.

LIST OF FIGURES

CHAPTER 1

PHARMACOLOGICALLY ACTIVE SUBSTANCES IN THE CENTRAL NERVOUS SYSTEM

The substances discussed in this chapter are differentiated from the other chemical constituents of the central nervous system by having powerful pharmacological actions on other organs which enable them to be identified and estimated. This may appear an artificial differentiation more especially since, with one exception, the actions used for their estimation are exerted on muscle in organs, such as the intestine and uterus, and on the cardiovascular system; actions which appear to have little in common with any possible function they may have in the brain. It is indeed likely that other techniques will reveal other, equally active, substances there. However, acetylcholine, adrenaline, noradrenaline, 5-hydroxytryptamine, γ-aminobutyric acid and substance P all probably exert actions on receptors on cell membranes; this distinguishes them from many other substances present in nervous tissue and makes them possible candidates in the search for substances concerned in the transmission of impulses at synapses.

Because of the complexity of the central nervous system, the direct investigation of the action of drugs at central synapses is more difficult than at autonomic ganglia or at the neuromuscular junction; and an insight into the role of naturally occurring substances depends, therefore, as much on a knowledge of their synthesis, storage, distribution and inactivation, and on the distribution and properties of enzymes concerned in their metabolism, as on the effects caused by varying their local concentrations. In recent years considerable progress has been made in this direction and will be summarized here. Injection into the blood stream, which has been helpful in investigating the physiological functions of such substances as acetylcholine and adrenaline in peripheral tissues, is often of little value when applied to the central nervous system because injected material often fails to pass from the blood into cerebral tissues. This has been ascribed to the existence of a blood-brain barrier and has been the subject of a recent review (Dobbing, 1961). Other methods of varying the local concentration of substances in the brain have therefore to be used: intracerebral injection, iontophoresis, injection into the cerebral ventricles, the use of the metabolic precursors of the substances, or of drugs modifying their synthesis or inactivation. These latter, indirect, methods often cause multiple changes, and interpretation of the results presents complexities which may only much later be appreciated. In the face of these difficulties it is not surprising

Table 1

Distribution in brain of various substances and of enzymes concerned in their synthesis and inactivation

(Species) (Reference)	choline acetylase (dog) (1)	acetyl-choline (cat) (2)	acetylcholine esterase (dog) (3)	dopa-5HTP decarboxylase (dog, cat) (a) (b) (4)	5-HT (dog, cat) (a) (b) (5)	dopamine (dog) (6)	noradrenaline (dog) (7)	amine oxidase (dog) (8)	catechol O-methyl transferase (monkey) (9)	histamine (dog) (10)	glutamic decarboxylase (monkey) (11)	γ-aminobutyric acid (rat) (12)	substance P (dog, man) (a) (b) (13)
Cerebral hemispheres													
Cortex	—	—	—	— / 51	0·2 / —	0·08	—	819	0·65	—	—	2·0	4·8 / 4·8
Rhinencephalon													
Olfactory bulb	1·15	1·3	197	7 / —	0·4 / —	—	—	573	—	—	—	—	— / —
Olfactory tract	3·75	—	—	5 / 69[1]	0·9 / —	—	0·05	—	—	50	—	} 3·2	5·5 / —
Pyriform area (51)	3·75	—	466	16 / 930[1]	— / 1·6	—	0·12	926	—	—	—		29 / —
Hippocampus (Ammon's horn)	2·60	—	238	16 / 159	0·6 / —	0·13	0·04	1,176	0·60[6]	80	9·9	—	15 / —
Neopallium													
Motor area (4)	3·00	—	178	— / 81	— / —	—	0·18	—	0·58	70	13·3	—	19 / 43
Somaesthetic area (3)	—	—	150	— / 39	— / 0·7	—	0·19	—	—	70	18·4	—	— / 39
Visual area (17)	1·33	—	107	— / 51	— / 1·4	—	0·04	—	—	70	—	—	7 / —
Acoustic area (20, 36a)	—	—	162	— / 69	— / 0·4	—	0·05	—	—	—	—	—	— / —
Cingulate gyrus (23, 24)	—	—	203	— / 51	— / —	—	0·09	—	—	70	—	—	— / 85
Basal ganglia													
Amygdaloid body	10·00	7·0	—	18 / 291	2·1 / —	—	0·06	968	0·37	140	14·7	—	— / —
Corpus striatum	13·25	2·7	—	306 / 1,260	0·7 / 1·6	5·90	0·06	935	0·78	140	16·2	—	46 / 85
Caudate nucleus	—	—	3,936	— / —	— / —	1·63	0·08[5]	—	—	—	—	—	— / —
Lentiform nucleus	—	—	2,606	— / —	— / —	—	—	—	—	—	—	—	— / 64
Putamen	—	—	—	— / —	— / —	—	—	—	} 0·82	—	16·4	—	— / 112
Globus pallidus	—	—	—	— / —	— / —	—	—	—		—	33·4	—	— / 2
White matter													
Corpus callosum	—	0·6	16	} 4 / 120	— / —	—	} 0·08	} 466	0·82	<50	0·1	—	6 / —
Internal capsule	3·10	2·1	—		— / —	0·09	0·17[5]		—	—	—	0·6	— / —
Diencephalon													
Thalamus	—	3·0	409	38 / 400	0·6 / 0·4	—	0·08	940	—	220	13·2	3·5[9]	12·5 / 12
Lat. nuclei	—	—	—	— / —	— / —	—	0·24	—	—	260	—	—	8·4 / —
Med. nuclei	—	—	230	— / 660	— / —	—	0·07	—	—	140	—	—	11 / 5
Lat. geniculate bodies	2·60	—	316	8 / 99	— / —	—	0·13	844	—	270	6·5	—	— / 37
Med. geniculate bodies	3·20	1·9	323	7 / 129	— / —	—	1·03	—	—	8	—	—	— / 102
Hypothalamus	2·00	—	—	117 / 750	1·7 / 2·5	0·26	0·41	1,624	0·73	740	20·5	3·5[9]	70 / 34
Mamillary body	—	—	—	— / —	— / —	—	0·28[4]	—	—	340	—	—	— / —
Supra-optic region	—	—	—	— / 780	— / —	—	—	—	—	—	—	—	— / —
Neurohypophysis	—	—	50	— / 159	— / —	—	—	—	1·46	11,400	—	—	— / —

(Species) / (Reference)	choline acetylase (dog) (1)	acetyl-choline (cat) (2)	acetylcholine esterase (dog) (3)	dopa-5HTP decarboxylase (dog, cat) (a) (4)	(cat) (b) (4)	5-HT (dog) (a) (5)	(cat) (b) (5)	dopamine (dog) (6)	noradrenaline (dog) (7)	amine oxidase (dog) (8)	catechol O-methyl transferase (monkey) (9)	histamine (dog) (10)	glutamic decarboxylase (monkey) (11)	γ-aminobutyric acid (rat) (12)	substance P (dog) (a) (13)	(man) (b) (13)
Optic nerve	0·00	0·3	11	7	—	—	—	—	0·02	701	—	<50	0·1	—	6	—
Optic tract	—	—	86	98	51	—	—	—	—	842	—	—	—	—	—	—
Midbrain																
Central grey matter	2·30	1·6	932	—	648	1·0	—	0·2	0·37	—	—	220	—	—	68	119
Sup. colliculi	1·40	1·7	364	—	522	—	—	—	0·40	—	0·96	218	21	—	76	55
Inf. colliculi	—	—	452	—	201	—	—	—	0·16	—	—	200	—	—	20	141
Red nucleus	—	—	—	—	201	—	0·76	—	0·11	—	—	215	—	—	—	30
Substantia nigra	0·09	0·2	1,075	<9	540	<0·1	—	0·03	0·26	—	—	<50	9·7	1·6	—	699
Cerebellum	—	—	—	—	—	—	—	—	—	—	—	—	1·0	—	1·6	—
Peduncles	0·33	3·2	290	28	21	0·4	0·33[3]	0·10	0·07	930	0·34	<15	0·1	1·7	41	3
Pons	—	—	—	—	300	0·6	0·13	0·13	0·41[5]	936	0·79	—	11·1	—	—	3
Brain stem reticular formation	—	—	—	—	[2]	—	—	—	0·35	—	—	—	4·8	1·5	25	—
Medulla oblongata	—	1·6	—	—	—	—	—	—	0·37[5]	1,117	—	<25	0·28	—	6	4
Pyramids	—	0·2	82	32	219	—	—	—	0·06	—	—	—	—	—	110	37
N. gracilis and cuneatus	—	—	477	—	—	—	—	—	0·11	—	—	—	—	—	—	—
Olivary nuclei	—	—	—	—	—	—	—	—	—	—	—	—	—	—	—	—
Hypoglossal triangle	—	—	—	—	90	—	—	—	—	—	—	53	—	—	—	—
Area acoustica	—	—	—	—	—	—	—	—	0·39	—	—	>30	—	—	—	—
Area postrema	—	—	—	—	—	—	—	—	1·04	—	0·94	920	1·4	—	290	248
Ala cinerea	—	—	—	—	—	—	—	—	—	—	—	—	—	—	—	—
Spinal cord																
Grey matter	—	1·6	611	—	—	—	—	—	—	—	—	<40	—	—	29	—
White matter (post. columns)	—	3·0	36	—	—	—	—	—	—	—	0·65	—	—	—	68	—
Post. roots	0·01	0·04	34	—	—	—	—	—	0·01	—	—	—	—	—	27	—
Ant. roots	11·05	0·04	149	—	—	—	—	—	0·06	—	—	—	—	—	40	—
Peripheral nerves	—	15·02	—	—	—	—	—	—	—	—	—	—	—	—	6	—
Sympathetic ganglia	—	33·0	—	—	—	—	—	—	—	—	0·99	—	—	—	6·5	—

(1) mg. acetylcholine formed/g./hr. (Hebb & Silver, 1956). (2) μg./g. (MacIntosh, 1941). (3) μl CO_2 evolved/g./10 mins. with acetyl-β-methylcholine as substrate (Burgen and Chipman, 1951). (4a) μg. 5-HT formed/g./hr. (Bogdanski et al., 1957). (4b) μg. dopamine formed/g./3 hrs.; [1] olfactory tubercle; [2] reticular formation: midbrain 810, pontile 383, medullary 351 (Kuntzman et al., 1961). (5a) μg./g. (Bogdanski et al., 1957). (5b) μg./g.; [3] reticular formation: midbrain 2·6, pontile 381 (Kuntzman et al., 1961). (6) μg./g. (Carlsson, 1959). (7) μg./g.; [4] pre-optic region (Vogt, 1957); [5] (Carlsson, 1959). (8) μg. 5-HT destroyed/g./hr. (Bogdanski et al., 1957). (9) μ moles metanephrine formed/kg./90 mins.; [6] hippocampus: ventral 0·46, dorsal 0·70; [7] sciatic 0·62, vagus 0·97, splenic 0·46 (Axelrod et al., 1959). (10) ng./g.; [8] hypothalamus: dorsal 900, ventral 460 (Adam, 1961). (11) μg. GABA formed/kg./hr. (Lowe et al., 1958). (12) μM/g.; [9] thalamus and hypothalamus together (Berl and Waelsch, 1958). (13a) units/g. (Amin et al., 1954). (13b) units/g. (Zettler and Schlosser, 1955).

that despite the accumulation of a great bulk of work on pharmacologically active substances in the brain, the function of these substances is in most cases still unknown.

ACETYLCHOLINE

The discovery of the transmission of impulses across synapses in the peripheral nervous system by acetylcholine led Dale in 1936 to suggest very tentatively that acetylcholine might have a similar function at some central synapses. Shortly afterwards interest in this conception received a further impetus by the independent discovery by Quastel *et al.* (1936) and by Stedman and Stedman (1937) that brain homogenates are able to synthesize acetylcholine. The early work on this subject has been reviewed by Feldberg (1945, 1954, 1957) and the present account will be mainly concerned with work published in the last five years.

SYNTHESIS AND DISTRIBUTION

The concentration of acetylcholine in different parts of the central nervous system has been determined by MacIntosh (1941), and from the values recorded in Table 1 it is apparent that some parts contain considerable quantities and others very little. Feldberg and Vogt (1948) measured the rate of synthesis of acetylcholine by homogenates of brain and concluded that acetylcholine synthesis is virtually confined to certain areas.

The final step in the synthesis of acetylcholine is the acetylation of choline. This is accomplished by the transfer of an acetyl group from acetyl-coenzyme A to choline by choline acetylase (Fig. 1) and coenzyme A so liberated combines with more acetate. Synthesis is depressed

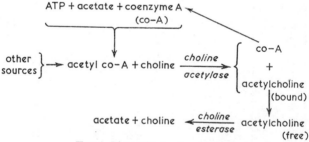

FIG. 1. Biosynthesis of acetylcholine.

by the administration of hemicholiniums (MacIntosh *et al.*, 1956) which probably interfere in the passage of choline into the neurones, where synthesis takes place. Under normal conditions adequate amounts of choline and coenzyme A are available in the brain, but in homogenates the rate of synthesis of acetylcholine will only give a measure of choline acetylase activity if an excess of the other components of the reaction is present. Hebb and Silver (1956) have found that the rate of acetylcholine synthesis can be much increased by the provision of acetyl-coenzyme A in addition to that initially there. They have re-examined the distribution of choline acetylase with this system and their results are given in Table 1. In effect they substantiate the earlier findings of Feldberg and Vogt on the localization of acetylcholine synthesis.

The highest concentrations of choline acetylase were found in the motor cortex, caudate nucleus, thalamus, medial and lateral geniculate bodies and the anterior spinal roots, while very low concentrations were found in the dorsal roots, optic nerves, cerebellum and cerebellar peduncles. The difference between these two groups of areas is even greater in the more recent estimations than in the earlier ones and this makes the explanation that they correspond respectively to areas containing preponderantly cholinergic neurones and non-cholinergic neurones even more likely. This view is now generally accepted and some progress has been made towards the classification of neurones: cholinergic neurones, like the preganglionic sympathetic neurones, transmitting impulses by the liberation of acetylcholine; non-cholinergic neurones, transmitting impulses by some other transmitter; and cholinoceptive neurones, like the postganglionic sympathetic neurones, which are activated by acetylcholine. The suggestion made by Feldberg and Vogt that there is evidence of an alternation of cholinergic and non-cholinergic (but cholinoceptive) neurones in some pathways, still appears likely. For example, in the retina and lateral geniculate body there are large amounts of choline acetylase while in the intervening part of the visual pathway, the optic nerve, there is little. Similarly, the anterior horns and roots contain much choline acetylase, which is to be expected as the lower motor neurone is known to be cholinergic, while the pyramidal tracts contain little, and are therefore presumably non-cholinergic. The motor cortex contains the cell bodies of these neurones and of the axons converging on them, and the intermediate concentration of choline acetylase in this region might then indicate that at any rate some of the latter are cholinergic, stimulating the non-cholinergic, upper motor neurones. That the latter are, in fact, cholinoceptive is supported by the result of the local application of acetylcholine and of eserine to the motor cortex: both cause an increase in activity in the pyramidal tracts. The Renshaw interneurones, occupying the ventro-medial part of the anterior horn, have been shown by Eccles *et al.* (1956) to be cholinoceptive. These neurones are stimulated by branches from lower motor neurones, and their axons end on anterior horn cells on which they have an inhibitory action. Repetitive firing of Renshaw cells was observed after the injection or local application (Curtis and Eccles, 1958) of acetylcholine and of anti-cholinesterases, and their activity was depressed by atropine and by dihydro-β-erythroidine, a drug which like atropine blocks the action of acetylcholine.

An insight into the intracellular distribution of acetylcholine and choline acetylase has been obtained by the high speed centrifugation of brain homogenates. Both are partly contained in the clear supernatant, but the larger part is found in a granular fraction containing mitochondria from which they can be separated by a sucrose gradient (Hebb and Whittaker, 1958; Whittaker, 1959). This is prepared by superimposing layers of sucrose solution of decreasing concentration on one another in a centrifuge tube. The fraction of the homogenate containing acetylcholine, choline acetylase and mitochondria was layered on top and centrifuged into the gradient and the contents of the layers subsequently analysed. Acetylcholine and choline acetylase were found together in the layer containing 0·8 to 1·0 M sucrose, while the mitochondria were in that containing 1·2 M sucrose. Mitochondria were identified by the presence of succinic dehydrogenase, recognized to be a mitochondrial enzyme elsewhere in the body, and by their heavy brown pigmentation.

Only part of the acetylcholine and choline acetylase in homogenates was in the free state, a much larger portion of both could be liberated by suitable treatment. For example part of each could be liberated by repeated freezing and thawing and about twice as much by treatment with ether. This suggested that the 'bound' part of each might be contained within a membrane and if this were so, since they were liberated by similar treatment, possibly both were contained within the same membrane. Work on cholinergic nerves in the peripheral nervous system and on sympathetic ganglia has led to the hypothesis that in these structures two forms of bound acetylcholine exist. This evidence is summarized by Birks and MacIntosh (1957) and will not be further discussed here, but the partial liberation of acetylcholine in brain homogenates by freezing and thawing and other mildly disruptive procedures may well also result from the presence of two forms of bound acetylcholine in the brain, one more easily liberated than the other.

The fraction of brain homogenate containing acetylcholine and choline acetylase also contains 5-hydroxytryptamine and this, like acetylcholine, is present partly in the free state and partly appears only after treatment with agents such as those used to liberate acetylcholine. With 5-HT too there is a graded release, less being released by the less violent forms of treatment.

De Robertis (1959, 1961) has described the *appearance of synapses*, as revealed by the electron microscope. In the mammalian central nervous system the synaptic surfaces are 1 to 5 μ in diameter and the membranes of the two neurones are thickened at these sites. Both pre- and post-synaptic membranes are about 60 Å thick and are separated

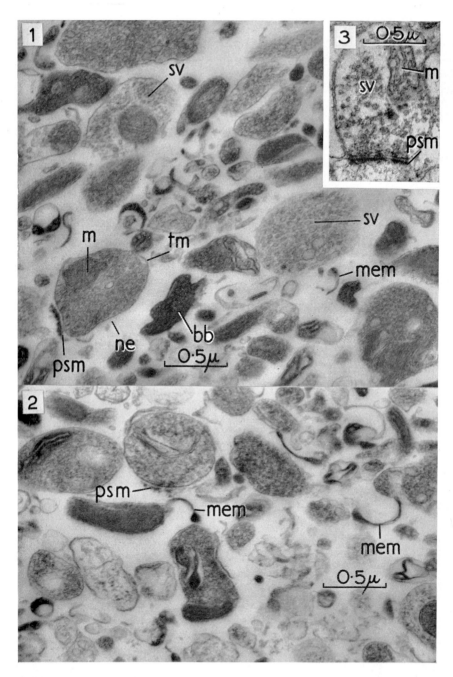

PLATE I Electron micrographs. (1, 2), Fraction of guinea-pig brain *homogenate* consisting
mainly of pinched-off nerve endings. (3) Section of *intact tissue* showing nerve ending
structures. Synaptic vesicles (sv); mitochondrion (m), within a thin outer membrane
(tm); post-synaptic membrane (psm) still adhering to the periphery. Isolated, horse-
shoe shaped membranes (mem) may be detached post-synaptic membranes. 'Black
bodies' (bb) are shrunken nerve-ending particles.

(Gray and Whittaker, 1962)

To face p. 7

by a space of 120 to 200 Å, the synaptic cleft, into which it is thought that the neurohormone is discharged. Eccles and Jaeger (1958) have discussed the microscopical appearance and dimensions of the synapse in relation to its electrical properties and have concluded that these fit well the purpose which it is thought to serve. In close proximity to the synapse, synaptic vesicles are to be seen. These are spherical or oval in shape, about 400 Å in diameter (range 200 to 650 Å) and with a dense membrane 40 to 50 Å thick. They are confined to the presynaptic side.

Examination with the electron microscope of the fraction of brain homogenate which contains the amines (Gray and Whittaker, 1960, 1962), revealed a structure (Plate I) already familiar from sections of the brain. Large bags, identified as pinched-off nerve endings, were seen and these contained smaller particles which had the same dimensions as synaptic vesicles. At places, attached to the larger bags, were thickened portions identifiable as presynaptic membranes. Thus acetylcholine and 5-HT are found in relation to structures known to be associated with the terminal parts of axons, and with a structure which has been identified as a synaptic site (Gray, 1959) but there is at present no direct evidence that transmitter substances are contained within the synaptic vesicles. Some smaller particles were also found and are still unidentified. More recently, using the same technique, Whittaker has found substance P associated with acetylcholine and 5-hydroxytryptamine in the same fraction.

Both acetyl- (or true) and non-specific (or pseudo-) cholinesterase are present in brain in considerable amounts, but the concentrations of the former are the higher. When brain homogenates are centrifuged acetylcholinesterase is found in all fractions, but Aldridge and Johnstone (1959) found the greatest concentration in particles which separate at a higher speed than mitochondria, and are distinct from them. Cholinesterase is more widely distributed than choline acetylase and some structures, like the cerebellum, are rich in it but have virtually no capacity for synthesizing acetylcholine.

The development of histochemical techniques has revealed a similar wide distribution in individual neurones. In known cholinergic neurones such as those of the hypoglossal nucleus and the Edinger-Westphal nucleus, which give origin to motor nerves and to presynaptic fibres of the parasympathetic system respectively, high concentrations of acetylcholinesterase are found; others contain practically none while still others contain intermediate amounts (Koelle, 1961). The concentration of acetylcholinesterase is thus less helpful in determining if a neurone is cholinergic than the concentration of choline acetylase (Hebb, 1961). Whether this wide distribution of cholinesterase serves to protect cholinoceptive neurones from acetylcholine not specifically liberated to stimulate them, whether in some neurones it is concerned with the destruction of acetylcholine set free as an intermediate step to the liberation of the actual transmitter, as suggested by Koelle (1961), or whether it has some other function unrelated to the destruction of acetylcholine, has still to be decided.

RELEASE OF ACETYLCHOLINE DURING CEREBRAL ACTIVITY

The amount of acetylcholine in the brain at different levels of cerebral activity has been estimated by a number of workers and it is now established that there is an inverse relationship. Crossland and Merrick (1954), for example, found that during both ether and barbiturate anaesthesia the amount of acetylcholine in mouse brain increased with increasing depth of anaesthesia. During convulsions the concentration fell to 55% below normal but after the convulsions had ended it took only 10 secs. to return to normal (Richter and Crossland, 1949). Synthesis *in vivo* is thus very rapid and the equilibrium between synthesis and destruction is displaced with changes in brain activity. To obtain these results the animals were killed and metabolism arrested suddenly by immersion in liquid air.

Further evidence of the association of activity with an increased turnover in acetylcholine has been obtained from experiments in which its release into perfusion fluids or C.S.F. has been measured. This can only be done in the presence of an anticholinesterase to prevent destruction. The stimulation of afferent nerves, asphyxia and the injection of adrenaline all cause an increased release of acetylcholine, and since both carbon dioxide and adrenaline are known to stimulate the reticular activating system, all three processes might be expected to lead to increased transmission in cerebral neurones. An ingenious method has been used by MacIntosh and Oborin (1953) to measure changing acetylcholine release. They found that when a small area of the cortex was covered by a little saline solution in a glass capsule, acetylcholine exuded into it and they measured the rate of exudation. During deep anaesthesia this was depressed and could be stopped altogether by undercutting the cortex and thus bringing electrical activity in this area to an end. Acetylcholine, released in the cerebrum of cats and sheep, has also been collected by Gaddum (1961) by means of his push-pull cannula. This consists of two fine concentric tubes, the inner a steel needle, the outer a thicker needle or a polythene tube. The tip is thrust into the tissue and Locke's solution run from a reservoir through the inner tube and, after washing the cells around the end of the cannula, escapes through the outer tube. It is collected and assayed on a suitable piece of plain muscle in a micro-bath, which has a capacity of 0·05 ml. (Gaddum and Szerb, 1961). By adapting the assay technique, other substances may be sought and the release of at least one other substance has been detected.

INJECTION OF ACETYLCHOLINE, ANTICHOLINESTERASES AND ATROPINE

The injection of acetylcholine and of anticholinesterases causes changes in the electrocorticogram which are best seen in preparations without anaesthesia in which the brain stem has been transected at the level of foramen magnum, that is in the *encéphale isolé* preparation described by Bremer; or in conscious animals with chronically implanted electrodes. When acetylcholine, eserine or dyflos is injected, the EEG becomes similar to that of an alerted animal, that is it consists of fast, unsynchronized low voltage waves (Fig. 2). However, according to

5 8/5O

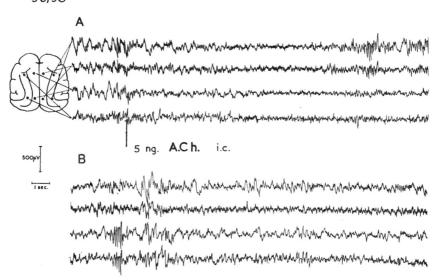

FIG. 2. Electrocorticogram of a cat (*encéphale isolé* preparation) showing (A) immediate effect of 5 ng. acetylcholine and (B) delayed effect of 5 μg. adrenaline. The adrenaline was injected 12 secs. before the beginning of (B). Both drugs were given by intracarotid injection. (Bradley, 1960.)

Bradley and Elkes (1957), after an intraperitoneal injection of eserine in a conscious cat there is a disparity between the behaviour of the animal, which is quiet and drowsy, and its EEG, which is alerted. The site of action of anticholinesterases for activation of the EEG has been studied by Desmedt and La Grutta (1955) and by Rinaldi and Himwich (1955). They found that activation occurs in preparations from which the reticular formation has been excluded by section of the brain stem above it, but not when connections between the thalamus and cortex are severed.

Large doses of dyflos cause epileptiform convulsions. The injection of atropine abolishes both the alerting reaction and the epileptiform discharge and if given alone, high amplitude slow waves appear, like those recorded during sleep, although the animals may show no signs of drowsiness.

The injection of acetylcholine or of an anticholinesterase into the cerebral ventricle of a cat causes ultimately the development of a catatonic state. Feldberg (1957) records three stages in the changes following the injection of dyflos. During the first stage there is intense and frequent scratching of the head and face which appeared to be due to severe itching; in the second, increased tone and reflex excitability of the leg muscles with quivering of the ears and head and in the last stage stupor and catatonia. Feldberg has suggested that some of the central effects of acetylcholine and anticholinesterases might be due to depolarization block, such as may be produced in the peripheral nervous system.

In conclusion, it may be said that recent work has accorded with the view that there are both cholinergic and cholinoceptive neurones in the central nervous system and that a tentative classification of a few of these may now be made but that the evidence for cholinergic transmission at any central synapse still falls short of that for the autonomic ganglion and the neuromuscular junction.

CATECHOL AMINES AND 5-HYDROXYTRYPTAMINE

These substances will be discussed together because their synthesis, inactivation, storage and distribution have much in common and are best described by comparison and contrast. Moreover, drugs which modify the concentrations of catechol amines often modify similarly those of 5-hydroxytryptamine.

The presence of adrenaline and noradrenaline in the brain was demonstrated first by Euler (1946) and later by Holtz (1950) who showed, by parallel bioassay on two test tissues, that brain sympathin is preponderantly noradrenaline. It was already known that this substance is present in some sympathetic nerves and it seemed at first possible that the small amounts in whole brain extracts came from the vasomotor nerves in brain and not from the brain substance itself. When the distribution of noradrenaline was worked out by Vogt (1954) it became apparent that in some parts of the brain the concentration was too high to be explained in this way, and the possibility arose that it might play a part in some cerebral neurones analogous to the part it plays in adrenergic nerves.

Amin, Crawford and Gaddum (1954) first found 5-hydroxytryptamine in brain in the course of experiments planned to determine the distribution of substance P (*v. infra*). They found that the guinea pig ileum and rat uterus used for the assay of substance P also contracted to another substance in brain extracts, and in a paper which provides a classical example of work of this kind they showed that the second substance was 5-hydroxytryptamine.

THE SYNTHESIS, METABOLISM AND STORAGE OF
CATECHOL AMINES AND 5-HYDROXYTRYPTAMINE IN THE BRAIN

The catechol amines found in the brain are dopamine (3, 4-dihydroxy-phenylethylamine), noradrenaline, and adrenaline; their synthesis and metabolism is described in Chapter 3 (page 98). Here only those aspects of special significance in the brain will be discussed.

Considerable amounts of dopamine and noradrenaline are found in mammalian brain and they are present in roughly equal amounts. There is much less adrenaline; the amount in different parts of dog brain varying from 6 to 30% (mean 15%) of the amount of noradrenaline (Vogt, 1957); in cat brain the proportion of adrenaline is about half this.

The *synthesis* of catechol amines is shown diagrammatically in Fig. 10 (page 98). It will be seen that the immediate precursor of dopamine is dihydroxyphenylalanine (dopa). The decarboxylation of this amino-acid with the formation of dopamine is definitely known to occur in the brain, and it is highly probable that the next step, the formation of noradrenaline from dopamine, also takes place there, but the capacity for dopamine synthesis appears to be far in excess of that required for noradrenaline formation.

The amount of 5-HT in brain is about the same as that of dopamine and noradrenaline and it too is formed in the brain by the decarboxyla-tion of an amino-acid, in this case 5-hydroxytryptophan (5-HTP) (see Fig. 13 page 126). The enzyme concerned in this change is the same as that decarboxylating dopa. Whether the brain is able to synthesize 5-HTP from tryptophan is not yet certain but from the results of Cooper and Melcer (1961) it seems possible that it may be dependent on supplies of 5-HTP reaching it from the small intestine (p. 126).

The decarboxylating enzyme is intracellular and is found in the cell sap. It is therefore probable that dopamine and 5-HT are synthe-sized within the cells in which they are subsequently stored; this is the more likely as they do not easily penetrate the blood brain barrier whereas the amino-acids, which are their precursors, pass through readily.

The *metabolism* of the catechol amines has been thoroughly investi-gated in recent years and is complex (see p. 103). The two most important mechanisms are the oxidative deamination of the side chain by amine oxidase and O-methylation by catechol-O-methyl transferase with the formation of the 3-methoxy derivative. The distribution of these enzymes is given in Table 1. While the amine oxidase activity of some parts of the brain is high compared with other tissues, the liver has nearly 10 times as much catechol-O-methyl transferase as the neurohypophysis, which contains more than any other neural tissue. O-methylation, and also the methylation of noradrenaline to adrenaline, is dependent on the presence of the co-enzyme, S-adenosyl methionine as a source of active methyl groups. Axelrod *et al.* (1959) have shown that the brain is able to synthesize this substance from adenosine triphosphate and methionine. Thus the brain is fitted to inactivate catechol amines by O-methylation but probably less well so than the liver. At present there is insufficient information to be dogmatic but, of the two inactivation reactions, oxidative deamination is probably the more important for dopamine, which is a better substrate than noradrenaline for amine oxidase, while O-methylation may be the more important for noradrenaline. However, Crout *et al.* (1961) found that in rats inhibition of amine oxidase caused a rise in brain noradrenaline, whereas inhibition of O-methyl transferase did not. Several other metabolic pathways exist for both substances and some lead to the formation of substances with pharmacological activity; so that the possibility that local concentrations of quite small amounts of active metabolites might lead to modification of cerebral function, must be kept in mind.

Amine oxidase readily oxidizes 5-HT (p. 128) and is probably the main means of inactivation of this substance in brain. Its distribution has been thoroughly investigated; that of catechol-O-methyl transferase, whose importance has only recently been discovered, much less so. Both enzymes are widely and comparatively uniformly distributed (see Table 1); the relative activity of the most active and least active parts of the brain being about 3 to 1. The wide distribution of these inactivating enzymes is similar to that of cholinesterase and it probably serves the same purpose, i.e. the protection of sensitive receptors from the action of circulating or diffusing active substances.

The *storage* of noradrenaline in rat brain has been studied by Green and Sawyer (1960). They separated rat brain homogenates in the ultracentrifuge into a clear supernatant and a sediment, and found an equal distribution of the amine between the two. Similar results were obtained by Weil-Malherbe and Bone (1959) in rabbit brain, while Bertler, Hillarp and Rosengren (1960), also working with rabbit brain, found about 70% bound. In peripheral nerves Euler and Hillarp (1956) found that part of the noradrenaline is contained in granules, from which it can be released by the action of acids and hypotonic solutions, and Euler (1957) has suggested that it may be bound to lecithin. Most of the 5-HT in the brain is also stored in intracellular particles, which are found in the same fraction as mitochondria after centrifugation of homogenates but can be separated from the mitochondria by a sucrose gradient (Whittaker, 1959). Reference to this work is made on page 6. During the preparation and fractionation of homogenates some liberation of bound amines is likely to occur so that, while it is clear that they are largely bound to intracellular particles, it is not yet certain what proportion, if any, is free in the cell sap.

Some progress has also been made in establishing the intra-cellular location of the synthesizing and inactivating enzymes. Dopa decarboxylase is found entirely in the supernatant of centrifuged brain homogenates (Blaschko *et al.*, 1955) and is therefore probably contained in the cytoplasm. O-methyl transferase is also a soluble enzyme (Axelrod, 1959) but according to Weiner (1960) amine oxidase is contained entirely in particles. These separate on centrifugation in the same fraction as mitochondria but, from observations on other organs, are probably distinct from them (Baker, 1959). In being particulate amine oxidase resembles, therefore, acetylcholinesterase (p. 7).

One function of inactivating enzymes is, no doubt, to remove an amine released during physiological processes when its function has been served. Spector *et al.* (1960) have suggested that if they are located within cells where amine synthesis is proceeding, they may also serve to maintain amine storage at a suitable level and prevent overflow from the cell on to receptor sites. Inhibition of amine oxidase upsets this balance: in the absence of normal destruction, it is probable that synthesized amines are stored until the sites are saturated and then escape from the cells and cause pharmacological effects.

DISTRIBUTION OF CATECHOL AMINES AND 5-HYDROXYTRYPTAMINE IN THE BRAIN

Reference to Table 1 reveals at once considerable variations in the concentrations of all three amines in different parts of the brain; high concentrations being 10 or 100 times low concentrations. When the distribution of the two catechol amines, noradrenaline and dopamine, is compared it is seen that there are similarities, but also striking differences. The highest concentrations of noradrenaline are in the hypothalamus but there are considerable amounts in the mid-brain, around the aqueduct, in the reticular formation, in the medial thalamic nuclei and even in some parts of the cortex. The quantities in these areas are much too great to be accounted for by the presence of adrenergic vasomotor fibres, but in those where there is less than 0·04 μg. noradrenaline/g., a large part may have this origin. Those parts of the brain, which when stimulated electrically (Ransom and Magoun, 1939), or by drugs (p. 25), give a generalized sympathetic discharge contain much noradrenaline.

There are large amounts of dopamine in the mid-brain, hypothalamus and pons but by far the highest concentration is in the caudate nucleus, which contains little noradrenaline.

The brain stem also contains high concentrations of 5-HT; the amygdala, hypothalamus and mid-brain being the richest parts. The cerebellum has little of any of these three amines.

The distribution of the synthesizing enzyme shows a general similarity. The concentration of 5-HTP decarboxylase (probably identical with dopa decarboxylase) is greatest in the caudate nucleus, hypothalamus and mid-brain with somewhat less in the thalamus, medulla and pons. In the auditory (cochlear nuclei, inferior colliculus, medial geniculates and acoustic cortex) and visual (optic nerve, superior colliculus, lateral geniculates and visual cortex) pathways there is little, and the cerebral cortex and cerebellum have virtually none.

No conclusions can be drawn at present about the function of the amines from these data. There is still much important information lacking: we have no knowledge, for example, of the distribution of noradrenaline synthesizing sites, nor do we know if dopamine has any function apart from that of a precursor of noradrenaline. Finally it must always be born in mind that comparisons of rates of synthesis are made on homogenized tissues and these may have little relation to the relative rates of synthesis *in vivo*, where differences in the concentration of substrates and of co-enzyme, as well as other factors, may considerably modify rates of synthesis.

ACTION OF ADRENALINE AND NORADRENALINE ON THE CENTRAL NERVOUS SYSTEM

The action of adrenaline and noradrenaline on peripheral autonomic synapses has been the subject of much work and the results obtained do not present a clear picture. It is not therefore surprising that in the central nervous system the position is in many respects confused; here, only some of the more important results can be summarized. Rothballer (1959) has recently reviewed this subject.

That the interpretation of the central effects of adrenaline and noradrenaline is complicated by their vascular actions, which cause changes in blood pressure and cerebral blood flow, has long been appreciated. More recently attention has been drawn (Bonvallet *et al.*, 1954) to an indirect action brought about by stimulation of the baroreceptors. Partly as a result of their pressor action, but also because of their action in sensitizing the carotid sinus by contracting smooth muscle fibres in it, adrenaline and noradrenaline reflexly depress the reticular activating system, causing deactivation of the EEG and inhibition of spinal motor mechanisms. A fall in blood pressure has the reverse effect. This action is thus analogous to the depression and stimulation of the vasomotor centre brought about by changes in blood pressure and, unless precautions are taken, it will complicate experiments designed to reveal direct actions on the central nervous system and confuse their interpretation.

The action on the brain of amines injected into the blood stream will be contingent on their passage through the blood-brain barrier, unless there are special receptors in the walls of the blood vessels. Of these there is at present no evidence. A number of observations have been made which indicate that adrenaline passes only with difficulty if at all from the blood into the brain. Raab and Gigee (1951) found no increase in brain adrenaline or noradrenaline after intravenous infusion of these substances in rats, and Schayer (1951) found little radio-activity in the brain of rats after infusion of ^{14}C labelled adrenaline, although considerable radio-activity was found in liver and kidney, and Axelrod, Weil-Malherbe and Tomchick (1959) using tritium labelled adrenaline found that small amounts will pass from the blood stream into the hypothalamus but not into other parts of the brain. Brodie *et al.* (1960b) have used infusions of sulphaguanidine and N-acetyl-aminoantipyrin, to investigate the blood-brain barrier. They found that certain areas— both lobes of the pituitary gland, the area postrema and the intercolumnar tubercle—absorb these substances and can be regarded therefore as being outside the blood-brain barrier, while the cortex and hypothalamus do not and are therefore inside the barrier. In the light of this evidence a general penetration of appreciable amounts of adrenaline into the brain seems unlikely.

The blood-CSF barrier is also resistant to the passage of adrenaline and noradrenaline, for it has been shown that injection of these substances into the cerebral ventricles, into the cisterna magna and by lumbar puncture into the subarachnoid space does not cause a rise in blood pressure if blood vessels are undamaged, and that the injected amine is still to be found in the CSF after many hours. In view of these findings the effects of adrenaline and noradrenaline described below, and apparently exerted directly on the brain after injection either into the blood stream or into the CSF, are the more remarkable. Penetration of the CSF-brain barrier probably explains those following the intraventricular injection of large doses, but the possibility that adrenaline and noradrenaline in the blood stream exert effects by acting at special sites where sensitive tissue is accessible to them without passing generally into the brain, must be kept in mind.

Intravenous injection of adrenaline into an unanaesthetized but sleeping cat results in the waking of the animal. Large doses of adrenaline or noradrenaline whether given by intravenous injection, by injection into the carotid artery, into a cerebral ventricle or into the cisterna magna cause the gradual development over 10 to 15 minutes of a stuperous condition. Feldberg and Sherwood (1955) found that 20 to 100 µg. of either adrenaline or noradrenaline injected into the lateral ventricle of a cat was followed in a few minutes by a state similar to light anaesthesia. The animal could be lifted and turned without struggling and when pricked, reacted slowly or not at all. The effect wore off after about $\frac{1}{2}$ hour. Animals rendered unconscious in this way however have a desynchronized EEG (Rothballer, 1959), that is to say, it is that of an alerted animal.

In 1954 Dell and his colleagues described the alerting by adrenaline of the EEG of the cat. To show this effect it is necessary that the animal should not be anaesthetized but that the EEG should be deactivated. This can be achieved by using a curarized animal, free from all discomfort and distraction; or by section of the brain stem. The intravenous injection of 2 to 8 µg. adrenaline/kg. body weight was followed after about 15 seconds by activation (desynchronization) of the EEG. Section of the brain stem at successively higher levels showed that the action was not affected by removal of the spinal cord and brain stem below the level of the 5th cranial nerve, but was lost when section reached the posterior level of the diencephalon. Electrical stimulation and the injection of adrenaline into the brain-stem reticular formation caused similar results. Noradrenaline and adrenaline both cause desynchronization and appear to be equally active. Dell *et al.* (1954) have also shown that adrenaline affects the descending reticulo-spinal system causing facilitation of mono- and poly-synaptic reflexes. Both ascending and descending actions are easily abolished by barbiturates. The sensitivity of the reticular formation to catechol amines is especially interesting when it is remembered that this region is particularly rich in noradrenaline, but there is at present no evidence as to the physiological function of the noradrenaline naturally present there.

Adrenaline has a number of other actions on the brain, which cannot here be discussed in detail; the evidence for these is given in Rothballer's review.

In large doses it causes changes in the transmission of impulses and in the excitability of the cortex, the significance of which is uncertain. Intravenous injection will block the release of antidiuretic hormone from the pituitary, provoked by an intravenous injection of acetylcholine; injected into the mamillary bodies it depresses the release of thyroxine from the thyroid gland, presumably by depressing the secretion of thyrotroptic hormone, and injection into the third ventricle in the rabbit can cause ovulation. The way in which these effects are caused is still quite unknown.

Intravenous infusion of adrenaline in man produce feelings of excitement, expectancy, apprehension and anxiety. There is an increase in rate and depth of respiration, palpitations and a coarse tremor of the extremities (Barcroft and Swan, 1953; Basowitz *et al.*, 1956). The symptoms following an infusion of noradrenaline are much less marked. Adrenaline increases Parkinsonian rigidity and tremor. It is probable that these effects are due to a central action but how much the emotional reaction to adrenaline is an indirect one, the result of palpitations and tachypnoea, cannot at present be decided. If it is central then it must be concluded that adrenaline has some central actions which noradrenaline does not have, although they are similar in their actions on the reticular formation.

ACTION OF 5-HT ON THE CNS

The blood-brain barrier is very resistant to penetration by 5-HT, as it is to catechol amines. For this reason large doses need to be given before any effect on the CNS is observed, and these doses produce violent effects on the cardiovascular system. Given intraperitoneally in mice, which are relatively insensitive to the vascular action, 5-HT is sedative in action, and Marrazzi (1957) found it to be more active than adrenaline in depressing transcallosal cortical responses, which he interprets as a depression of synaptic transmission. On the other hand the electro-corticogram is desynchronized, thus resembling that of an alerted animal. Using electrodes placed deep in the brain of cats, Vogt *et al.* (1957) found however that, while there is evidence of activation of the cortex and reticular formation, electrical activity in the medial hypo-thalamic and thalamic nuclei is depressed.

Failure to penetrate the blood-brain barrier has been circumvented by Curtis and Davis (1961) by the electrophoretic application of 5-HT and some related substances to single neurones, through an electrode inserted into the lateral geniculate body. They found the transmission of impulses, evoked by stimulation of the optic nerve, was depressed, and suggested that depression of excitatory receptors on the neurone was the most likely explanation of this action. Another approach has been used by Feldberg and Sherwood (1954) and Domer and Feldberg (1960), who injected 5-HT through a cannula implanted through the skull of a cat and leading into a lateral ventricle. An animal treated in this way develops a tremor, tends to lie down and to be unwilling to move about; if forced to do so it appears to suffer from muscular weak-ness and its movements are awkward and clumsy. It tends to remain in positions in which it is put; that is it is catatonic but not sleepy or drowsy.

SUBSTANCES CHANGING THE CONCENTRATION OF CATECHOLAMINES AND OF 5-HT IN THE BRAIN

Dopa and 5-hydroxytryptophan

The amino-acids dopa and 5-hydroxytryptophan penetrate the blood-brain barrier much more readily than the corresponding amines and with them a considerable rise in the concentration of dopamine and 5-HT respectively in the brain can be achieved. Bertler and Rosengren (1959) found that after the administration of dopa to rabbits the greatest increase in concentration of dopamine was in the caudate nucleus, and was associated with an increase in motor activity. No change in the concentrations of adrenaline or of noradrenaline occurred. The rise in brain 5-HT which follows the administration of 5-HTP is associated with evidence of stimulation of cerebral centres. The animals develop excitement, tremors, ataxia, hyperthermia, pupillary dilatation, piloerection, tachycardia and increased salivation (Udenfriend, Weissbach and Bogdanski, 1957). These effects are enhanced by pretreatment with iproniazid.

Inhibitors of dopa and 5-HTP decarboxylase

A number of substances which inhibit the decarboxylation of dopa and 5-HTP *in vitro* are known (p. 128) but little work has been done with them *in vivo*. The concentration of dopamine, noradrenaline and 5-HT in brains of experimental animals is depressed by α-methyldopa, but probably this is not entirely due to decarboxylase inhibition and release of noradrenaline from binding sites (Hess *et al.*, 1961), and possibly other actions, are involved. Smith (1960) has shown that mice become sedated and hypothermic and that there is narrowing of the palpebral fissure and constriction of the pupil. In man there is a fall in blood pressure. The relation of these changes to amine depletion needs further investigation.

Pyridoxal deficiency causes a fall in the amount of 5-HT in the brain, intestine, liver and blood of chicks (Weissbach *et al.*, 1959) and rats (Yeh *et al.*, 1959). This is due to the necessity for pyridoxal phosphate as a co-enzyme in the decarboxylation of 5-HTP. It must be remembered, however, that there are a number of other pyridoxal dependent reactions which may also be affected in pyridoxal deficiency and which may be partly responsible for the neurological changes in this condition.

Inhibitors of amine oxidase

The first potent amine oxidase inhibitor to be used was iproniazid. It was prepared in 1951 as a variant of isoniazid, and while being used in the chemotherapy of tuberculosis it was noticed that there was often an improvement in the mood of patients given it. At the same time inhibition of amine oxidase by iproniazid *in vitro* was reported by Zeller and Barsky (see Zeller *et al.*, 1955). Subsequent work on amine oxidase inhibitors has followed two main directions: (a) their pharmacological effects and their relationship to changes in the metabolism and tissue concentrations of catechol amines and 5-hydroxytryptamine and (b) their clinical evaluation in the treatment of depressive states. It was at first assumed that the therapeutic effect of iproniazid is due to inhibition of amine oxidase and in recent years a number of other inhibitors have been synthesized. Many of these are hydrazides and are closely related to iproniazid chemically, but a number of non-hydrazide inhibitors are also known. The more important members of the group are classified in Table 5 (p. 58) and their structure given in Fig. 6 (p. 59). An account of their metabolism and properties will be found in Chapter 2 (p. 57).

Effect of amine oxidase inhibitors on the concentration of brain amines. After a single dose of iproniazid (100 mg./kg. body wt.) to rats, mice or

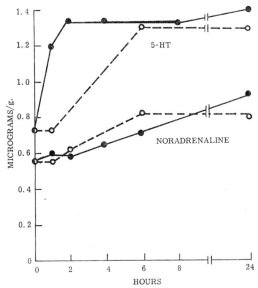

FIG. 3. Concentration of 5-HT and noradrenaline in rabbit brain stem after single subcutaneous doses of iproniazid o– – – –o (100 mg./kg.) and pheni-prazine ●——● (2 mg./kg.) (Spector *et al.*, 1960).

rabbits there is a rise in the brain concentration of dopamine, noradrena-line and 5-hydroxytryptamine (Holzer and Hornykiewicz, 1959; Spector *et al.*, 1960) but this rise differs both in speed and extent with the different amines (Fig. 3). The concentrations of dopamine and of 5-hydroxy-tryptamine rise most rapidly and reach values about double their initial

TABLE 2

Concentrations of catechol amines and of 5-HT in rat brain after iproniazid and harmine.
(Concentrations in µg./g. brain; the time in brackets is the interval between injection and estimation.)

	Dopamine[1]	Noradrenaline[2]	5-HT[2]
Control	0·66	0·4	0·4
After iproniazid (100 mg./kg. i.p.)	1·09 (16 hrs.)	0·8 (24 hrs.)	1·30 (24 hrs.)
After harmine (30 mg./kg. i.p.)	0·87 (½ hr.)		

[1] Holzer and Hornykiewicz (1959).   [2] Procop *et al.* (1959).

values six hours after the injection. The concentrations of noradrenaline increases more slowly and after the same interval is only about 25% above its initial value. Some results of estimations 16 to 24 hours after iproniazid are given in Table 2. Very similar changes are seen after injections of pheniprazine and JB 835, two other hydrazine amine oxidase inhibitors. With these substances, however, the rise in 5-hydroxytryptamine concentration is even more rapid than with iproniazid (Fig. 3). However, when the amine oxidase activity of brain homogenates of animals treated with these three drugs is estimated, it is found that with all there is almost complete inhibition shortly after the injection, indicating that although all are capable of reaching the substance of the brain rapidly, iproniazid is slower *in vivo* in inactivating amine oxidase than the others; presumably because there is an obstruction to its access to the enzyme and that this is removed during homogenization. This illustrates the fallacy of using the results of enzyme inhibition studies *in vitro* to assess the degree of inhibition of an enzyme *in vivo*.

On discontinuing daily injections of iproniazid, brain 5-hydroxytryptamine concentration may remain elevated for a fortnight or longer (Green and Erickson, 1960) but the brain noradrenaline concentration returns to normal in the course of a few days. This more rapid fall in noradrenaline may perhaps be due to its removal by another pathway. Iproniazid is quite quickly eliminated and Hess *et al.* (1958) found no trace in the tissue 24 hours after an intraperitoneal dose. The prolonged effect of iproniazid on the concentration of 5-hydroxytryptamine in the brain is therefore not due to persistence of the drug in the brain and suggests that its action results in the destruction of amine oxidase, resembling in this respect the action of the organic phosphorus anti-cholinesterases rather than eserine, and that recovery depends on re-synthesis of the enzyme. However, the recent observation that some amine oxidase inhibitors inhibit the release of noradrenaline from storage sites (Axelrod *et al.*, 1961), necessitates a reassessment of the mechanism by which these substances raise brain amine concentrations.

In the rat and rabbit the administration of a single large dose of pheniprazine causes excitement of sudden onset and short duration similar to that caused by amphetamine (Eltherington and Horita, 1960) of which this compound is the hydrazine analogue (p. 61). Smaller doses of iproniazid, pheniprazine and JB 835 have no effect on behaviour unless they are repeated daily; then, after 4 or 5 days the animal becomes hyperactive. This change appears some time after brain 5-hydroxytryptamine has reached a maximum and on discontinuing the drug is lost before an appreciable fall in brain 5-hydroxytryptamine has occurred. The period of excitement fits much more closely the changes in brain noradrenaline than brain 5-hydroxytryptamine concentration. This association is further seen with cats and dogs. In these species iproniazid and pheniprazine do not cause excitement and although there is a considerable rise in 5-hydroxytryptamine, brain noradrenaline is not raised (Spector *et al.*, 1960).

Since the hydrazine amine oxidase inhibitors affect a number of metabolic processes (p. 61) it is of importance to compare their actions with inhibitors of this enzyme which are chemically dissimilar. Harmaline (Udenfriend *et al.*, 1958) and tranylcypromine (Green and Erickson, 1960) are both considerably more potent than iproniazid when tested *in vitro* (p. 64). After both, brain 5-hydroxytryptamine and adrenaline concentrations rise more rapidly (Holzer and Hornykiewicz, 1959) but return to normal more rapidly also and with both there is evidence of cerebral stimulation, as there is also with α-methyl and α-ethyl tryptamine, which *in vitro* are comparable to iproniazid in potency (Greig *et al.*, 1959).

The availability of potent amine oxidase inhibitors makes it possible to estimate the rate of synthesis of 5-hydroxytryptamine if certain assumptions are made. If it is assumed that removal of 5-hydroxytryptamine from the brain is entirely due to amine oxidase, and that 100% inhibition of brain amine oxidase is achieved *in vivo*, then the rate of rise of brain 5-hydroxytryptamine concentration is equal to its rate of synthesis. By making the further assumptions that neither the inhibitor nor the elevation of brain 5-hydroxytryptamine affect the rate of 5-hydroxytryptamine synthesis, an estimate of the half life can be made. It is necessary to appreciate, however, that any or all of these assumptions may be found to be unjustified. Using pheniprazine and JB 835, Spector *et al.* (1960) reached a figure of 15 mins. for the half life of 5-hydroxytryptamine in the brain; this is in agreement with the conclusion previously reached by Udenfriend and Weissbach (1958) using harmaline. Holzer and Hornykiewicz (1959) concluded that the rate of turnover of dopamine in brain is of the same order as that of 5-hydroxytryptamine. While it is reasonable to suppose that the removal of a large proportion of both dopamine and 5-hydroxytryptamine can be blocked by amine oxidase inhibitors, this assumption could at present not be justified for noradrenaline, since much may be removed by catechol-O-methyl transferase. The slow rise in brain noradrenaline after amine oxidase inhibitors may partly be due to its metabolism along other pathways, but there is also reason to believe that the formation of noradrenaline from dopamine proceeds relatively slowly and this may also be partly responsible for these slow changes.

Reserpine

The administration of reserpine (formula p. 49) to an animal is followed by a release of catechol amines and of 5-HT from all storage sites throughout the body. That the brain participates in this has been

2

shown for dopamine by Carlsson (1959), for noradrenaline by Holzbauer and Vogt (1956) and for 5-HT by Pletscher, Shore and Brodie (1956). The loss is progressive over several hours (Fig. 4) and follows a similar course with respect to all three amines though dopamine is lost somewhat more rapidly than the others (Bertler, 1961). Depletion is prolonged and continues long after the disappearance from the tissue of all detectable reserpine and appears to be due to an impairment of the storage capacity of the brain for these amines. The rate of amine synthesis is unaffected. In most species tested (see below), if the animals are pre-treated with an amine oxidase inhibitor, the fall in amines is delayed until the action of the inhibitor has passed off (Spector *et al.*, 1960). From this it is concluded that after reserpine alone, the liberated amines are destroyed intracellularly, but that if amine oxidase is inhibited they are not destroyed, and because of their failure to pass the blood brain barrier, are not removed.

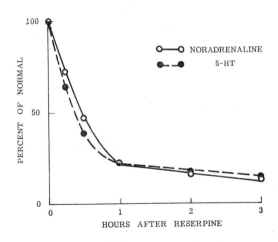

FIG. 4. Noradrenaline and 5-HT content of rabbit brain stem after the intravenous injection of reserpine (5 mg./kg.). (Shore *et al.*, 1957.)

After reserpine animals are sedated and hypothermic; there is narrowing of the palpebral fissure, relaxation of the nictitating membrane, constriction of the pupil, lachrymation and salivation; hypotension, bradycardia and diarrhoea. There are also behavioural changes which are described on p. 48.

The explanation of these effects is still very incomplete. Hypotension, bradycardia and relaxation of the nictitating membrane are probably the result of peripheral depletion of catechol amines (p. 23), and diarrhoea may be due in part to the action of liberated 5-HT on the intestine

(p. 133). The following evidence is in agreement with the view that miosis and salivation are the result of increased central parasympathetic activity. Bogdanski *et al.* (1961) found that miosis is unaffected by sympathetic section but prevented by parasympathetic section and by atropine; salivation is prevented by atropine and by general anaesthesia; both miosis and salivation are prevented by the previous administration of ganglion blocking agents. Parasympathetic stimulation reaches a maximum 2 to 6 hours after an intravenous injection of reserpine and then diminishes but the sedative effect is still marked after 24 hours. The relation of these centrally mediated effects to depletion of brain amines must now be considered.

Attempts have been made to obtain depletion of one amine, without appreciable changes in others, by the use of other rauwolffia alkaloids and of synthetic derivatives of reserpine. At present there is some disagreement as to the results of experiments of this kind. The subject is discussed by Brodie *et al.* (1960a) who have shown that the substance dimethylaminobenzoyl methylreserpate (Su 5171) can, in suitable

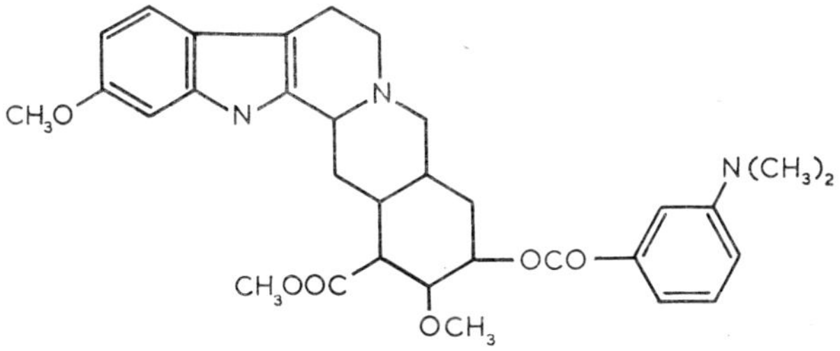

dimethylaminobenzoyl methylreserpate (Su 5171)

dosage, give a 50% reduction in the noradrenaline content of rabbit brain stem with only a slight reduction in its 5-HT content (Fig. 5). Animals so treated were not sedated though they had slight miosis. Brodie *et al.* (1960a) have also found that when reserpine is given to rats or rabbits which had been 'cold stressed' by being placed in a cold room at 4°C. for 4 hours, although there is a marked fall in brain noradrenaline concentration, there is little reduction in the amount of 5-HT in the brain. These animals also are not sedated and show no enhanced salivation though again there is some miosis. From these experiments it would appear that release of brain noradrenaline is not, by itself, associated with sedation though there is no positive evidence that release of brain 5-HT is associated with it. Should this be proved there will still remain the question as to whether the changes are brought about by a diminution of the stores or to local increase in concentration of unbound 5-HT, as has been suggested by Brodie *et al.* (1960a). The fact that α-methyldopa, a decarboxylase inhibitor, causes sedation, narrowing of the palpebral fissure and miosis (p. 128) would imply that if they are produced by the same mechanism, this would be by depletion of the stores, for it is unlikely that this substance could lead to an accumulation of unbound 5-HT.

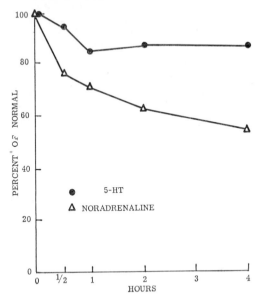

FIG. 5. Noradrenaline and 5-HT content of rabbit brain stem after the intravenous injection of dimethylaminobenzoyl methylreserpate (0·25 mg./kg.). (Brodie *et al.*, 1960.)

When rats and rabbits pretreated with iproniazid are given reserpine the results are quite different. Not only is the fall in brain amines much reduced, as has been mentioned above, but the animals become more active than normal and hyperthermic, their pupils become dilated and there is piloerection. How far these effects are due to excess free amines cannot be decided until there is reliable evidence of the relative amounts of bound and free amines under different conditions. In cats, iproniazid does not prevent the depletion of brain noradrenaline by reserpine and there is also no excitement or increased activity (Vogt, 1959).

Brodie, Shore and Pletscher (1956) compared the sedative action and amine releasing capacity of a number of substances related to reserpine and found that only those having a sedative action released amines.

Tetrabenazine and other synthetic benzoquinolizine derivatives (formula p. 50) were found by Pletscher (1957) to deplete the brain of noradrenaline and 5-HT. The action of tetrabenazine resembles that of reserpine but differs from it in certain important respects. Brain noradrenaline is more affected than brain 5-HT and recovery of both amines is more rapid. After a single intravenous dose of 50 mg./kg.,

Quinn *et al.* (1959) found that the noradrenaline content of rabbit brain reached a minimum of 15% in 4 hours but after 24 hours was 70% of the normal. This dose caused a maximum loss of only 50% brain 5-HT and after 24 hours it had returned to normal. Sedation is much less marked with tetrabenazine than with reserpine and this accords with the view discussed above that noradrenaline depletion is not the cause of sedation. That these two compounds act at the same receptors is suggested by the antagonism of tetrabenazine given immediately before reserpine to the sedative effects of this substance.

Tetrabenazine causes some depletion of noradrenaline in the adrenal medulla but little change in the concentration of catechol amines or of 5-HT in the peripheral tissues. In conformity with this, blood pressure is not appreciably lowered nor is there diarrhoea.

Other substances. Vogt (1959) found a group of drugs with diverse central actions which lowered hypothalamic noradrenaline in the cat and dog. This group contained ether, nicotine, picrotoxin, morphine, β-tetrahydronaphthylamine and insulin. On the other hand leptazole, caffeine, ephedrine and chlorpromazine caused no reduction. She pointed out that both groups contained both convulsants and cerebral depressants but that the group of active drugs contained members known to act on cerebral sympathetic centres; and she showed that drugs which deplete the hypothalamus of noradrenaline all cause sympathetic stimulation, measured by the discharge of catechol amines from the adrenal medulla. Drugs which fail to deplete the hypothalamus also fail to cause a sympathetic discharge. This suggests that the noradrenaline of the hypothalamus has a functional significance. It was also noticed that drugs depleting hypothalamic noradrenaline also depleted mesencephalic noradrenaline but did not change that of the area postrema. None of the above active drugs changed brain 5-HT. Amphetamine depleted dog brain of noradrenaline and, in much larger doses, of 5-HT also (Paasonen and Vogt, 1956).

A rise in the amount of 5-HT in the brain has been found by Bonnycastle *et al.* (1957) and Anderson and Bonnycastle (1960) after the administration to rats of barbiturates, ether and a variety of anticonvulsants belonging to several different chemical groups. Cerebral depression, as measured by the animals' activity and righting reflexes, preceded the rise in brain 5-HT concentration and it was therefore concluded that depression was not the result of the rise but might be the cause of it. These results recall those of Crossland and others, referred to on page 8, in which a reciprocal relationship between cerebral activity and acetylcholine concentration in the brain was found. No rise in the concentration of 5-HT in other organs was found nor did amine oxidase inhibitors, which also raise brain 5-HT concentration, protect rats from the convulsant effects of leptazole.

TRYPTAMINE

Tryptamine like 5-HT is a substrate for amine oxidase. It has been found in normal human urine (Rodnight, 1956) and, after the administration of amine oxidase inhibitors, in brain and other organs (Hess *et al.*, 1959). It is formed when homogenates of rat kidney are incubated with tryptophan (Weissbach *et al.*, 1959) which has itself been identified in brain (Price and West, 1960). The pharmacological actions of tryptamine are, in general, similar to those of 5-HT but considerably weaker, though they are powerfully potentiated by amine oxidase inhibitors (Vane, 1959 and page 143). It is not known if it is normally present in brain but its actions may be of importance in special circumstances.

PHENYLETHYLAMINE

Phenylethylamine and its three hydroxyderivatives, *ortho-*, *meta-* and *para-tyramine* have all been found in normal human urine (Jepson *et al.*, 1960). They are presumably formed in the body from the corresponding amino-acids, phenylalanine and ortho-, meta- and para-tyrosine since the appropriate decarboxylases are present (Blaschko, 1950). The amines have not so far been found in the brain, but it is not unlikely that they are there in small quantities and when metabolism is disturbed by disease or by the action of drugs, might accumulate. Their pharmacological actions are weak when tested by classical methods but they might well have significant actions, either directly or by competition with more active amines, if synthesized in the neighbourhood of suitable receptors.

SUMMARY

With the information at present available an accurate summary of the foregoing detail is impossible but some aspects are well worked out and from them the following picture emerges. Dopamine and 5-hydroxytryptamine are synthesized in the brain from the corresponding amino acids dopa and 5-hydroxytryptophan by an intra-cellular enzyme free in the cytoplasm; the resulting amines are stored in the cells in which they are synthesized, mainly in granules. Noradrenaline is formed from dopamine but little is known about the site of this synthesis. All three amines are formed and stored mainly in the brain stem but there are differences in their distribution: for example the high concentration of dopamine in the caudate nucleus is striking. Dopamine and 5-hydroxytryptamine are probably mainly inactivated in the brain by amine oxidase; this enzyme may also be important in the inactivation of noradrenaline but catechol-O-methyl transferase also plays a part.

The amines do not easily pass through the blood-brain barrier and their central actions after systemic administration are slight compared with their peripheral actions; but when dopa or 5-hydroxytryptophan is injected there is an increase in brain dopamine and 5-hydroxytrypt-amine respectively. Amine oxidase inhibitors cause a rise in the concentrations of all three amines. Both treatments are followed by cerebral stimulation. Reserpine, which releases all three amines and causes a reduction in their concentrations in the brain, and α-methyldopa which also lowers brain 5-HT and probably also noradrenaline and depresses 5-hydroxytryptophan decarboxylase, have a sedative action. The relative importance of the amines and of their 'bound' and 'free' forms in producing these effects is uncertain. Other amines, not normally found in the brain or present in small amounts may, because of high local concentrations resulting from disease or the administration of drugs, also affect cerebral function.

Amine oxidase inhibitors, of which there is now a considerable number, are useful not only in experimental pharmacology but also in the therapy of mental disease (p. 73), but at present it is not possible to explain the clinical effects in terms of depressed amine inactivation, and since they exert actions on other enzyme systems these too must be taken into account.

GAMMA-AMINOBUTYRIC ACID, FACTOR I AND RELATED SUBSTANCES

Gamma-aminobutyric acid (GABA) has been known to exist in living matter (bacteria, yeasts, fungi, *chlorella* and higher plants) for a number of years but it was first identified in mammalian brain in 1950 by Roberts and Frankel and by Awapara, Landua, Fuerst and Seale. The concentration in biological material may be estimated colorimetrically by the method of Berl and Waelsch (1958) after chromatographic separation.

Its synthesis and metabolism in mammalian brain is illustrated in Fig. 6. It is formed by the decarboxylation of L-glutamic acid and removed by transamination with α-ketoglutarate yielding succinic semial-dehyde. Pyridoxal-5-phosphate is the co-enzyme for both reactions but it appears to be more tightly bound to the apo-enzyme in the transaminase than in the decarboxylase. Pyridoxal deficiency will therefore tend to depress synthesis more than destruction. Another result of the participation of pyridoxal in these reactions is that carbonyl trapping agents (e.g. hydrazides) lower the concentration of GABA in brain. On the other hand the administration of hydroxylamine raises the concentration of GABA in brain (Roberts, 1961) by depressing transamination. The concentration of GABA in brain, as well as being modified by substances affecting its synthesis and metabolism, is diminished by reserpine (Balzer, Holtz and Palm, 1961).

Brain homogenates are not only able to convert GABA into succinic semialdehyde *in vitro* but also form γ-amino-β-hydroxybutyric acid and γ-guanidinobutyric acid from it, and Udenfriend *et al.* (1961) have found considerable amounts of γ-aminobutyryl-histidine (homocarnosine) in brain though its origin has not yet been established. The two

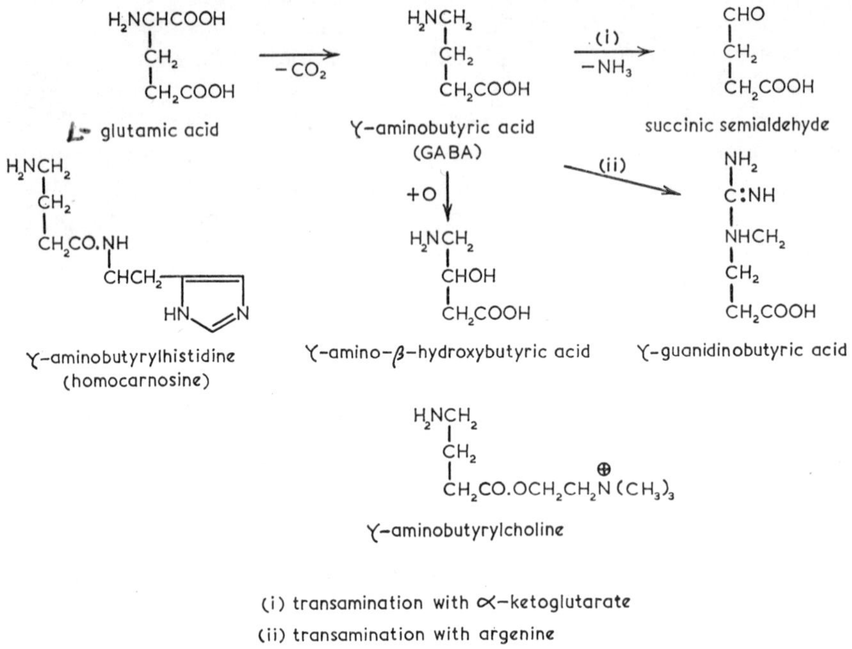

(i) transamination with α−ketoglutarate

(ii) transamination with arginine

FIG. 6. Metabolism of γ-aminobutyric acid. Some related substances.

butyric acids, the quaternary ammonium compound γ-aminobutyrylcholine (Fig. 6) and several related substances have pharmacological properties resembling GABA though their relative potency and their physiological significance is not yet clear (see Honour and McLennan, 1960). The further history of GABA is entangled with that of factor I.

Factor I was first detected by Florey (1954), in extracts made from mammalian CNS, by its action on crustacean stretch receptors. This action has been utilized (Elliott and Florey, 1956) for a sensitive and convenient bioassay method. Stretch receptors of the abdominal muscle of the crayfish each have two sensory neurones; one of these gives a brief discharge on stretching the muscle, the other gives a continuous discharge as long as the stretch is maintained. It is the rate of discharge of this second neurone which is used for the assay; application of solutions of factor I reduce the rate of discharge or may stop it completely. Recently Florey (1961) has developed a second method of assay which is simpler to use and more sensitive. It depends on inhibition by factor I of contractions of the isolated hind gut of the crayfish stimulated by acetylcholine. Gamma-amino butyric acid has similar actions.

Factor I is dialysable and thermostable and can be distinguished from potassium, acetylcholine, substance P, adrenaline, noradrenaline and histamine. Only about 34% of that contained in brain can be extracted with unheated saline, the remainder can be extracted by heat, by hypotonic solutions or by weak acid or alkali. This portion would therefore appear to be either loosely bound or contained within a membrane. These two fractions are referred to respectively as 'free' and 'occult'. The relative amounts of them obtained from brain are not appreciably affected by the period of homogenization of the tissue, by grinding with sand or by the volume of saline used for extraction (Elliott and van Gelder, 1960). They probably therefore represent fractions which actually exist *in vivo*. Moreover when GABA is incubated with brain slices there is an increase in occult factor I, but no such increase follows incubation of it with brain homogenates.

Bazemore, Elliott and Florey (1957) prepared a crystalline material from beef brain with high stretch receptor activity which they demonstrated to be GABA. More recently Levin, Lovell and Elliott (1961) have compared the stretch receptor activity of extracts prepared by two different methods from the brains of three mammalian species with their GABA content. They calculated that all this activity could be accounted for by the GABA present. On the other hand McLennan (1959) has separated factor I by paper chromatography into two fractions, both of which inhibit the stretch receptors, and has compared (Honour and McLennan, 1960) the pharmacological actions of these fractions with those of GABA and some related substances: β-guanidinopropionic acid, γ-guanidinobutyric acid and γ-aminobutyrylcholine. These substances all inhibited the stretch receptor (Table 3) but differed from factor I in their action on certain other mammalian synapses: both fractions of factor I were found to inhibit monosynaptic reflexes

TABLE 3

Inhibitory activity of various organic acids on crayfish stretch receptors.

	Inhibitory activity on crayfish stretch receptors.
γ-aminobutyric acid	1[1]
γ-amino-β-hydroxybutyric acid	$\frac{1}{2}$[1]
carnitine chloride	$\frac{1}{8}$[2]
β-alanine	$\frac{1}{20}$[1]
δ-aminovaleric acid	$\frac{1}{20}$[1]
α, γ-diaminobutyric acid	$\frac{1}{60}$[1]
γ-guanidinobutyric acid	some activity[2]
β-guanidinopropionic acid	some activity[2]

[1] Elliott and Jasper (1959).   [2] Honour and McLennan (1960).

elicited by electrical stimulation of a dorsal root, and to block transmission through the inferior mesenteric ganglion, but none of the pure substances had either action. The other substances in Table 3 could be excluded on chromatographic evidence or on their pharmacological properties. It seems likely that factor I is closely related to GABA but further work is needed to establish its chemical identity and to decide whether more than one substance is responsible for the factor I activity of brain extracts.

According to Purpura *et al.* (1958) a number of ω-amino-*n*-aliphatic acids have synaptic activity. Those with chains containing 2 to 5 carbon atoms have an action similar to GABA but weaker, while the 6 and 8 carbon compounds have an apparently excitatory action; of these the latter (ω-aminocaprylic acid) causes sustained seizures when applied to the brain.

Hayashi (1959) has reported that γ-amino-β-hydroxybutyric acid is about 20 times as potent in preventing convulsions as GABA and has found it in dog brain. Haloperidol (p. 51) is structurally similar to GABA: it has a sedative action and causes extrapyramidal symptoms.

DISTRIBUTION OF GLUTAMIC ACID DECARBOXYLASE, GABA AND FACTOR I IN MAMMALIAN BRAIN

There is at present little detailed information about the distribution of glutamic acid decarboxylase (Table 1) and therefore of the sites of GABA synthesis, but the enzyme appears to be widely distributed in the grey matter of the brain with very little in the white matter. The globus pallidus is reported as being especially rich (Lowe, Robins and Eyerman, 1958).

Both GABA (estimated colorimetrically) and factor I (estimated biologically) are found throughout the brain. There is a wide variation in the concentration found in the same area in different animals, but in general the values for grey matter are higher than those for white matter and those for GABA and factor I are of the same order (Table 1). The spinal cord contains relatively little, and peripheral nerves and sympathetic ganglia none. Traces of GABA, but not of factor I, have been found in the cerebrospinal fluid (Elliott and Jasper, 1959; Florey and Florey, 1958).

ACTIONS OF GABA AND FACTOR I

Crustacea. In the crayfish, the cell body of the sensory nerve transmitting impulses from stretch receptors in an abdominal muscle fibre, lies on the fibre and sends short dendrites into it. An inhibitory nerve also runs into the muscle and its axon forms synapses on the dendrites of the sensory neurone. If the inhibitory nerve is stimulated while the muscle is stretched, impulses in the axon of the sensory nerve are suppressed; the application of a weak solution of GABA (10^{-5}M) to the muscle fibre has a similar effect. Kuffler and Edwards (1958) have investigated this mechanism and compared the action of GABA with that of stimulation of the inhibitory nerve. They have proposed the following scheme to explain the sequence of events. Stretching the muscle leads to deformation and depolarization of the dendrites and an impulse is set up in the axon near the cell body. Both GABA and stimulation of the inhibitory nerve increase conductance within the cell and this serves to attenuate the stretch depolarization of the dendrites so that impulses are not set up in the axon. While there is a striking parallel between the action of GABA and of an inhibitory transmitter, they conclude that there is as yet insufficient evidence to prove that GABA is this transmitter.

Further evidence is provided by the action of picrotoxin. This blocks both the inhibitory action of GABA on stretch receptor impulses and the effect of stimulation of the inhibitory nerve. There is also good evidence that the transmitter released by the inhibitory nerve to the crayfish heart is similar to factor I and to GABA (Florey, 1957).

Mammals. Investigation of the action of GABA on peripheral structures and isolated organs has revealed no clear picture. Neuro-muscular transmission in the mammal is not affected by GABA or factor I but the latter substance has been found to depress conduction through the inferior mesenteric and stellate ganglia and to inhibit monosynaptic spinal reflexes in the cat (Florey and McLennan, 1955). GABA may either stimulate or relax the isolated guinea pigs ileum; it diminishes contractions elicited by acetylcholine, histamine, 5-HT and nicotine. With other species the effects are less marked and less consistent (Hobbiger, 1958).

The topical application to mammalian cortex of solutions containing 0·2 to 1·0% GABA cause the following reversible effects:

1. Spontaneous cortical activity is changed from predominantly surface negative to surface positive waves.

2. Surface negative post-synaptic potentials evoked by electrical stimulation of the cortex are abolished and replaced by surface positive potentials.

3. The surface negative component of the cortical response to thalamic stimulation is suppressed, but neither the preceding surface positive component nor the associated negative wave recorded by electrodes inserted 1 mm. into the cortex, are appreciably changed.

These and other observations on the cortex have been explained by the selective blockade of surface cortical elements or apical dendrites (Elliott and Jasper, 1959).

The results of the application of GABA and of other amino-acids by iontophoresis to spinal neurones has been summarized by Curtis (1961). Some, like GABA, depress the excitability of the neurones both to chemical stimuli and to antidromic stimulation and appear to have a postsynaptic action; others, of which L-aspartic acid, L-glutamic acid and L-cysteic acid are normally present in the CNS, cause membrane depolarization and excitation of the cell. The concentrations reached in the vicinity of the cell by the method of application used is uncertain, so that the likelihood of these actions occurring *in vivo* is unknown, but the possibility that disturbances of metabolism, either general or local, might result in disturbances of function due to the accumulation of certain amino-acids remains, and makes the interpretation of the action of drugs modifying metabolism still more hazardous.

Roberts (1961) has found that in mice the rise in brain GABA concentration which follows the administration of the GABA transaminase inhibitor, hydroxylamine, is accompanied by a diminished sensitivity of the animals to leptazol convulsions. Although the two changes follow the same time course it must not at once be assumed that the one is the cause of the other.

ACTION OF DRUGS ON THE CONCENTRATION OF
FACTOR I IN THE BRAIN

Elliott and van Gelder (1960) have estimated the amount of free and occult factor I in the cerebral hemispheres of rats after various forms of treatment. A convulsant dose of insulin caused a fall, mainly due to a reduction in the occluded form, and this they suggest may result from the reduction in brain glutamate which follows insulin administration. Exposure to 5% oxygen in nitrogen for 30 minutes caused a rise, mainly due to an increase in free factor I, and might be ascribed to a reduction in α-ketoglutarate required for removal of GABA. Hydroxylamine, which inhibits α-ketoglutarate transaminase, also led to a rise in free factor I while carbazides led to a decrease in occult factor I presumably by inactivation of pyridoxal phosphate. After iproniazid and other amine oxidase inhibitors there was a rise in free factor I, though whether GABA or factor I is a substrate of amine oxidase is not known. In general substances which reduced total factor I mainly affected the occult form, whereas those which raised total factor I mainly affected the free form. Since the changes appear to be brought about by inhibition of enzymes synthesizing and destroying it, this has led to the suggestion that factor I is synthesized into the occult form and that it is the free form which is metabolized.

Insulin, hydroxylamine and hydrazide have been shown to cause changes in the total amount of GABA in brain similar to those described above.

SUBSTANCE P

Substance P is a polypeptide of unknown composition first found in intestine and brain by Euler and Gaddum in 1931. Its extraction, assay and properties are described in chapter 5 (p. 167). The material extracted from brain has been shown to be different from all other known substances and to be identical with substance P extracted from intestine.

There is some slender evidence that in the intestine substance P may be associated with nervous tissue. In dogs, pigs and horses the highest concentrations are found in the muscularis mucosa which also contains Meissner's plexus, but in cats there is more in the external muscles of the gut. Moreover in Hirchsprung's disease there is little in the inactive aganglionic part and more than normal in the hyperactive part (Ehrenpreis and Pernow, 1953).

Published estimations of the concentration of substance P in the brain vary very considerably. This is no doubt partly due to the presence in the extracts of substances interfering with the bioassay. Laszlo (1960) found considerable amounts of adenosine monophosphate in extracts prepared by the customary methods. This substance relaxes plain muscle preparations on which the assay is made.

Two sets of figures for the distribution of substance P in the CNS of man and the dog respectively are given in Table 1. The highest concentration reported is in the substantia nigra of man but the nearby and related red nucleus contains very little. After the substantia nigra the next highest concentration is found in an area adjacent to the 4th ventricle which contains the area postrema and ala cinerea; it is not yet decided which of these two structures is responsible for the high figures. The hypothalamus, which contains much acetylcholine, dopamine, noradrenaline and 5-HT, also contains much substance P. The medial geniculates and inferior colliculi, both with acoustic connections, contain more than the lateral geniculates and superior colliculi which have optic connections. The visual cortex, optic nerve, corpus callosum, pons, pyramids and cerebellum all have very little while the corpus striatum is rich. There is also a striking difference between the motor and sensory roots; the latter, together with the dorsal columns which contain fibres from them, and the nuclei gracilis and cuneatus to which they run, contain considerable amounts. This provoked the suggestion, still unsubstantiated, that substance P might be the transmitter of the first sensory neurone, which is known not to be cholinergic (Lembeck, 1953).

The effect of administration of amphetamine, ephedrine, insulin, β-tetrahydronaphthylamine, caffeine, ether and reserpine on the concentration of substance P in the brain has been tested but no change has been found (Paasonen and Vogt, 1956). These substances reduce the concentration of noradrenaline in the hypothalamus (p. 25).

The central nervous system of fish also contains substance P: there are high concentrations in the telencephalon and medulla and low concentrations in the cerebellum and spinal cord (Dahlstedt and Euler, 1959).

The distribution of substance P in centrifuged homogenates of brain has been investigated by Whittaker and is referred to on page 7.

THE ACTIONS OF SUBSTANCE P ON THE CNS

The investigation of the actions of substance P have been hampered by lack of pure preparations of high potency. Zettler (1956) found that the subcutaneous injection of 2800 units/kg. into mice reduced their spontaneous activity after 10 minutes to 50% and that when their activity had been increased by previous injections of amphetamine or morphine, this also was reduced; but the other actions he reported were only manifest against the background of the effect of another drug. He found that the hypnotic action of hexobarbitone and catatonia caused by bulbocapnine were both potentiated and that the tremor caused by harmine and the convulsions caused by strychnine and picrotoxin were antagonized. Protection against leptazol convulsions needed very much larger doses and there was no protection at all against electro-shock convulsions. Whether the anticonvulsant action of substance P can be explained by its hypotensive action has not been investigated. Zettler has also found that after doses of 8,500 units/kg. the pain threshold of mice to electric shocks is depressed and that morphine analgesia is antagonized. Neither Angelucci (1956) who perfused the frog's spinal cord with substance P nor Kissel and Domino (1959) who injected it intravenously into spinal cats found any change in spinal reflexes.

The effect of intracarotid injection of 30 to 100 units substance P on the EEG of conscious rabbits has been reported by Lechner and Lembeck (1958). In the majority of experiments there was an increase in frequency and a decrease in amplitude of the waves recorded from cortical electrodes, and an increase in frequency and of synchronization of those recorded from the hippocampus. This, the authors suggest, probably indicates alerting by stimulation of an activating system.

The injection of 10 to 20 units substance P intracisternally or into the lateral ventricle of cats (Euler and Pernow, 1956) leads to effects such as licking and swallowing which have been found by Feldberg (1957a) to follow the administration by this route of a number of drugs, but there were also changes in the behaviour of the animal. Most animals showed a 'lack of spontaneity' but one, previously friendly, became fierce and angry.

Work on the pharmacological effects of substance P gives no indication as to what part if any it plays in the central nervous system, but its irregular distribution suggests that further investigation would be well worth while. It would be much facilitated by the availability of a pure preparation and a reliable assay method.

The first estimates of histamine in nervous tissue were made by Kwiatowski (1943) who showed that although considerable amounts are present in some peripheral nerves, the amounts in the central nervous system are relatively low. Harris, Jacobsohn and Kahlson (1952) found high concentrations in the pituitary gland and measurable amounts in the hypothalamus and medial eminence, but elsewhere in the brain amounts were too small to estimate. A more complete survey using a more sensitive method of estimation has recently been carried out by Adam (1961). He has confirmed the previous findings of high concentrations in the pituitary and found the highest in the stalk and posterior lobe. The pituitary gland and its stalk contain considerable numbers of mast cells, which elsewhere in the body are able to synthesize (Shayer, 1956) and store histamine, and the concentrations of histamine appeared to vary with the number of mast cells present. The hypothalamus contained less than a tenth of the amount in the neurohypophysis and the highest concentrations were found in those parts adjacent to the hypophyseal stalk. No mast cells were found in the hypothalamus or elsewhere in brain tissue. In general there was a rough correspondence between the amounts of histamine, 5-hydroxytryptamine and noradrenaline. The area postrema was particularly rich and the lowest concentrations were found in white matter and in the cerebral cortex. There is some evidence that in peripheral nerves histamine may be associated with Swann cell cytoplasm rather than axons, and Paton (1958) has suggested that if glia is in part related to Swann cells this may account for the presence of histamine in brain.

Histamine is formed by the decarboxylation of histidine and both Holtz and Westermann (1956) and Clouet, Gaitonde and Richter (1957) have found histidine decarboxylase in rat brain. White (1959) using ^{14}C-labelled histidine has determined the rate of decarboxylation *in vitro* by minced portions of cat, dog and pig brain. This was greatest with hypothalamus and much lower rates were found with cortex and area postrema. The area postrema formed histamine so slowly compared with the amount of pre-formed histamine found in it by Adam, that it is likely that it collects histamine synthesized elsewhere, as it probably does 5-hydroxytryptamine and noradrenaline.

There is at present no evidence that brain histamine has any function in nervous transmission, but in the cervical sympathetic ganglion of the cat, Trendelenberg (1955) found that histamine potentiated the effects of submaximal preganglionic stimulation; that is to say, it facilitated transmission through the ganglion.

ADENOSINE DERIVATIVES

No systematic analysis of the distribution of adenosine compounds (adenosine tri- di- and mono-phosphates and adenosine itself) in the brain appears to have been made. Considerable amounts are present and are to be found in the bodies of neurones and in both myelinated and non-myelinated fibres (Lowry *et al.*, 1954). Adenosine triphosphate (ATP) is a high energy compound and concerned with a variety of metabolic processes but it may have other functions as well. Holton (1959) has demonstrated its liberation from sensory nerves during antidromic stimulation and has suggested that it may be responsible for antidromic vasodilatation. This discharge may however be incidental to permeability changes in the nerve fibre during conduction, and it cannot be assumed without further evidence that it is the chemical transmitter of these neurones. In the adrenal medulla and possibly also in platelets, amines are bound to ATP, and Schümann (1958) has suggested that it may be concerned in the binding of noradrenaline in adrenergic nerves, so the possibility that it is combined with an active substance within the nerve and that its appearance is incidental to the release of this substance, must also be kept in mind.

Intravenous injections of adenosine compounds or their application to the cerebral cortex modifies EEG spikes induced by the previous administration of convulsants, but has little effect on the normal EEG.

Estimation. Adenosine triphosphate may be estimated by the firefly luminescence method of Strehler and Totter (1954) which depends on the fact that the emission of light by extracts of the dried lanterns of the firefly *Photinus pyralis* varies with the concentration of ATP in the solution. The enzymatic estimation of adenosine phosphates is described by Kalckar (1947) and by Bücher (1953).

CEREBELLAR FACTOR

The identification and estimation of most of the substances described in this chapter has depended on some action on an isolated organ or on the peripheral circulation of an experimental animal. Crossland and Mitchell (1956) have examined extracts of brain for their ability to change the electrical activity recorded from electrodes placed on the cerebellar cortex of a decerebrate rabbit. Injections were made into the carotid artery. Extracts of cerebral hemisphere, midbrain and cerebellum all increased electrical activity, but the action of cerebral and midbrain extracts was lost if the extracts were made alkaline and boiled, and appeared to be due to acetylcholine. The action of cerebellar extracts was however resistant to this treatment. No change in electrical activity was recorded after injections of 5-HT, adrenaline, substance P or ATP in doses which might be present in the extracts, but 0·05 µg. histamine produced a change similar to that seen with cerebellar extracts. Histamine however had a much longer latent period and its action was abolished by chlorcyclizine.

The cerebellar factor, as it has been called, is a basic substance soluble in water, ethanol and butanol but insoluble in acetone, ether and chloroform. It is stable at room temperature but rapidly destroyed by boiling in acid solution but not by trypsin or chymotrypsin. Incubation with homogenates of nervous tissue leads to its destruction probably enzymatically: this destruction is prevented by strychnine but not by picrotoxin. It has no action on any of a number of smooth muscle preparations on which it has been tested.

The cerebellum of all mammalian species so far examined have been found to contain it (Crossland, 1960) and it has also been found in other parts, both white and grey, of the central nervous system (optic nerves and tracts, dorsal roots, spino-cerebellar tracts, cerebellar peduncles, internal capsule, lateral geniculate bodies, thalamus and sensory cortex).

CHEMICAL TRANSMISSION IN THE CENTRAL NERVOUS SYSTEM
In the peripheral nervous system of mammals two substances are known which transmit nervous impulses at synapses; and in invertebrates there is evidence of the liberation, as well, at some nerve endings of an inhibitory substance which depresses synaptic conduction. Attempts have therefore been made to identify local neuro-hormones in the central nervous system. Such a substance must be one that can be rapidly liberated from a source where it is held inactive and as rapidly inactivated, after it has served its purpose, by an enzyme easily available. Acetylcholine and noradrenaline, the only mammalian peripheral transmitters so far identified, fulfil these two requirements centrally as they do peripherally. Certain neurones in the central nervous system can be classified as cholinergic with some degree of certainty but identification of adrenergic neurones is far less certain. No adrenergic nerves have been found issuing from the spinal cord and although there are parts of the brain with a high concentration of noradrenaline, it is there associated with dopamine and 5-hydroxytryptamine, which appear to be equally easily liberated and inactivated. All three amines are found in centres associated with the autonomic system and changes in their concentration lead to effects which are partly mediated through this system, but it is not known what part they play in this.

There is evidence that activity of some neurones, as for example the Renshaw cells and those of the descending reticular formation, results in inhibition of the neurones to which they run. The actions of γ-aminobutyric acid and factor I, in both mammals and invertebrates, make these the most likely of known substances in the brain to have an inhibitory action, but there is no reason at present to associate them with any inhibitory tracts and some evidence that in mammals the action of γ-aminobutyric acid is not exerted at the synapse but postsynaptically (Curtis, 1961).

The sensory nerves and their continuation in the posterior columns are neither cholinergic nor adrenergic; the high concentration of substance P in them has led to the suggestion that it might be a transmitter; but nothing is at present known about its synthesis, storage or release, nor is it known to be able to stimulate any neurones.

Though it seems likely that there are non-cholinergic neurones in the CNS, probably of more than one kind, and there are several possible candidates for the role of transmitter, the evidence does not yet indicate any one of these as actually functioning as one.

REFERENCES

* Denotes review

ADAM, H. M. (1961). In 'Regional Neurochemistry'. Ed. Kety, S. S. and Elkes, J. Pergamon Press

ALDRIDGE, W. N. and JOHNSON, M. K. (1959). *Biochem. J.* **73**, 270

AMIN, A. H., CRAWFORD, T. B. B. and GADDUM, J. H. (1954). *J. Physiol.* **126**, 596

ANDERSON, E. G. and BONNYCASTLE, D. D. (1960). *J. Pharmacol. exp. Ther.* **130**, 138

ANGELUCCI, L. (1956). *Brit. J. Pharmacol.* **11**, 161

AWAPARA, J., LANDUA, A. J., FUERST, R. and SEALE, B. (1950). *J. biol. Chem.* **187**, 35

AXELROD, J. (1959). *Physiol. Rev.* **39**, 751

AXELROD, J., ALBERS, R. W. and CLEMENTS, C. D. (1959). *J. Neurochem.* **5**, 68

AXELROD, J., HERTTING, G. and PATRICK, R. W. (1961). *J. Pharmacol. exp. Ther.* **134**, 325

AXELROD, J., WEIL-MALHERBE, H. and TOMCHICK, R. (1959). *J. Pharmacol. exp. Ther.* **127**, 251

BAKER, R. V. (1959). *J. Physiol.* **145**, 473

BALZER, H., HOLTZ, P. and PALM, D. (1961). *Experientia*, **17**, 38

BARCROFT, H. and SWAN, H. J. C. (1953). 'Sympathetic Control of Human Blood Vessels.' London: Edward Arnold

BASOWITZ, H., KORCHIN, S. J., OKEN, D., GOLDSTEIN, M. S. and GUSSAK, H. (1956) *Arch. Neurol. Psychiat. (Chicago)*, **27**, 98

BAZEMORE, A. W., ELLIOTT, K. A. C. and FLOREY, E. (1957). *J. Neurochem.* **1**, 334

BERL, S. and WAELSCH, H. (1958). *J. Neurochem.* **3**, 161

BERTLER, A. (1961). *Acta physiol. scand.* **51**, 75

BERTLER, A. and ROSENGREN, E. (1959). *Experientia*, **15**, 382

BERTLER, A., HILLARP, N. A. and ROSENGREN, E. (1960). *Acta physiol. scand.* **50**, 113

BIRKS, R. I. and MACINTOSH, F. C. (1957). *Brit. Med. Bull.* **13**, 157

BLASCHKO, H. (1950). *Biochem. et Biophys. Acta*, **4**, 130

BLASCHKO, H., HAGEN, P. and WELCH, A. D. (1955). *J. Physiol.* **129**, 27

BOGDANSKI, D. F., WEISSBACH, H. and UDENFRIEND, S. (1957). *J. Neurochem.* **1**, 272

BOGDANSKI, D. F., SULSER, F. and BRODIE, B. B. (1961). *J. Pharmacol. exp. Ther.* **132**, 176

BONNYCASTLE, D. D., GIARMAN, N. J. and PAASONEN, M. K. (1957). *Brit. J. Pharmacol.* **12**, 228

BONVALLET, M., DELL, P. and HIEBEL, G. (1954). *Electroenceph. clin. Neurophysiol.* **6**, 119

BRADLEY, P. B. (1960). In Ciba Foundation Symposium on 'Adrenergic Mechanisms'. Ed. Vane. London: Churchill

BRADLEY, P. B. and ELKES, J. (1957). In 'Metabolism of the Nervous System'. Ed. Richter, D. London: Pergamon Press

BRODIE, B. B., SHORE, P. A. and PLETSCHER, A. (1956). *Science*, **123**, 992

BRODIE, B. B., FINGER, K. F., ORLANS, F. B., QUINN, G. P. and SULSER, F. (1960a). *J. Pharmacol. exp. Ther.* **129**, 250

BÜCHER, T. (1953). *Advances in Enzymology*, **14**

BURGEN, A. S. V. and CHIPMAN, L. M. (1951). *J. Physiol.* **114**, 296

*CARLSSON, A. (1959). *Pharm. Rev.* **11**, 490

CLOUET, D. J., GAITONDE, M. K. and RICHTER, D. (1957). *J. Neurochem.* **1**, 228

COOPER, J. R. and MELCER, I. (1961). *J. Pharmacol. exp. Ther.* **132**, 265

*CROSSLAND, J. (1960). *J. Pharm (Lond.)*, **12**, 1

CROSSLAND, J. and MERRICK, A. J. (1954). *J. Physiol.* **125**, 56

CROSSLAND, J. and MITCHELL, J. F. (1956). *J. Physiol.* **132**, 391

CROUT, J. R., CREVELING, C. R. and UDENFRIEND, S. (1961). *J. Pharmacol. exp. Ther.* **132**, 269

CURTIS, D. R. (1961). In 'Regional Neurochemistry'. Ed. Kety and Elkes. London: Pergamon Press

CURTIS, D. R. and ECCLES, R. M. (1958). *J. Physiol.* **141**, 446

CURTIS, D. R. and DAVIS, R. (1961). *Nature (Lond.)*, **192**, 1083

DAHLSTEDT, E., EULER, U. S. v., LISHAJKO, F. and ÖSTLUND, E. (1959). *Acta physiol. scand.* **47**, 124

DALE, H. H. (1936–37). 'The Harvey Lectures.' **32**, 229

DELL, P., BONVALLET, M. and HUGELIN (1954). *Electroenceph. clin. Neurophysiol.* **6**, 119 and 599

DE ROBERTIS, E. (1959). *Int. Rev. Cytol.* **8**, 61

DE ROBERTIS, E. (1961). In 'Regional Neurochemistry'. Ed. Kety and Elkes. London: Pergamon Press

DESMEDT, J. E. and LA GRUTTA, G. (1955). *Boll. Soc. ital. biol. sper.* **31**, 913

*DOBBING, J. (1961). *Physiol. Rev.* **41**, 130

DOMER, F. R. and FELDBERG, W. (1960). *Brit. J. Pharmacol.* **15**, 578

ECCLES, J. C., ECCLES, R. M. and FATT, P. (1956). *J. Physiol.* **131**, 154

ECCLES, J. C. and JAEGER, J. C. (1958). *Proc. Roy. Soc. B.* **148**, 38

EHRENPREIS, T. and PERNOW, B. (1953). *Acta physiol. scand.* **27**, 380

ELLIOTT, K. A. C. and FLOREY, E. (1956). *J. Neurochem.* **1**, 181

*ELLIOTT, K. A. C. and JASPER, H. H. (1959). *Physiol. Rev.* **39**, 383

ELLIOTT, K. A. C. and VAN GELDER, N. M. (1960). *J. Physiol.* **153**, 423

ELTHERINGTON, L. G. and HORITA, A. (1960). *J. Pharmacol. exp. Ther.* **128**, 7

EULER, U. S. v. (1946). *Acta physiol. scand.* **12**, 73

EULER, U. S. v. (1957). In 'Metabolism of the Nervous System'. Ed. Richter. London: Pergamon Press

EULER, U. S. v. and GADDUM, J. H. (1931). *J. Physiol.* **72**, 74

EULER, U. S. v. and HILLARP, N. Å. (1956). *Nature (Lond.)*, **177**, 44

EULER, U. S. v. and PERNOW, B. (1956). *Acta physiol. scand.* **36**, 265

*FELDBERG, W. (1945). *Physiol. Rev.* **25**, 596

*FELDBERG, W. (1954). *Pharm. Rev.* **6**, 85

FELDBERG, W. (1957a). In 'Psychotropic drugs'. Ed. Garattini and Ghetti. Elsevier

FELDBERG, W. (1957b). In 'Metabolism of the Nervous System'. Ed. Richter. London: Pergamon Press

FELDBERG, W. and SHERWOOD, S. L. (1954). *J. Physiol.* **123**, 148

FELDBERG, W. and SHERWOOD, S. L. (1955). *Brit. J. Pharmacol.* **10**, 371

FELDBERG, W. and VOGT, M. (1948). *J. Physiol.* **107**, 372

FLOREY, E. (1954). *Arch. internat. physiol.* **62**, 33

FLOREY, E. (1957). *Naturwiss.* **44**, 424

FLOREY, E. (1961). *J. Physiol.* **156**, 1

FLOREY, E. and McLENNAN, H. (1955). *J. Physiol.* **129**, 384 and **130**, 446

FLOREY, E. and FLOREY, E. (1958). *J. Physiol.* **144**, 220

GADDUM, J. H. (1961). *Biochem. Pharmacol.* **8,** 81
GADDUM, J. H. and SZERB, J. C. (1961). *Brit. J. Pharmacol.* **17,** 451
GRAY, E. G. (1959). *J. Anat (Lond.)*, **93,** 420
GRAY, E. G. and WHITTAKER, V. P. (1960). *J. Physiol.* **153,** 35P
GRAY, E. G. and WHITTAKER, V. P. (1962). *J. Anat (Lond.).* **96,** 79
GREEN, H. and ERICKSON, R. W. (1960). *J. Pharmacol. exp. Ther.* **129,** 237
GREEN, H. and SAWYER, J. L. (1960). *J. Pharmacol. exp. Ther.* **129,** 243
GREIG, M. E., WALK, R. A. and GIBBONS, A. J. (1959). *J. Pharmacol. exp. Ther.* **127,** 110
HARRIS, G. W., JACOBSOHN, D. and KAHLSON, G. (1952). Ciba Foundation Colloquia on Endocrinology, No. 4. London: Churchill
HAYASHI, T. (1959). *J. Physiol.* **145,** 570
HEBB, C. O. (1961). *Nature (Lond.)*, **192,** 527
HEBB, C. O. and SILVER, A. (1956). *J. Physiol.* **134,** 718
HEBB, C. O. and WHITTAKER, V. P. (1958). *J. Physiol.* **142,** 187
HESS, S., WEISSBACH, H., REDFIELD, B. G. and UDENFRIEND, S. (1958). *J. Pharmacol. exp. Ther.* **124,** 189
HESS, S., REDFIELD, B. G. and UDENFRIEND, S. (1959). *Fed. Proc.* **18,** 402
HESS, S., CONNAMACHER, R. H., OZAKI, M. and UDENFRIEND, S. (1961). *J. Pharmacol. exp. Ther.* **134,** 129
HOBBIGER, F. (1958). *J. Physiol.* **144,** 349
HOLTON, P. (1959). *J. Physiol.* **145,** 494
HOLTZ, P. (1950). *Acta physiol. scand.* **20,** 354
HOLTZ, P. and WESTERMANN, E. (1956). *Arch. exp. Path. Pharmak.* **227,** 538
HOLZBAUER, M. and VOGT, M. (1956). *J. Neurochem.* **1,** 8
HOLZER, G. and HORNYKIEWICZ, O. (1959). *Arch. exp. Path. Pharmak.* **237,** 27
HONOUR, A. J. and MCLENNAN, H. (1960). *J. Physiol* **150,** 306
JEPSON, J. B., LOVENBERG, W., ZALTZMAN, P., OATES, J. A., SJOERDSMA, A., UDENFRIEND, S. (1960). *Biochem. J.* **74,** 5P
KALCKAR, H. M. (1947). *J. biol. Chem.* **167,** 461
KISSEL, J. W. and DOMINO, E. F. (1959). *J. Pharmacol. exp. Ther.* **125,** 168
KOELLE, G. B. (1961). *Nature (Lond.)*, **190,** 208
KUFFLER, S. W. and EDWARDS, C. (1958). *J. Neurophysiol.* **21,** 589
KUNTZMAN, R., SHORE, P. A., BOGDANSKI, D. and BRODIE, B. B. (1961). *J. Neurochem.* **6,** 226
KWIATOWSKI, H. (1943). *J. Physiol.* **102,** 32
LASZLO, I. (1960). *J. Physiol.* **153,** 69P
LECHNER, H. and LEMBECK, F. (1958). *Arch. exp. Path. Pharmak.* **234,** 419
LEMBECK, F. (1953). *Arch. exp. Path. Pharmak.* **219,** 197
LEVIN, E., LOVELL, R. A. and ELLIOTT, K. A. C. (1961). *J. Neurochem.* **7,** 147
LOWE, I. P., ROBINS, E. and EYERMAN, G. S. (1958). *J. Neurochem.* **3,** 8
LOWRY, O. H., ROBERTS, N. R., LEINER, K. Y., WU, M-L., FARR, A. L. and ALBERS, R. W. (1954). *J. biol. Chem.* **207,** 39
MACINTOSH, F. C. (1941). *J. Physiol.* **99,** 436
MACINTOSH, F. C. and OBORIN, P. E. (1953). Abstr. XIX Int. Physiol. Congr. 380
MACINTOSH, F. C., BIRKS, R. I. and SASTRY, P. B. (1956). *Nature (Lond.)*, **178,** 1181
*MCILWAIN, H. and RODNIGHT, R. (1961). *Practical Neurochemistry*. London: Churchill
MCLENNAN, H. (1959). *J. Physiol.* **146,** 358
MARRAZZI, A. S. (1957). *Ann. N.Y. Acad. Sci.* **66,** 496
PAASONEN, M. K. and VOGT, M. (1956). *J. Physiol.* **131,** 617
*PATON, W. D. M. (1958). *Ann. Rev. Physiol.* **20,** 431
PLETSCHER, A. (1957). *Science*, **126,** 507
PLETSCHER, A., SHORE, P. A. and BRODIE, B. B. (1956). *J. Pharmacol. exp. Ther.* **116,** 84
PRICE, S. A. P. and WEST, G. B. (1960). *Nature (Lond.)*, **185,** 470
PROCKOP, D. J., SHORE, P. A. and BRODIE, B. B. (1959). *Experientia*, **15,** 145
PURPURA, D. P., GIRADO, M. and GRUNDFEST, H. (1958). *Science*, **127,** 1179

QUASTEL, J. H., TENNENBAUM, M. and WHEATLEY, A. H. M. (1936). *Biochem. J.* **30,** 1668

QUINN, G. P., SHORE, P. A. and BRODIE, B. B. (1959). *J. Pharmacol. exp. Ther.* **127,** 103

RAAB, W. and GIGEE, W. (1951). *Proc. Soc. exp. Biol. N.Y.* **76,** 97

RANSON, S. W. and MAGOUN, H. W. (1939). *Ergebn. Physiol.* **41,** 56

RICHTER, D. and CROSSLAND, J. (1949). *Amer. J. Physiol.* **159,** 247

RINALDI, F. and HIMWICH, H. E. (1955). *Arch. Neurol. Psychiat.* **73,** 387 and 396

ROBERTS, E. (1961). In 'Regional Neurochemistry'. Ed. Kety and Elkes. London: Pergamon Press

ROBERTS, E. and FRANKEL, S. (1950). *J. biol. Chem.* **187,** 55

RODNIGHT, R. (1956). *Biochem. J.* **64,** 621

*ROTHBALLER, A. B. (1959). *Pharmacol. Rev.* **11,** 494

SCHAYER, R. W. (1951). *J. biol. Chem.* **189,** 301

SCHAYER, R. W. (1956). *Amer. J. Physiol.* **186,** 189

SCHÜMANN, H. J. (1958). *Arch. exp. Path. Pharmak.* **233,** 296

SHORE, P. A., MEAD, J. A. R., KUNTZMAN, R. G., SPECTOR, S. and BRODIE, B. B. (1957). *Science,* **126,** 1063

SMITH, S. E. (1960). *Brit. J. Pharmacol.* **15,** 319

SPECTOR, S., SHORE, P. A. and BRODIE, B. B. (1960). *J. Pharmacol. exp. Ther.* **128,** 15

STEDMAN, E. and STEDMAN, E. (1937). *Biochem. J.* **31,** 817

STREHLER, B. C. and TOTTER, J. R. (1954). In 'Methods of Biochemical Analysis'. **1,** 341. Ed. Glick. London: Interscience

TRENDELENBERG, U. (1955). *J. Physiol.* **129,** 337

UDENFRIEND, S., WEISSBACH, H. and BOGDANSKI, D. F. (1957). *Ann. N.Y. Acad. Sci.* **66,** 602; *J. biol. Chem.* **224,** 803

UDENFRIEND, S., WITKOP, B., REDFIELD, B. G. and WEISSBACH, H. (1958). *Biochem. Pharmacol.* **1,** 160

UDENFRIEND, S. and WEISSBACH, H. (1958). *Proc. Soc. exp. Biol. N.Y.* **97,** 748

UDENFRIEND, S., PISANO, J. J. and WILSON, J. D. (1961). In 'Regional Neurochemistry'. Ed. Kety and Elkes. London: Pergamon Press

VANE, J. R. (1959). *Brit. J. Pharmacol.* **14,** 87

VOGT, M. (1954). *J. Physiol.* **123,** 451

VOGT, M. (1957). *Brit. Med. Bull.* **13,** 166

*VOGT, M. (1959). *Pharmacol. Rev.* **11,** 483

VOGT, M., GUNN, C. G. and SAWYER, C. J. (1957). *Neurology,* **7,** 559

WEIL-MALHERBE, H. and BONE, A. D. (1959). *J. Neurochem.* **4,** 251

WEINER, N. (1960). *J. Neurochem.* **6,** 79

WEISSBACH, H., BOGDANSKI, D. D., REDFIELD, B. G. and UDENFRIEND, S. (1957). *J. biol. Chem.* **227,** 617

WEISSBACH, H., KING, W., SJOERDSMA, A. and UDENFRIEND, S. (1959). *J. biol. Chem.* **234,** 81

WHITE, T. (1959). *J. Physiol.* **149,** 34

WHITTAKER, V. P. (1959). *Biochem. J.* **72,** 694

WILSON, C. W. M. and BRODIE, B. B. (1961). *J. Pharmacol. exp. Ther.* **133,** 332

YEH, S. D. J., SOLOMON, J. D. and CHOW, B. F. (1959). *Fed. Proc.* **18,** 357

ZELLER, E. A., BARSKY, J. and BERMAN, E. R. (1955). *J. biol. Chem.* **214,** 267

ZETTLER, G. and SCHLOSSER, L. (1955). *Arch. exp. Path. Pharmak,* **224,** 159

ZETTLER, G. (1956). *Arch. exp. Path. Pharmak.* **228,** 513

CHAPTER 2

PSYCHOTROPIC DRUGS

A large number of drugs have been introduced recently which have an action on the central nervous system and are used in patients with abnormal mental processes, with the object of restoring these to normal. These drugs are not just sedatives, hypnotics, analgesics or anticonvulsants, but are believed to act more specifically on certain mental processes. Since so little is known about the pharmacology of mental activity, it is no wonder that the mode of action and even clinical significance of these newer drugs are difficult to evaluate. A number of them have essentially depressant effects and have been called, amongst other names, tranquillizers or ataractics, the idea being that they calm patients without making them drowsy as sedatives sometimes do; whilst others, such as some amine oxidase inhibitors, have mainly stimulant effects. All of them, however, are used in an attempt to restore normality in various 'psychotic' and 'neurotic' conditions and they have thus been called psychotropic or psycho-active drugs. In the same group is another series of drugs, of which lysergic acid diethylamide (LSD) and mescaline are the most important examples, which produce various disturbances in thought, including hallucination and delusions, and have been called hallucinogens as well as psychotomimetic or psychodysleptic drugs. Their effect is rather similar to those observed in certain mental diseases, especially schizophrenia, and their action has been studied in the hope of elucidating the mechanism responsible for these mental diseases (see discussion by Beecher, 1959).

Because of difficulties in classification, the Council on drugs of the American Medical Association has indeed abandoned the section on ataractics in 'New and nonofficial drugs' and has decided 'to describe agents proposed for use for their particular effect on the central nervous system, in accordance with their fundamental pharmacological classification, in so far as this is known', and they give a classification under many headings and subheadings (J. Amer. med. Ass., 1958). This classification lists most of the groups of depressant drugs, though it makes little attempt to deal similarly with central nervous stimulants. Any satisfactory classification of all these drugs is in fact very difficult in the present stage of our knowledge. A thoughtful discussion on psychopharmacological drugs is given by Himwich (1958), and in the Symposium on 'Brain mechanisms and drug action' (1957).

Brodie and his co-workers (1959) have made a bold attempt to contribute to this question by invoking the work of Hess on the integration of the autonomic nervous system, central and peripheral, with other brain functions and trying to correlate this with the distribution of pharmacologically active substances in the brain. On the basis of results obtained by stimulating various parts of the brain electrically in unanaesthetized cats, Hess postulated that reactions of the organism to environmental changes are affected by a *subcortical system which co-ordinates autonomic, somatic* and *psychic* functions. He further proposed that the subcortical system, like the peripheral autonomic system, consists of separate and antagonistic divisions, the ergotropic and trophotropic.

According to Hess, the *ergotropic* division produces behaviour patterns which prepare the body for positive action, i.e. arousal and an activated psychic state, increased sympathetic activity and enhanced skeletal muscle tone and activity and contains at least part of the reticular activating system. The *trophotropic* division, in contrast, controls behaviour patterns that are recuperative in nature, i.e. increased parasympathetic activity, drowsiness and sleep with lowered response to external stimuli and decreased muscle tone and activity.

Brodie *et al.* (1959) have sought to explain the central actions of a number of drugs in terms of their actions on the two divisions of the central autonomic system and have tentatively discussed the possibility that these actions might be exerted by potentiating or blocking neurohormones or, in the case of reserpine and amine oxidase inhibitors, in lowering or raising the concentrations of brain amines. However, at present this must be considered as largely speculative and the various substances which in recent years have been used in the treatment of mental disorders will be classified here rather arbitrarily as (1) major tranquillizers, i.e. chlorpromazine and other phenothiazines, and reserpine and related substances, (2) minor tranquillizers, e.g. meprobamate and (3) essentially stimulant substances like amphetamine, iproniazid (and other amine oxidase inhibitors) and imipramine.

PHENOTHIAZINE DERIVATIVES

The discovery of these compounds arose out of a search for new and better antihistamines. The first phenothiazine derivative found to be of general value in medicine was *promethazine* (Phenergan) which is still widely used, essentially as an antihistamine, though it has quite a marked sedative action (see Robson and Keele, 1950 and 1956 for review of action of histamine and anti-histamine drugs). Chlorpromazine was introduced in 1951 and has a wide variety of actions, described in detail by Robson and Keele (1956). Since then many new phenothiazines have been introduced (see Friend, 1960; Rees, 1960) and in this section the action of chlorpromazine will be briefly reviewed in comparison with the newer compounds. These have in general been made in an attempt to produce

Table 4

Phenothiazine derivatives

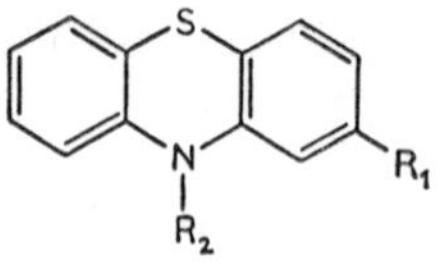

*Dimethylaminopropyl
side chain*

Name	Trade Name	Chemical Structure	Remarks
Promethazine	Phenergan	$R_1 = H$ $R_2 = CH_2.CH.NH(CH_3)_2CH_3$	Anti-histamine.
Chlorpromazine	Largactil Thorazine	$R_1 = Cl$ $R_2 = (CH_2)_3.N(CH_3)_2$	
Promazine	Sparine	$R_1 = H$ $R_2 = (CH_2)_3N(CH_3)_2$	Weaker than chlorpromazine.
Trifluopromazine	Vespral	$R_1 = CF_3$ $R_2 = (CH_2)_3N(CH_3)_2$	Fairly potent.
Acepromazine (Acetylpromazine)	Notensil	$R_1 = OC.CH_3$ $R_2 = (CH_2)_3.N(CH_3)_2$	Weaker than chlorpromazine.
Methotrimeprazine (Levopromazine)	Veractil	$R_1 = OCH_3$ $R_2 = CH_2.CH(CH_3).CH_2.N(CH_3)_2$	Similar in potency to chlorpromazine.
Methoxypromazine	Tentone	$R_1 = OCH_3$ $R_2 = (CH_2)_3.N(CH_3)_2$	Weak.
Trimeprazine	Temaril	$R_1 = H$ $R_2 = CH_2.CH.CH_3.N(CH_3)_2$	Antipruritic.

Piperidine side chain

Name	Trade Name	Chemical Structure	Remarks
Mepazine	Pacatal	$R_1 = H$ 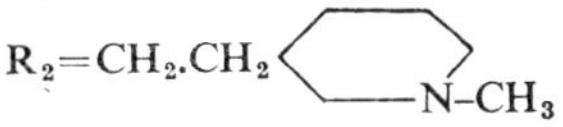 $R_2 = CH_2.CH_2$ —N–CH$_3$	Weak and still toxic.
Thioridazine	Melleril	$R_1 = S.CH_3$ 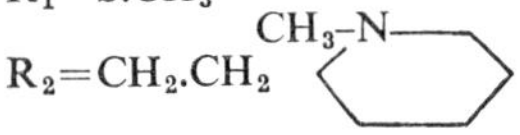 $R_2 = CH_2.CH_2$ CH$_3$–N—	Weak but little toxicity.
Pipamazine	Mornidine	$R_1 = Cl$ 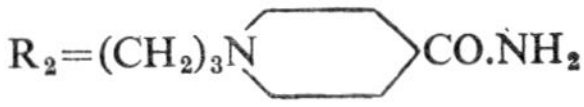 $R_2 = (CH_2)_3N$ CO.NH$_2$	Anti-emetic.

Piperazine side chain

Name	Trade Name	Chemical Structure	Remarks
Prochlorperazine	Stemetil	$R_1 = Cl$ 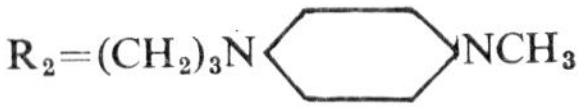	Potent.
	Compazine	$R_2 = (CH_2)_3N$ NCH$_3$	
Perphenazine	Fentazine	$R_1 = Cl$ 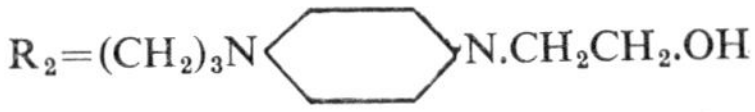	Potent.
	Trilafon	$R_2 = (CH_2)_3N$ N.CH$_2$CH$_2$.OH	
Trifluoperazine	Stelazine	$R_1 = CF_3$ $R_2 = (CH_2)_3N$ N.CH$_3$ 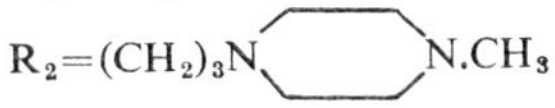	Very potent severe extra-pyramidal effects.
Thiopropazate	Dartalan	$R_1 = Cl$ 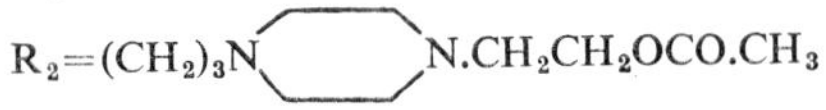 $R_2 = (CH_2)_3N$ N.CH$_2$CH$_2$OCO.CH$_3$	Potent.
Thioperazine	Vontil	$R_1 = SO_2N(CH_3)_2$ 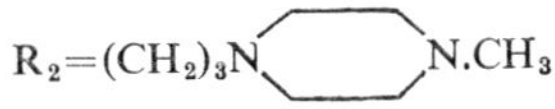 $R_2 = (CH_2)_3N$ N.CH$_3$	Very potent anti-emetic.
Fluphenazine	Moditen	$R_1 = CF_3$ 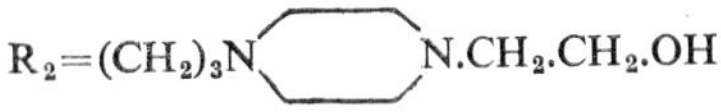 $R_2 = (CH_2)_3N$ N.CH$_2$.CH$_2$.OH	Very potent.

a potent and selective action, particularly 'tranquillizing' and anti-emetic, trying to avoid certain toxic effects, notably on the liver and haemopoetic system and avoiding stimulation of the extra-pyramidal part of the central nervous system leading to Parkinsonism. The names and formulae of various phenothiazines are shown in Table 4. It will be seen that chemical substitution has been affected in two positions (R_1 and R_2) and the drugs so made can be classified into three groups, according to the substituent at R_2 which may be:

1. A dimethylaminopropyl side chain, e.g. chlorpromazine and trifluopromazine.

2. A piperidine side chain, e.g. mepazine and thioridazine.

3. A piperazine side chain, e.g. trifluoperazine.

The substituents at R_1 include halogens, methoxy, thiomethyl and other organic radicals.

Chlorpromazine

In general it can be said that chlorpromazine inhibits the hypothalamus, the reticular formation, the chemoreceptor trigger zone and to some extent the vomiting centre. As a result a number of psychological effects are produced which have been analysed in a variety of ways. The drug also produces a weak anticholinergic, antihistamine, antispasmodic and hypotensive action. The action of narcotic analgesics and some barbiturates is potentiated, although there is no interference with their metabolism. The pressor response to adrenaline and noradrenaline is reduced. Body temperature is altered by two mechanisms: by an action on the diencephalon and by peripheral vasodilation, both tending to a lowering of body temperature. Some of the recent work on the action of chlorpromazine on the central nervous system is reviewed by Werner (1959); he stresses how difficult it is at present to explain the widespread effects of the drug in normal and pathological conditions in terms of its sites of action. A few investigations will be quoted to illustrate this. Krivoy (1957) found that chlorpromazine and reserpine inhibit reflex activity in the cat, the effect being predominantly on monosynaptic reflex pathways. De Maar et al. (1958) obtained evidence that chlorpromazine acts selectively by depressing the frequency response of neurones responsible for the 'slow' potentials recorded in the medial reticular formation. Papatheodorou et al. (1958) investigated the effects of chlorpromazine in normal monkeys and in monkeys with brain stem lesions. They found that the drug decreased motor activity and responsiveness to all stimuli and produced a picture suggesting catatonia. Signs of permanent neurological defects following brain stem lesions were rendered less apparent by chlorpromazine. Given over several days there were tremor, rigidity and some EEG changes. The authors suggest that chlorpromazine may have a generalized effect on the central nervous system upon which may be superimposed further actions on specific structures or functions of the system. Interesting effects have also been observed on the sexual apparatus though again the site of action requires further investigation. It has been found that chlorpromazine (as well as perphenazine and reserpine) will induce pseudo-pregnancy in rats (Barraclough and Sawyer, 1959; Velardo, 1958) and will also produce menstrual abnormalities in women (Clark and Johnson, 1960).

The main *clinical uses* of the drug are (1) in psychiatry to reduce and control agitation, tension, anxiety and other abnormal mental states. Highly successful results have been obtained (see p. 68). (2) As an anti-emetic where it may be very valuable, though not in travel sickness. (3) As part of anaesthesia and in the control of body temperature in anaesthesia. (4) In a variety of other conditions, e.g. pruritis and hiccough.

Toxic effects are not uncommon. An obstructive type of jaundice occurs in about 2% of cases, but usually clears up when the drug is discontinued. It is probably allergic in nature and sensitivity to the drug may be retained for long periods. Agranulocytosis occurs, though fortunately rarely. Extra-pyramidal nervous system activity occurs and ranges from mild loss of skilled muscle movements to frank Parkinsonism. Other toxic effects include rashes, light sensitivity, pruritis and very rarely gynecomastia. Adrenergic blocking effects leading to postural hypotension may also occur. These toxic effects are further discussed on p. 69.

Chlorpromazine sulphoxide is a major metabolite of chlorpromazine in dogs and though there are both quantitative and qualitative differences in their actions, the metabolite is on the whole pharmacologically less active than the parent compound (Moran and Butler, 1956).

Newer Phenothiazines

It is difficult to estimate the value of the many new compounds in comparison with chlorpromazine, and claims made for some substances are not supported by the available evidence. At present it appears that the piperazine derivatives are the most potent and that, unless the dose is carefully controlled, severe extrapyramidal effects may occur with these compounds. These include not only rigidity, tremor and loss of associated movements, but also uncontrolled motor activity, oculogyric crises and spasms of the neck, tongue and pharyngeal muscles. On the other hand these compounds are less liable to produce the other major toxic effects of chlorpromazine (Friend, 1960; Hollister, 1958). Various aspects of the pharmacology and therapeutic use of trifluoperazine are discussed by Brill (1959). Amongst the piperidine derivatives, mepazine is weaker than chlorpromazine and still liable to produce toxic effects while thioridazine is also rather weak but is less toxic (Kinross-Wright, 1959). Taeschler and Cerletti (1959) have investigated the effect of various phenothiazines in rats and found that the sedative effects and the decrease in emotional behaviour caused by these drugs seem to be independent of each other, a conclusion similar to that reached for chlorpromazine by Miller *et al.* (1957). In agreement with previous work by Courvoisier (which they quote) Taeschler and Cerletti found that there is a parallelism between the cataleptic effect of these drugs in animals and the incidence of extrapyramidal side effects in man. Piala *et al.* (1959) using several tests in various animals including monkeys, found that trifluopromazine was more active than chlorpromazine as a tranquillizer and anti-emetic and was less likely to cause cardio-vascular reactions. The relation of chemical structure to activity among the phenothiazines is also discussed by High *et al.* (1960) and their tests show that fluphenazine is a highly potent compound. Further work with the newer compounds is badly needed. They are discussed from a clinical point of view on p. 69.

RAUWOLFIA ALKALOIDS

These have been used in a crude form for many centuries in popular medicine and the main compounds and preparations available are given by Robson and Keele (1956), although the discussion there is essentially on hypotensive drugs. A large number of alkaloids have been extracted from Rauwolfia, which are discussed by Bein (1956). The main alkaloids are reserpine, riscinnamine and canescine (deserpidine) (see p. 49). The differences between their actions are not marked. The sites of action of reserpine on the central nervous system, like those of chlorpromazine, are chiefly subcortical; unlike chlorpromazine, reserpine however stimulates the reticular activating system, rather than depressing it and is thus not as powerful a sedative as chlorpromazine (Hollister, 1958). A number of effects of reserpine using tests as discussed on p. 78 have been described. Amongst these the following are of particular interest. Reserpine was apparently found to have a taming effect on rhesus monkeys resulting in easier handling and a behaviour which was characterized as 'insulation from environment', a condition which is different from that obtained with barbiturates where reflexes are lost and the animal cannot be roused (Schneider and Earl, 1954). Weiskrantz and Wilson (1955) tested avoidance behaviour in monkeys, using an apparatus in which the animals could avoid shock by pushing a panel; impairment of the previously established avoidance behaviour started 2–3 hours after administration of reserpine and the avoidance response was eventually blocked in all animals. They eliminated various portions of the brain by operation and concluded from their observations that reserpine protects the hypothalamus from activating impulses, its site of action being probably situated somewhere in the region of the orbito-insulatemporal areas. This question of the site of action of reserpine is, however, far from settled, and in a more recent discussion,

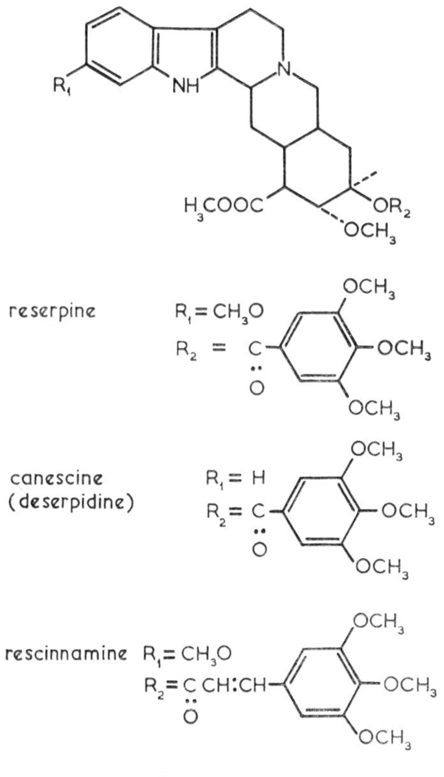

reserpine $R_1 = CH_3O$

$R_2 = $ C

caneseine
(deserpidine) $R_1 = H$

$R_2 = $ C

rescinnamine $R_1 = CH_3O$

$R_2 = $ C CH:CH—

Rauwolfia Alkaloids

Weiskrantz (1957) concludes that the drug serves to block incoming sensory information; the animal becomes non-reactive and non-attentive except to very strong stimulation.

The action of reserpine on the brain is no doubt partly, if not entirely, brought about by the release of dopamine, noradrenaline, adrenaline and 5-hydroxytryptamine which it causes. This is described in chapter 1, p. 21. It is part of a general release of amines from stores throughout the body (see chapter 3, p. 110 and chapter 4, p. 147).

Fate in Body. The action of reserpine comes on slowly and is prolonged, and the smaller the dose, the longer the latent period. This is seen even if the drug is given intravenously.

The drug is an ester and can thus be split into its component parts—
methyl reserpate and trimethoxy-benzoate. Other metabolic products
have also been described (Plummer, Sheppard and Schulert, 1957). The
metabolism of reserpine differs in various animal species and the drug
is particularly rapidly hydrolyzed by the intestine of the rat (Glazko
et al., 1956). The reason for the prolonged action of reserpine is not
completely explained. Hess, Shore and Brodie (1956) could find no trace
of it in the brain 2 to 4 hours after an injection though Plummer *et al.*
(1957), using tritium labelled reserpine, found appreciable amounts of
radio-activity in the brain of guinea pigs up to 48 hours after the
administration of 100 μg./kg. Some effects of reserpine may therefore
be due to the survival of small amounts but there seems little doubt that
reserpine damages the storage mechanism of brain amines and that this
is only slowly repaired. Robison *et al.* (1961) have described derivatives
of methyl reserpate which act rapidly and show no cumulation.

TETRABENAZINE (Nitoman)

This is a benzoquinolizine (formula below) which has properties
similar to reserpine, though it does not contain an indole group. Its
properties are described by Quinn, Shore and Brodie (1959). It is rapidly
metabolized when administered to rabbits. It has a selective action on
brain 5-HT and noradrenaline, though more on the latter than on the
former. It releases little or none of these amines peripherally; it does not

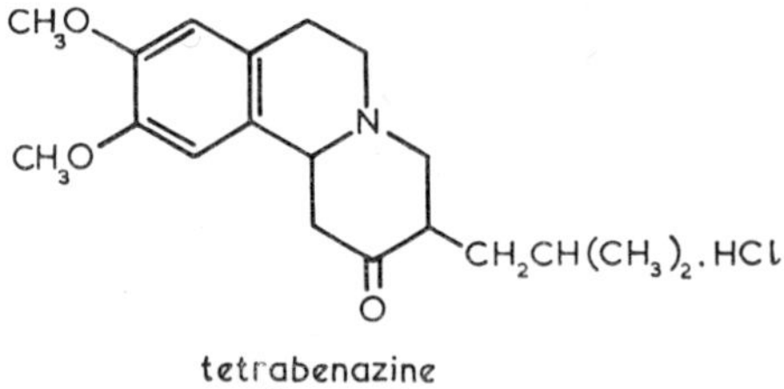

tetrabenazine
(Nitoman)

tend to cause diarrhoea or hypotension. The sedative effect of the drug
seems to be related to the change in brain 5-HT rather than noradrenaline. There is some evidence that it competes with reserpine for brain
receptors.

Preliminary clinical trials suggest that tetrabenazine is effective in the
psychiatric conditions for which reserpine is used. It differs from
reserpine in having a shorter duration of action and having only weak
peripheral effects. Side effects are common and include Parkinsonism
and loss of equilibrium, hypotonia, and hormonic disturbances, viz.,
metrorrhagia and spontaneous lactation (Diseases Nervous System,
1960).

HALOPERIDOL

This is a substituted butyrophenone with a structure resembling γ-aminobutyric acid (see below), the pharmacology of which is discussed in chapter 1 (p. 27).

Haloperidol is a white microcrystalline powder, poorly soluble in water, and has actions similar to the phenothiazines. It is one of many

$$HO-OC-CH_2-CH_2-CH_2-NH_2$$

γ-aminobutyric acid

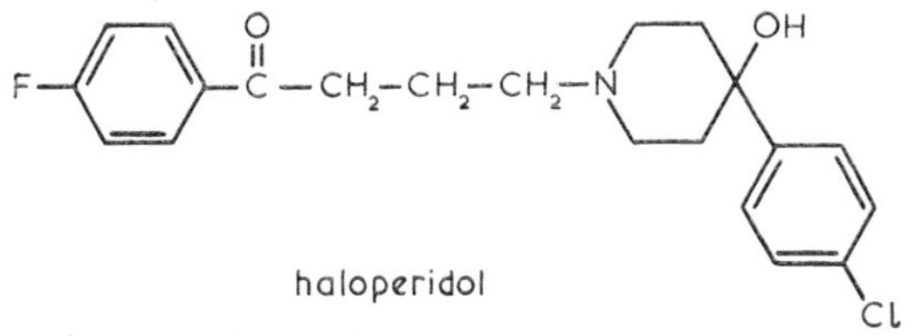

haloperidol

similar compounds synthesized by Janssen and his co-workers (1959). A number of pharmacological investigations have been performed with it and there is good evidence that it produces marked effects on the central nervous system (see Niemegeers and Janssen, 1960; Janssen, Jageneau and Niemegeers, 1960). It has been used in a variety of psychiatric conditions and also in anaesthesia. It may be given orally or by intramuscular or intravenous injection. It has marked anti-emetic properties. Like the phenothiazines it can produce extrapyramidal effects, and motor restlessness may occur during its administration. It has been used fairly extensively on the continent. It is clear that though the drug may have marked sedative effects which come on 10 to 20 minutes after intravenous injection, it can also produce side effects, which can be severe, e.g. tremor, rigidity, oculogyric crises and nystagmus. Some fall in blood pressure may occur.

There is at present no information about the fate of the drug in the body. Much further information will have to be obtained before its value can be assessed.

MEPROBAMATE (Equanil, Miltown, Mepavlon)

This drug was developed from the parent compound, mephenesin, which was introduced in 1946 as a muscle relaxant. It is a simple aliphatic substance with a low solubility in water, but readily soluble in most organic solvents. Its chemical structure, together with that of mephenesin, is shown below. The properties of meprobamate are discussed in the Annals of the New York Academy of Sciences (1957) and by Berger (1956).

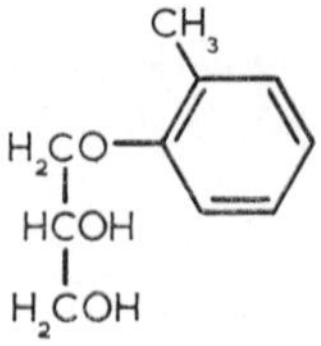

mephenesin 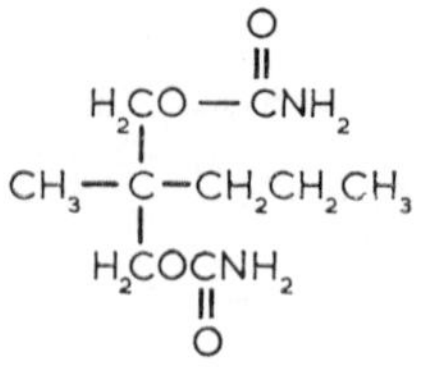   meprobamate

Fate in body. Meprobamate is well absorbed when given orally and about 10% is excreted unchanged in the urine. The bulk of the remaining 90% of the drug is apparently excreted as two metabolites, including a gluconate (Berger, 1956). This has been demonstrated both in experimental animals and in man. Experiments with labelled meprobamate (^{14}C) show that a maximum blood level is reached in 1–2 hours and that very little is left in the blood after 24 hours (Carlo, 1957). The liver is the main site of metabolism of the drug (Agranoff, Bradley and Axelrod, 1957). The major metabolite in dogs is hydroxymeprobamate, and this has no meprobamate-like activity (Walkenstein *et al.*, 1958).

Pharmacological effects. Meprobamate has a muscle relaxant action, anticonvulsant action, and also apparently a 'taming effect' best observed in monkeys. The muscle relaxant effect is similar to that observed with mephenesin, but of greater potency and longer duration. The drug shows good protection of mice against the convulsant action of leptazol and strychnine and effectively modifies electroshock seizures in animals. According to Berger (1956), monkeys on a suitable dose of meprobamate lose their fear and hostility, become tame and friendly and retain full interest in their environment. Experiments on normal human subjects show that meprobamate produces no abnormalities of behaviour, as measured by tests of driving, steadiness and vision. The experiments with meprobamate in man show that the drug is capable of checking emotional responses without interfering with skill, rational behaviour and adequate responses to environmental stimuli. As to the site of action, the drug has a marked blocking effect on interneurones which can be easily demonstrated at the level of the spinal cord and has also a selective action on the thalamus producing a marked synchronization of activity. It does not seem to affect the autonomic nervous system.

Toxicity. This is low when tested in animals, as is also shown by the fact that subjects who have taken large numbers of tablets in attempted suicide have become somnolent but quickly recovered.

Nevertheless, as the drug has been increasingly used clinically, it has become evident that a variety of toxic effects can occur and that it can do serious harm: habituation and addiction, occasionally with a typical withdrawal syndrome; various symptoms of idiosyncrasy; and even a fatal case of aplastic anaemia. Death following attempted suicide has also been reported (Annotation, 1958).

METHYLPENTYNOL (methylparafynol, Oblivon, Dormison) and *methyl pentynol carbamate*

Both these substances have been used as hypnotics and as minor tranquillizers. Their formulae are shown below. Methylpentynol is an unsaturated tertiary alcohol which was introduced into therapeutics by Margolins *et al.* (1951) while the carbamate has been investigated more recently by Halpern (1956) who concluded from his results that the drug acts on mesencephalic and subcortical parts of the brain.

The distribution of these drugs is similar to that of ethyl alcohol, i.e. they are distributed throughout the body fluid, enter cells, cross the blood brain barrier and the placenta. They are, however, rather slowly metabolized or excreted (Marley and Vane, 1958) and it has in fact been found in man that both drugs will accumulate in the blood and body tissues when given in a dose of 0·5 G. four times daily for 5 days (Bartholomew, Bourne and Marley, 1958). After cessation of such a treatment the drug can be found in the blood for up to three days.

The pharmacological properties of the compounds are described by Marley (1959) and compared with those of alcohol and barbiturates. The pentynols depress monosynaptic and polysynaptic reflexes and

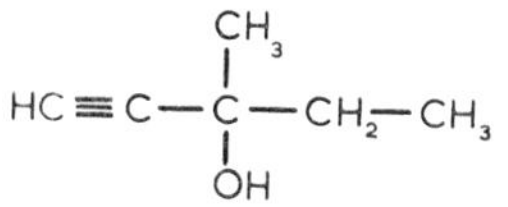

$$HC \equiv C - \overset{\overset{\displaystyle CH_3}{|}}{\underset{\underset{\displaystyle OH}{|}}{C}} - CH_2 - CH_3 \qquad\qquad HC \equiv C - \overset{\overset{\displaystyle CH_3}{|}}{\underset{\underset{\displaystyle COONH_2}{|}}{C}} - CH_2 - CH_3$$

methylpentynol 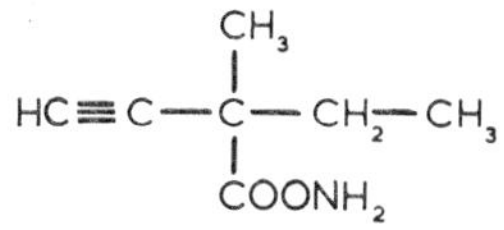   methylpentynol carbamate

produce a number of pharmacological effects, including weak ganglion and neuromuscular blocking actions and transitory hypotension. Dicker and Steinberg (1957) investigated the effect of methylpentynol in man in an exacting test, and found that it depressed the autonomic reaction to a difficult motor task but also impaired performance. The results suggest that the modes of action of methylpentynol and hexobarbitone are different.

The drugs have been used as tranquillizers because of the results obtained in animal experiments and clinically. Thus methylpentynol appears to reduce fear in rats (Dicker, Steinberg and Watson, 1957) and can allay anxiety in human subjects (Bourne, 1954). The drug is by no means free from side effects similar to those seen in barbiturate and

3

alcoholic intoxication (Marley and Chambers, 1956). They usually occur with doses greater than 1·0 G. per day and are much more liable to occur in patients with psychiatric disorders. Mild disturbance of hepatic function may also occur with the larger doses (Bartholomew *et al.*, 1958).

CHLORDIAZEPOXIDE (Methaminodiazepoxide, Librium)

This is a new type of compound synthesized by Sternbach and Reeder (see Randall *et al.*, 1960) with the structure shown below. It is highly soluble in water, unstable in solution and the powder must be protected from light. Its pharmacological properties have been investigated by Randall *et al.* (1960). It produces a loss of aggressive behaviour in monkeys in doses which do not depress general activity or avoidance behaviour; it has a calming effect on rats made hyperactive by lesions in the septal area of the brain. It shows muscle relaxant, sedative and anticonvulsant activity in mice. Additional effects observed were antiinflammatory effects in rats and a remarkable stimulation of appetite in

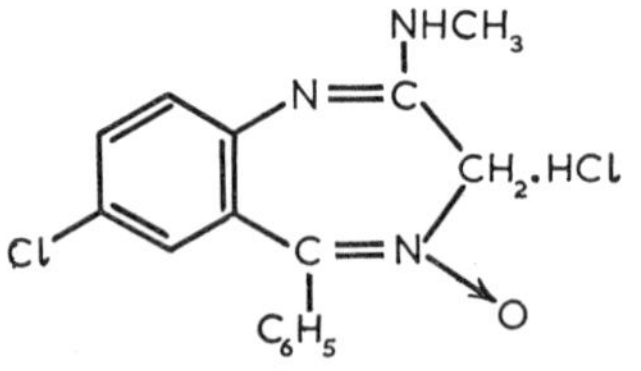

chlordiazepoxide

rats and dogs. There were no autonomic blocking effects. In chronic toxicity tests in rats and dogs no abnormal effects or evidence of cumulation were seen. There are at present no data about the fate of this drug in the body. Clinical results show that chlordiazepoxide is by no means free from toxic effects and suggest that it should be used carefully. Among the side effects observed are drowsiness, ataxia, dizziness, muscle tenderness and spasm, constipation, loss of libido and menstrual abnormalities, and increased appetite with excessive gain of weight. Transient macular rashes have also occurred (see Diseases of the Nervous System, 1960).

METHYLPHENIDATE (Ritalin)

This is a central stimulant developed in the Ciba Laboratories. It is a water soluble substance, methyl-α-phenyl-2-piperidine acetal hydrochloride and the formula is shown on p. 55.

Its pharmacological properties in animals have been investigated by Meier, Gross and Tripod (1954). It is described by them as having an effect intermediate between amphetamine and caffeine. It stimulates co-ordinated motor activity. It also stimulates respiration and produces a moderate but prolonged hypertension. Drassdo and Schmidt (1954) investigated its cardiovascular effect in man and found that it could produce a rise in blood pressure and increase in pulse rate, though in some subjects a fall in blood pressure was observed. A dose of 10 mg. produced an effect lasting for 4–6 hours. Methylphenidate will reverse the depressant effect of promazine in man. It has been suggested that it has a stimulant effect in both cortical and subcortical centres (Ehrmantraut *et al.*, 1957). Antagonism of the depressant action of reserpine has also been shown in a variety of animals, including monkeys (Plummer, Maxwell and Earl, 1957; Cole and Glees, 1956). Little is known about its fate in the body. The distribution and elimination of methylphenidate

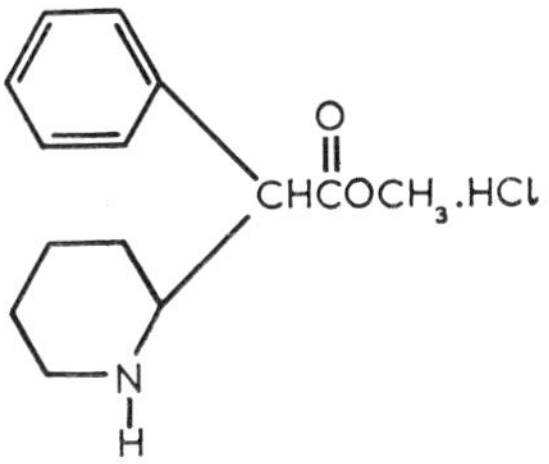

methylphenidate (Ritalin) 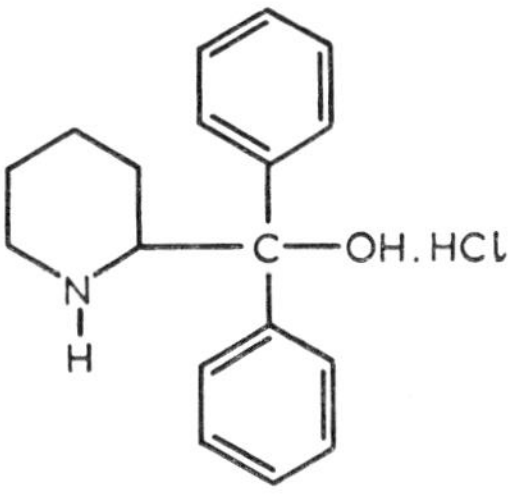   pipradol (Meratran)

(labelled with ^{14}C) have been studied by Sheppard *et al.* (1960). About 70% of the dose injected into guinea pigs appears in the urine, within 24 hours, mostly as degradation products.

The drug has been used as a mild cortical stimulant in various types of depression (see p. 73) as well as for counteracting the manifestations of depression produced by phenothiazine derivatives, Rauwolfia alkaloids, barbiturates, anticonvulsants and other sedative drugs. It has a low toxicity, but may produce nervousness, insomnia, anorexia, dizziness, palpitation, headache and nausea. Appreciable cardiovascular stimulation is not infrequent when the drug is given parenterally, particularly intravenously.

PIPRADOL (Meratran)

This is also a central stimulant and was developed by the Merrell Laboratories. It is both water and alcohol soluble. It is α-(2-piperidyl)-benzhydrol hydrochloride and its formula is shown above.

Pharmacological experiments with the drug are reported by Blohm, Summers and Greenwood (1954) and by Brown and Werner (1954). It induces co-ordinated hyperactivity in animals; these do not become hypersensitive to stimuli and appetite is not affected. Convulsions do not occur with a dose less than the L.D.50, nor does depression follow the administration of the drug (as is found with amphetamine). After oral dosage to rats it is rapidly absorbed and rapidly eliminated from the body, about equally in the urine and faeces. According to NND (1961) pipradol seems to have a wide margin of safety and appears to be relatively non-toxic.

AZACYCLONOL (Frenquel)

This is α-(4-piperidyl)-benzhydrol hydrochloride and is thus clearly related to pipradol. Azacyclonol will protect human volunteers against the acute effect of intoxication with lysergic acid diethylamide (Fabing, 1955). Gray and Forrest (1958) investigated the compound in cases of chronic schizophrenia and concluded that the drug was not of any great value.

BENACTYZINE (Suavitil)

This is the hydrochloride of the diethylaminoethyl ester of benzilic acid. It is one of a series of related compounds which have sedative and hypnotic actions and, peripherally, atropine-like actions (Holten and Sonne, 1955). The clinical results are not impressive (Davies, 1956).

IMIPRAMINE (Tofranil)

This is a compound rather similar chemically to the phenothiazines, but with somewhat different biological properties. Its structure is shown below. Its pharmacological properties have been investigated by Domenjoz and Theobald (1959). It is noteworthy that these particular

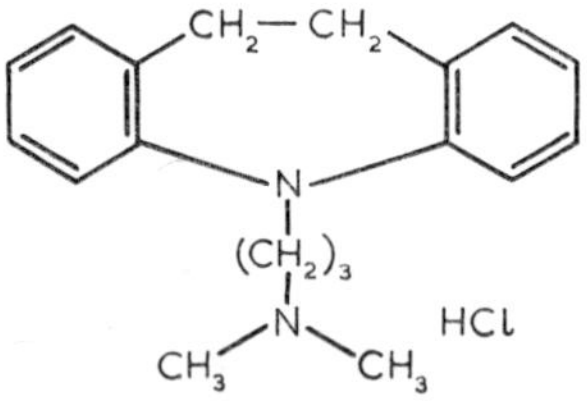

imipramine

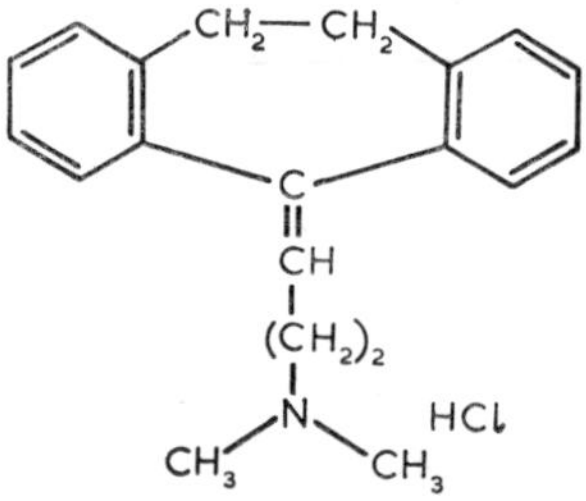

amitriptyline

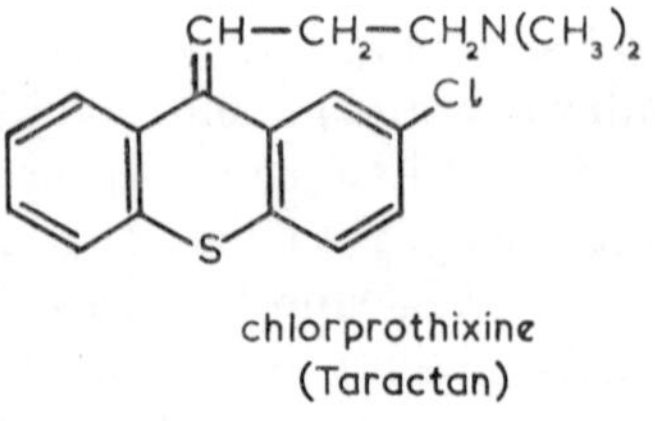

chlorprothixine
(Taractan)

investigators were unable to demonstrate any clear cut 'psychotropic effects' in animal experiments. Imipramine is well absorbed when given orally; it is rapidly metabolized and also quickly taken up by various organs. In a case of suicide, large amounts of the drug or its metabolites were demonstrated in the liver, spleen, adrenals and brain (Herrmann and Pulver, 1960). There is evidence that the effect of imipramine on the brain is mediated by a metabolic product, desmethyl-imipramine (Gillete et al., 1961).

In non-toxic doses imipramine has no depressant effect on motor behaviour. It intensifies the central depressant properties of narcotics, yet it has a marked antagonistic action against the central inhibitory effects of reserpine and bulbocapnine. Antagonism to a number of actions of histamine, acetylcholine, adrenaline, noradrenaline, and 5-hydroxytryptamine has been demonstrated, but further analyses of these seem desirable. A marked anti-anaphylactic action in the sensitized guinea pig has also been demonstrated.

An interesting action of imipramine is that it markedly lowers the 5-HT content of blood platelets, in contrast to iproniazid which causes a rise. Imipramine suppresses the in vitro uptake of 5-HT by human platelets; it has no inhibitory effect on 5-hydroxytryptophan decarboxylase (Marshall et al., 1960).

In patients with cardiovascular disease, imipramine may cause severe postural hypotension and even myocardial infarction and great caution should therefore be used in the administration of the drug to such patients (Muller et al., 1961). Other ill effects are described on p. 75.

AMITRIPTYLINE (Tryptizol)

This has a structure and properties similar to imipramine. Some aspects of its metabolism are described by Hucker and Porter (1961), and its pharmacology is described by Vernier (1961); further details are given in a memorandum prepared by Stone (1961).

CHLORPROTHIXINE (Taractan)

This is a thioxanthine derivative (see p. 56) with properties rather similar to chlorpromazine. Allgén et al. (1960) describe its elimination in man and rats. Its pharmacological properties have been investigated by Pellmont et al. (1960) who find that in both central and peripheral actions it is more potent than chlorpromazine, though there is also evidence that it is more toxic in mice. Its anti-serotonin effects are quite striking. Further clinical investigation of this substance is required, though it has already been found that side effects may occur, particularly hypotension and extra-pyramidal disturbances, the former being more common than with chlorpromazine (Hoffet and Cornu, 1960).

INHIBITORS OF AMINE OXIDASE (Mono-amine oxidase)

In 1938 Gaddum and Kwiatkowski described the potentiation by ephedrine of the cardiovascular effects of injected adrenaline and of sympathetic stimulation, and suggested that this might be explained if ephedrine inhibited the breakdown of adrenaline. Shortly afterwards, the inhibition of amine oxidase by ephedrine was described by Richter and Tingey (1939) but it soon became apparent that this inhibition would be very weak in the concentrations of ephedrine with which potentiation was obtained, and for this and other reasons this explanation of the potentiation of adrenaline by ephedrine was abandoned.

In 1952 Zeller reported that iproniazid, which had shortly before been introduced for the chemotherapy of tuberculosis, is a powerful amine

Table 5

Classification of inhibitors of amine oxidase

1. Hydrazines:
   Iproniazid [Marsalid]
   Phenelzine [phenethylhydrazine, Nardil]
   Pheniprazine [α-methylphenethylhydrazine, Cavodil, Catron, P I H, JB 516]
   α-methylphenpropylhydrazine [JB 835]
   Phenoxypropazine [(1-methyl-2-phenoxyethyl) hydrazine, Drazine]
   Nialamide [N - (2 - benzylcarbamoylethyl) - N' - isonicotinoyl hydrazine, Niamid]
   Isocarboxazid [3 - N - benzylhydrazinocarbonyl - 5 - methyl*iso*oxazole, Marplan]
   Pivazide [N-benzyl-N'-pivaloylhydrazine, Tersavid]
   2-benzyl-l-picolinylhydrazine [RO 5–0700]
2. Harmala alkaloids
3. Tryptamine derivatives:
   α-methyl tryptamine
   α-ethyl tryptamine [etryptamine, Monase]
4. Others:
   Choline *p*-tolyl ether [TM 6]
   Tranylcypromine [± *trans*-2-phenyl*cyclo*propylamine, Parnate, SKF 385]
   Pargyline [N-benzyl-N-methyl-2-propynylamine, A 19120]
   Amidines
   Amphetamine, ephedrine, cocaine, procaine, antihistamines, methylene blue, sulphydryl reagents.

oxidase inhibitor (see Zeller *et al.*, 1955); since then many more have been described. Some of these are given, classified according to their chemical structure, in Table 5 and the structure of representatives of each group is shown in Table 6.

The very extensive work on amine oxidase inhibitors since then (see Davison, 1958; Symposium, 1959) has been conducted for two principal reasons: because it has been hoped that the inhibition of an enzyme destroying catechol amines and 5-hydroxytryptamine might lead to valuable information about the function and mode of action of these substances, and because amine oxidase inhibitors were early found to have important therapeutic properties.

Table 6

Structure of inhibitors of amine oxidase

iproniazid $\quad R - CO.NHNHCH \begin{cases} CH_3 \\ CH_3 \end{cases}$

nialamide $\quad R - CO.NHNHCH_2CH_2CO.NHCH_2C_6H_5$

phenelzine $\quad \phi - CH_2CH_2NHNH_2$

pheniprazine $\quad \phi - CH_2CHNHNH_2$
$\qquad\qquad\qquad\; | $
$\qquad\qquad\qquad CH_3$

JB 835 $\quad \phi - CH_2CH_2CHNHNH_2$
$\qquad\qquad\qquad\qquad\; |$
$\qquad\qquad\qquad\qquad CH_3$

phenoxypropazine $\quad \phi - OCH_2CHNHNH_2$
$\qquad\qquad\qquad\qquad\quad |$
$\qquad\qquad\qquad\qquad\; CH_3$

pivazide $\quad \phi - CH_2NHNHCO.C \begin{cases} CH_3 \\ CH_3 \\ CH_3 \end{cases}$

pargyline $\quad \phi - CH_2N \begin{cases} CH_2C{\equiv}CH \\ CH_3 \end{cases}$

isocarboxazid $\quad \phi - CH_2NHNHCO-$

tranylcypromine $\quad \phi - CH - CHNH_2$
$\qquad\qquad\qquad\quad \backslash \;\; /$
$\qquad\qquad\qquad\quad\; CH_2$

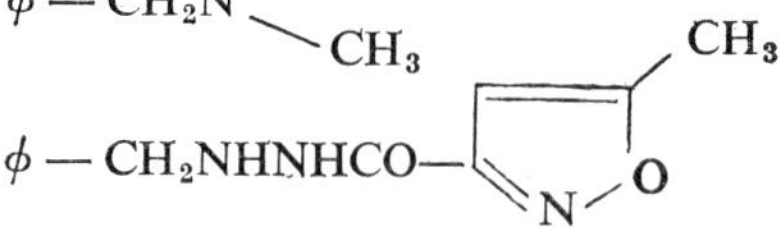

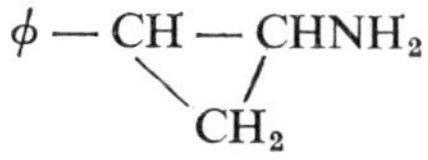

amphetamine $\quad \phi - CH_2CHNH_2$
$\qquad\qquad\qquad\qquad |$
$\qquad\qquad\qquad\; CH_3$

choline p – tolyl ether $\quad CH_3 - \phi - OCH_2CH_2\overset{\oplus}{N} \begin{cases} CH_3 \\ CH_3 \\ CH_3 \end{cases}$

$\underline{R} : $ $\qquad\qquad \phi :$

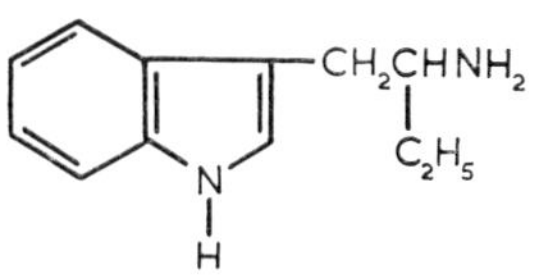

etryptamine
(α-ethyl tryptamine)

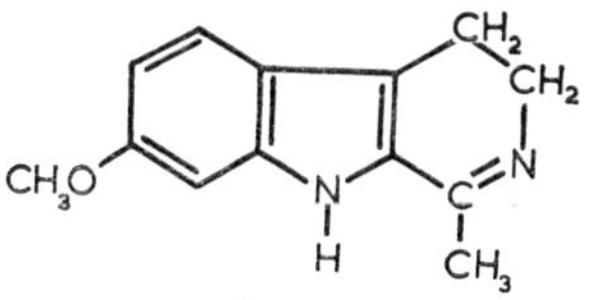

harmaline

In assessing an amine oxidase inhibitor the following information should be available:

1. The effect of the addition of the substance *in vitro* on the amine oxidase activity of tissue homogenates (brain, liver, kidney, etc.). The activity is measured either by following the disappearance of the added substrate (e.g. 5-hydroxytryptamine), the consumption of oxygen or the formation of the aldehyde (Green and Haughton, 1961) or of NH_3 resulting from the oxidative deamination reaction:

$$R—CH_2NH_2+O_2 \longrightarrow R—CHO+NH_3$$

2. The amine oxidase activity of homogenates of organs removed from animals to which the substance had previously been administered.

3. The effect of administration of the substance on the tissue concentrations of naturally occurring amines which are substrates for it. Increases in the concentrations of dopamine, noradrenaline, adrenaline, 5-HT and tryptamine have been observed in many tissues after a single large dose or repeated small doses of potent amine oxidase inhibitors. These changes have been mostly investigated in the brain and are discussed on p. 19.

4. The effect of administration of the substance on the excretion of substrates of amine oxidase and of their metabolites. These substrates may be normally present in the body or may be administered for the purpose of the test. For example the daily excretion of tryptamine in the urine (Sjoerdsma *et al.*, 1959, 1960) and the percentage conversion of orally administered 5-hydroxytryptamine into urinary 5-HIAA (Sjoerdsma *et al.*, 1958) have been used for this purpose in man.

5. Modification of the pharmacological action of substrates. The potentiation by ephedrine of the action of adrenaline on the rabbit's ear has been referred to above and shows that this action cannot be accepted alone as evidence of amine oxidase inhibition.

Since amine oxidase is contained in intracellular granules (p. 13) there are at least two, and more probably three, barriers between a drug circulating in the blood stream and the enzyme: the capillary wall (or blood-brain barrier), the cellular membrane and probably the membrane of the granule. The preparation of tissue homogenates abolishes two of these and will abolish the third as well if the treatment leads to the liberation of the enzyme from its intracellular granules. Evidence of amine oxidase inhibition obtained from experiments *in vitro* (categories 1 and 2 above) must not therefore be taken as evidence of *in vivo* inhibition.

The interpretation of the pharmacological actions of amine oxidase inhibitors is by no means simple. Not only are there a number of naturally occurring amines which are substrates for amine oxidase and whose concentration may be increased, and may be responsible for some of the effects observed, but none of the inhibitors so far described has an action confined to mono-amine oxidase. Many inhibit a number of other enzymes as well. Iproniazid has, for example, been reported to inhibit the liver enzymes which metabolize hexobarbitone (Laroche and Brodie, 1960), diphosphopyridine nucleotidase (Zeller *et al.*, 1959), spermine oxidase (Tabor *et al.*, 1954), succinic dehydrogenase (Pletscher and Pellmont, 1958), guanidine deaminase (Zeller *et al.*, 1952) and histaminase (Cohn and Shore, 1960). Recently, Axelrod *et al.* (1961) have found that some amine oxidase inhibitors inhibit the release of noradrenaline from storage sites. It is therefore necessary to be very cautious in attributing a certain action to inhibition of amine oxidase and even more cautious in attributing it to the accumulation of any particular amine. At present there is no action of these substances which can, with certainty, be attributed to a rise in concentration in the brain of one particular substance to the exclusion of all others. In addition there are considerable species differences in reactions to these drugs.

Much of the work on this subject has been done with iproniazid, or more recently with more potent members of the hydrazine group to which iproniazid also belongs, but comparison of these results with those obtained with inhibitors structurally different may help to decide which actions are due to inhibition of amine oxidase and which are not. *Iproniazid* injected intraperitoneally into rats or mice reaches maximum tissue concentrations within an hour and is then rapidly eliminated (Fig. 7). After 24 hours Hess *et al.* (1958) could detect none in brain or liver, although amine oxidase inhibition persisted for 5 or 6 days. The principal metabolite, isonicotinic acid, is also rapidly excreted. Acetone, formed by splitting off the terminal isopropyl group is formed as well and Koechlin and Iliev (1959) found evidence of the formation of isoniazid and isopropylhydrazine.

Pheniprazine is both more potent and longer acting than iproniazid (Horita, 1958). Structurally it is related to amphetamine (Table 6) and this may explain the excitement, restlessness and hypertension (p. 66) which follow immediately on the administration of large doses. *Phenoxypropazine* has a similar potency with both *in vitro* and *in vivo* tests, and a similar duration of action, but little amphetamine-like activity. *Isocarboxazid* is also more potent than iproniazid and is also rapidly excreted. Schwartz (1960) found that after the injection into rats of the ^{14}C-labelled compound, 75% of the radioactivity was excreted in the urine and 7% in the faeces in 24 hours, whereas inhibition of the enzyme persisted for up to three weeks. With all hydrazide amine oxidase inhibitors there is a disparity between their prolonged action and rapid elimination. This might be due either to the persistence of an active metabolite or to a long lasting, possibly irreversible, change in the structure of the enzyme. Evidence for the persistence of a metabolite is at present lacking and the observation of Zeller *et al.* (1955) that iproniazid inhibition of amine oxidase *in vitro* is non-competitive and irreversible is in favour of the second alternative.

Evidence that these substances inhibit amine oxidase *in vivo* has been obtained by Sjoerdsma *et al.* (1960) who found that iproniazid, pheniprazine, phenelzine, nialamide and tranylcypromine (see below) depress 5-hydroxyindole acetic acid excretion and increase tryptamine excretion

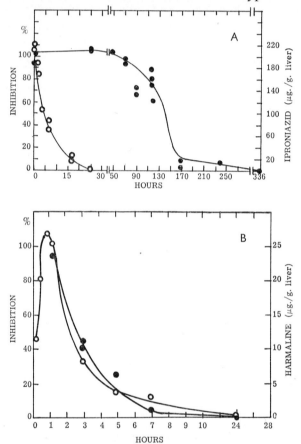

FIG. 7. Amine oxidase inhibition ●———● and drug concentration ○———○ in rat liver homogenates at intervals after the intraperitoneal injection of (A) iproniazid (195 mg./kg.) (Hess *et al.*, 1958) and (B) harmaline (5 mg./kg.) (Udenfriend *et al.*, 1958).

in man, and by the finding that they raise brain 5-hydroxytryptamine concentrations in experimental animals (Zbinden *et al.*, 1960).

The seeds of *Peganum harmala* have been used medicinally since the days of Dioscorides in the first century A.D. Several alkaloids (harmaline, harmine, harmalol) and a number of derivatives with similar properties are known. These are referred to collectively as the *harmala alkaloids* and it is of interest, in view of the recent similar use of iproniazid, that they were administered some 30 years ago in the treatment of angina pectoris (Bramwell *et al.*, 1933). Their inhibitory action on amine oxidase has been described by Udenfriend *et al.* (1958). Harmaline (see p. 59), tested *in vitro* on rat liver homogenates, will cause 50% inhibition of amine oxidase at a molar concentration 1/300 of that required by iproniazid. When given by intraperitoneal injection, a maximum effect is found, on homogenates, in an hour and this then diminishes with the decreasing concentration of the drug in the body (Fig. 7). The action of harmaline, unlike that of iproniazid, is thus reversible. Brain 5-hydroxytryptamine (Fig. 8) and dopamine (Holzer and Hornykiewicz, 1959) rise more rapidly after harmaline than after iproniazid but also fall more rapidly. Thus, though potent, rapid acting

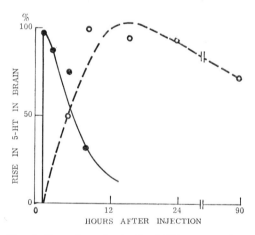

FIG. 8. Percentage rise in the 5-HT content of rat brain after the injection of harmaline (30 mg./kg.) ●———● and iproniazid (100 mg./kg.) o–––––o. (Pletscher, 1961.)

amine oxidase inhibitors, the harmala alkaloids are short lasting and have other actions which limit their clinical value. They have not been used as anti-depressives.

Pletscher and Besendorf (1959) noticed that if iproniazid is given to rats one hour after harmaline, brain noradrenaline and 5-hydroxytryptamine concentrations first rise and then return to normal as the harmaline action passes off; there is no subsequent rise due to iproniazid. Holzer and Hornykiewicz (1959) have made the same observation with respect to dopamine. This effect would be explained by the protection of amine oxidase from iproniazid by harmaline already attached to it, and it therefore appears likely that these two inhibitors have the same point of attachment on the enzyme. A similar protection of cholinesterase by eserine from the action of organic phosphorus inhibitors has been described by Koelle (1946).

Both α-*methyl* and α-*ethyl tryptamine* (etryptamine, Monase) cause a reversible inhibition of amine oxidase and *in vitro* have about the same potency as iproniazid (Greig *et al.*, 1959). Inhibition is of short duration and is competitive. They also inhibit 5-hydroxytryptophan decarboxylase. Animals into which they have been injected become restless and irritable and it would thus appear that oxidase inhibition predominates, as decarboxylase inhibitors cause sedation.*

Choline p-tolyl ether (see p. 59) is one of a group of choline phenyl ethers whose inhibitory action was described by Brown and Hey (1956). *In vitro* it is three times as potent as amphetamine and, according to Corne and Graham (1957), about equal in activity to iproniazid. When it is injected into guinea pigs or cats there is little effect on the amine oxidase activity of the animals homogenized livers; but Schayer *et al.* (1954) found that injection into mice reduced the rate of metabolism of injected tryptamine, and that, when a similar test was done with noradrenaline, the pattern of excreted metabolites was changed. These results they attributed to amine oxidase inhibition.

Tranylcypromine is of particular interest. It is not a hydrazide but yet has a powerful action, rapid in onset, with a duration intermediate between that of harmaline and iproniazid. Its action has been described by Maas and Nimmo (1959), who found it to be non-competitive, and by Green and Erickson (1960). According to the latter investigators it is about 860 times as potent as iproniazid on rat brain homogenates *in vitro*. The oral administration of 5 mg./kg. to rats is followed 1 hour afterwards by complete inhibition of the amine oxidase of brain homogenates; this persists for 15 hours and normal enzyme activity is only restored after 5 days. Brain 5-hydroxytryptamine and noradrenaline concentrations are both raised, the increases being more rapid than with iproniazid. The highest concentration of noradrenaline was reached in 5 hours and declined to normal in 7 days; whereas after 40 mg. iproniazid/kg. the maximum was reached only after 8 hours. The dose response curves for the two compounds, both for the *in vitro* experiments and for the rise in brain noradrenaline concentration, were parallel suggesting a similar mode of action. Tranylcypromine is the only non-hydrazine inhibitor used to any extent in man. Its central action according to Kinross-Wright (1959) is complicated by amphetamine-like actions, like that of pheniprazine, and its value in the treatment of depression is still uncertain; on the circulation it has sympathomimetic actions which can be antagonized by dibenyline (Spencer *et al.*, 1960). Zeller *et al.* (1960) have pointed out that there is considerable steric similarity between tranylcypromine and the hydrazine inhibitors and

---

* Monase has now been withdrawn by the manufacturers following reports of cases of agranulo cytosis.

that both have a benzene group attached to a two-membered chain with an amino group. From a comparison of related compounds they have made deductions about the structure of the active centre of amine oxidase.

A still more recent non-hydrazine compound, about which there is at present little experimental data, is *pargyline* (A19120) (Taylor *et al.*, 1960). This appears to have a long action which *in vitro* cannot be reversed by washing. The remaining members of group 4 in Table 5 do not need comment as their action has been known for some years and they have been discussed in the review by Blaschko (1952).

Biochemical and pharmacological effects of amine oxidase inhibitors

1. The *rise in concentration of certain endogenous amines*, dopamine, noradrenaline, adrenaline and 5-hydroxytryptamine, which occurs in the brain, heart, blood and intestine after the administration of amine oxidase inhibitors, has been referred to above, and is presumably due to diminished breakdown and increased storage of the amines. With some substances, and in some species, it is accompanied by excitement, and attempts have been made to correlate the changes in the concentration of particular amines with behaviour. This is of considerable interest in relation to the clinical use of amine oxidase inhibitors in the treatment of depressive conditions and is discussed on p. 73. A rise in the brain concentrations of dopamine and 5-hydroxytryptamine also follows the administration of the amino-acid precursors of these amines, namely dopa and 5-hydroxytryptophan; and this is accompanied by characteristic pharmacological effects. Both the tissue concentrations and the pharmacological effects are increased by the previous administration of an amine oxidase inhibitor (Udenfriend *et al.*, 1957). On the other hand, the fall in brain noradrenaline and 5-hydroxytryptamine which follows the administration of reserpine and tetrabenazine (p. 22) is diminished, and the sedation and pupillary constriction they cause are changed to excitement and dilatation.

2. The *sleeping time* of mice given hexobarbitone is prolonged by the previous administration of certain amine oxidase inhibitors (Fouts and Brodie, 1956). Laroche and Brodie (1960) have now shown that iproniazid, pheniprazine and nialamide inhibit the metabolism of hexobarbitone by liver microsomes and that potentiation of hexobarbitone is not due to amine oxidase inhibition, the time course of which is much longer.

3. Costa *et al.* (1961) have described *desynchronization of the EEG* after injection of pheneprazine and tranylcypromine. These are compounds with amphetamine-like actions. Changes in the EEG could only be produced with iproniazid when lethal doses were used.

4. *Anticonvulsant action.* Prockop *et al.* (1959) have shown that certain hydrazide amine oxidase inhibitors protect mice and rats against electroshock and leptazol convulsions.

5. *Ganglionic blockade*. The effect of amine oxidase inhibitors on transmission through the superior cervical ganglion of the cat has been studied by Gertner (1961). Perfusion of the ganglion with iproniazid, pheniprazine, phenelzine, nialamide, tranylcypromine and harmine caused a slowly developing block as measured by the response of the nictitating membrane to preganglionic stimulation. This was largely reversible on discontinuing the infusion but complete recovery was only obtained with harmine. The response to postganglionic stimulation and to injections of acetylcholine into the perfusing solution, and the release of acetylcholine into the perfusate on preganglionic stimulation was unaffected by amine oxidase inhibitors. The means by which the blockade is brought about is at present unexplained but it is clearly different from that of other ganglion blocking drugs. Since a similar result was obtained with inhibitors chemically very dissimilar, and blocking potency varied with the potency of the amine oxidase inhibitor, it seems likely that blockade is brought about by some mechanism dependent on amine oxidase inhibition.

6. *Cardio-vascular action*. Goldberg and Sjoerdsma (1959) investigated the action of a number of amine oxidase inhibitors on the blood pressure and contractile force of the dog's heart, using a strain gauge stitched into the wall of the right ventricle for the latter measurement. They found that iproniazid and harmaline caused a fall in blood pressure and that harmaline reduced the contractile force of the heart and markedly slowed the rate. Pheniprazine and to a less extent JB 835, on the other hand, raised the blood pressure and increased the rate of the heart. The pressor action of pheniprazine can be blocked by dibenyline and by rendering the animal tachyphylactic to amphetamine (Eltherington and Horita, 1960) and is thus a manifestation of sympathomimetic properties due to its amphetamine-like structure (Table 6). The use of certain amine oxidase inhibitors in the treatment of hypertension is referred to on p. 318. Whether the hypotensive action is entirely explicable by ganglion blockade has not yet been determined, but both effects develop gradually.

The effect of amine oxidase inhibitors on the cardiovascular actions of amines which are substrates for this enzyme has been the subject of a number of investigations. Goldberg and Sjoerdsma (1959) found that they potentiate the action of tyramine, dopamine and tryptamine (but not of noradrenaline) on the blood pressure and on the contractile force of the dog's ventricle, and Furchgott *et al.* (1955) and Helmer (1957) found that they potentiate the contraction of rabbit aortic strips by tyramine and dopamine. The pressor action of dopamine in the cat is also potentiated (Corne and Graham, 1957; Balzer and Holtz, 1956). In the guinea pig, dopamine has a depressor action; this too is potentiated by iproniazid (Hornykiewicz, 1958). These results accord with the view that amine oxidase is of major importance in the inactivation of tyramine, dopamine and tryptamine and of minor importance in that of noradrenaline.

7. Pletscher and Bernstein (1958) found that the daily oral administration of 5 to 8 mg. iproniazid/kg. in man caused a steady increase in *the 5-hydroxytryptamine content of platelets*; after 10 days they contained more than twice as much as initially and the number of platelets in the blood had also increased. A thrombocytosis has also been observed in animals after the daily injection of a large dose of 5-hydroxytryptamine.

8. An increase in the *concentration of lactic and pyruvic acid* in the blood after administration of amine oxidase inhibitors has recently been reported by Pletscher (1961) but the cause is at present unknown.

9. *Fertility.* The interruption of pregnancy in rats and mice by amine oxidase inhibitors is referred to on p. 287.

Toxic effects in man

The administration to man of the hydrazide amine oxidase inhibitors causes 'psychic' stimulation, euphoria and an increase in appetite. These changes develop gradually during the course of about two weeks and take a similar period to disappear when the drug is discontinued. A number of ill effects have been reported, particularly with iproniazid, and of these liver damage is the most serious. It has been estimated that this complication occurs in only 1 in 2,000 patients treated with iproniazid but it has a bad prognosis and a mortality of about 15%. At post-mortem acute hepatic necrosis is found. Cases have been described by Kahn and Perez (1958) and by Pare and Sandler (1959), who advocate routine weekly serum glutamic-oxaloacetic transaminase tests for patients on iproniazid. The newer hydrazide amine oxidase inhibitors cause liver damage more rarely, but cases have been described with both pheniprazine (Holdsworth *et al.*, 1961) and isocarboxazid (Benack, 1961). Pheniprazine may also cause red-green colour blindness. Recently Shee (1960) has reported two cases where the administration of pethidine to patients on iproniazid was followed by deep coma. Within 5 to 10 minutes of giving 25 mg. prednisolone hemisuccinate intravenously, both patients became rousable and were completely recovered in 24 hours. However, in another case (Palmer, 1960) in which pethidine was given to a patient on phenelzine and not subsequently treated with prednisolone, the patient died. There is no satisfactory explanation of these reactions, but the giving of pethidine to patients who have recently taken an amine oxidase inhibitor should be avoided. Other effects ascribed to this group of drugs are oedema, anaemia and thrombocytopaenia, headache and vertigo, peripheral vasodilitation, orthostatic hypotension, diminished palmar sweating, dysuria and constipation, decreased libido, insomnia, tremor, hypoglycaemia and bone decalcification (Kline, 1958; Dewar, Horler and Newall, 1959; Scherbel, 1961).

Use in medicine

As well as being used in mental disease (p. 73), amine oxidase inhibitors have been used in the treatment of hypertension (p. 318). They have been advocated in the symptomatic treatment of ischaemic heart disease, but more critical assessment in this latter condition has lead to unfavourable reports (Dewar *et al.*, 1959; Snow and Anderson, 1959); and they have been said to have an analgesic action and to potentiate analgesics, anaesthetics and a variety of other drugs, but further evidence for these actions is needed.

CLINICAL USE OF PSYCHOTROPIC DRUGS

The biochemical basis of mental illness is largely unknown and drugs are usually used empirically. Although many of the drugs are undoubtedly of great value, the present popularity of pharmacotherapy must be seen partly as a general dissatisfaction with the older methods of psychiatric treatment, either because of their crudity or relative ineffectiveness.

In this section the drugs have been classified into major tranquillizers, minor tranquillizers and other drugs used in the treatment of anxiety, and the antidepressants, and in general these groups of drugs are mainly used in schizophrenic and manic patients, anxiety neuroses and depressive states respectively. However, in small doses the major tranquillizers are often used to allay anxiety in neurotic conditions (Rees and Lambert, 1955; Hinton, 1959). The space allocated in this account to a particular group of drugs does not necessarily correspond to its clinical efficacy or popularity. Very roughly the sale in Great Britain of major tranquillizers: minor tranquillizers: antidepressants is in the ratio 5:3:5. Of the antidepressants, imipramine has as big a sale as all the mono-amine oxidase inhibitors combined, while that of the stimulants is about half as great. The pharmacology of these compounds is discussed in the first part of this chapter.

MAJOR TRANQUILLIZERS

Since Delay *et al.* (1953) introduced it into psychiatry, *chlorpromazine* has stood the test of time and of extensive trials in all parts of the world and is now established as the standard for comparing the efficacy of newer drugs of this type (Rees, 1960). All investigators agree that it is most effective in psychotic patients who are excited, disturbed or who have exhibited psychotic symptoms such as delusions and hallucinations. In other words it is used to relieve symptoms rather than in the treatment of a specific diagnostic entity. Furthermore, when used in isolation it tends to lose its effectiveness and the aim should be to use it as a means of obtaining the patient's co-operation in psychotherapy, occupational therapy and general resocialization (Rathod, 1958).

The dosage used varies from 150 mg. to over 1,000 mg. daily and although improvement usually occurs in the first week, it is best to persist with the drug for at least 6 weeks before assuming it is ineffective. When improvement is attained, dosage may be reduced to a maintenance level which should be continued for at least 3 months and in the chronic schizophrenic, indefinitely.

Toxic effects are common but not usually serious. Typical figures are those of Denber and Bird (1957) who, using doses of about 300 mg. a day in 1,523 patients, noted extrapyramidal symptoms in 7·6%, skin rashes in 4·6%, cardiovascular (mainly hypotensive) effects in 1·8%, oedema in 1·7%, jaundice in 1·2% and convulsions in 1·1%. Blood dyscrasias are uncommon, but well recognized, occurring in about 0·3% of treated patients (Kurtz, 1958). When jaundice and skin reactions occur it is almost always in the first few weeks of treatment (Doughty, 1955; Lomas et al., 1955). These side effects are not entirely related to dosage; individual susceptibility and perhaps hypersensitivity are also factors. Although liver function tests and biopsy material suggest that liver dysfunction occurs in up to 50% of patients (Waitzkin, 1958), this is often reversible even while the drug is continued (Bartholomew et al., 1958; Waitzkin, 1958) and more serious disturbances may be on a background of previous hepatic damage (Roizin et al., 1959). An interesting but unexplained finding is the higher incidence of blood dyscrasias in females and to a lesser extent this holds for the incidence of extrapyramidal symptoms (Roizin et al., 1959).

It is convenient to compare the newer phenothiazine derivatives (see classification p. 44) with chlorpromazine as a standard. Ayd (1960) compared the clinical potency of some of these newer drugs and the results are summarized in Table 7. However, the fact that a drug is potent at a lower dosage does not necessarily mean that it is more useful clinically. Although acetyl promazine and promazine have been found less effective than chlorpromazine as major tranquillizers and have fallen off in popularity, other drugs, such as thioridazine (Melleril) and methotrimeprazine (Veractil) are widely used though only equipotent to chlorpromazine.

The definitive role of this new range of drugs has yet to be determined but it may well be that the various 'target symptoms' will yield better to individual compounds. Thus it has been claimed that the more apathetic and withdrawn patients are best treated by those phenothiazines with a piperazine side chain such as trifluoperazine and prochlorperazine (Hollister et al., 1960; Weckowicz and Ward, 1960).

On the other hand, the drowsiness which may occur with compounds without a piperazine chain (Freyhan, 1959) can be of use in patients with an associated agitation, and are particularly useful in elderly psychotic patients in whom they are preferable to barbiturates, which often tend to make these patients more confused.

These newer drugs have an advantage over chlorpromazine as they have less tendency to cause jaundice. However, on the whole, they have

Table 7

Relative potency of various phenothiazines

(Chlorpromazine = 1)

	Potency	Reference
Mepazine (Pacatal)	½	Lomas, 1957; Klett and Lasky, 1960.
Promazine (Sparine)	½	Fazekas *et al.*, 1956; Gilmore and Shatin, 1959.
Acetylpromazine (Notensil)	<1	Simpson, 1958.
Thioridazine (Melleril)	1	Kinross-Wright, 1959; Sandison *et al.* 1960.
Methotrimeprazine (Veractil)	1	Baker and Thorpe, 1958; Quin *et al.*, 1960.
Trifluopromazine (Vespral)	>1	Goldman, 1958; Hanlon *et al.*, 1958; Klett and Lasky, 1960.
Prochlorperazine (Stemetil)	3–5	Goldman, 1958; Freyhan, 1959; Klett and Lasky, 1960.
Thiopropazate (Dartalan)	4–7	Hamilton *et al.*, 1960.
Perphenazine (Fentazine)	5–10	Cahn and Lehman, 1957; Goldman, 1958.
Trifluoperazine (Stelazine)	8–12	Freyham, 1959; Hollister *et al.*, 1960; Klett and Lasky, 1960.
Fluphenazine (Moditen)	10–20	Ayd, 1959.

a much greater tendency to produce extrapyramidal symptoms and this is particularly so with the drugs with a piperazine side chain. The extrapyramidal symptoms include not only Parkinsonism, but also dyskinetic syndromes with bizarre spasms of the perioral, facial, neck and back musculature. These manifestations develop early in the treatment and can be promptly terminated by a reduction of the dose and the administration of anti-Parkinson agents. Another syndrome is akathisia. This was described by Sicard (1921, 1923) as occurring in epidemic encephalitis and paralysis agitans and denotes an 'impatience musculaire' or forced restlessness. The severity of this syndrome ranges from a feeling of inner restlessness associated with a restless feeling in the legs, to a severe agitation and hyperactivity (Edison and Samuels, 1958; Freyhan, 1959; Hollister *et al.*, 1960).

Although the more potent drugs have an increased tendency to produce extrapyramidal symptoms, most authorities deny that there is any relation between improvement in the mental state and the occurrence of extrapyramidal symptoms in the individual patient. However, others believe that there is such an association (Delay *et al.*, 1959) and avoid the use of anti-Parkinson drugs for this reason (Denham and Carrick, 1961).

The *rauwolfia alkaloids* have also been extensively used as major tranquillizers. Following their introduction into psychiatry by Kline in 1954, their value has been confirmed and generally accepted (Shepherd and Watt, 1956; Wing, 1956; Mielke, 1957). On the whole they act less quickly than the phenothiazines which are generally preferred by English psychiatrists. However, patients failing to respond to phenothiazines may improve with rauwolfia alkaloids; before the advent of the new phenothiazines, this applied particularly to the apathetic withdrawn type of patient (Delay *et al.*, 1959). The dose of *reserpine* recommended varies from 4–15 mg. a day (Malamud *et al.*, 1957; Kline, 1958; Turner *et al.*, 1958) and should be continued for several months before failure is accepted (Kline, 1958). Extrapyramidal symptoms, hypotension and depression (Lemieux *et al.*, 1956; Deshaies *et al.*, 1957) are all relatively common side effects.

Haloperidol is a substituted butyrophenone which deserves comment as early reports suggest that, while having general properties of a major tranquillizer, it has a particularly beneficial effect in mania (Delay *et al.*, 1960; Divry *et al.*, 1960).

Although the major tranquillizers have an undoubted effect in composing the disturbed patient and in reducing or abolishing delusions and hallucinations, it is by no means easy to assess their overall value in relation to other methods of treatment (Lewis, 1959). It is doubtful whether the social emancipation of chronic patients, the passing of the disturbed ward atmosphere and the disuse of maintenance E.C.T., leucotomy and mechanical restraints can be attributed entirely to the new drugs. Nor can the major tranquillizers be given all the credit (Brill and Patton, 1957, 1959; Delay, 1959) for the recent dramatic fall in the rate of increase in the mental hospital population (Shepherd, 1957, 1961). Other powerful changes in outlook and practice had been taking place at the same time and even earlier. This is not to belittle the therapeutic value of the major tranquillizers. Particularly in acute cases, the drugs abolish or greatly reduce hallucinations and delusions making the patient more available to psychotherapy and social therapies. Patients can be discharged from hospital earlier on a maintenance dose of the drug and no longer suffer the very real dangers of institutionalization. Indeed, hospitalization may often be avoided and a feature of the 'tranquillizer era' has been the ability to treat schizophrenics as outpatients, in day hospitals and in general hospitals.

MINOR TRANQUILLIZERS, TRANQUILLOSEDATIVES AND OTHER DRUGS USED IN STATES OF ANXIETY AND TENSION

It is particularly the relatively mild psychoneuroses which can be readily influenced by changes in the environment and especially by a change in the therapeutic enthusiasm of the doctors and nurses (Feldman, 1956; Eison *et al.*, 1959). Thus a survey of the Anglo-American literature carried out by Foulds (1958) revealed that although the 'success' rate claimed for psychiatric drugs in uncontrolled trials is 85%, in controlled trials it is as low as 19%. In the last 10 years there has been a succession of drugs for which extravagant claims were at first made, and which have since quickly fallen into disrepute.

Mephenesin (see p. 51) was introduced as a specific for the relief of tension and the early uncontrolled trials reported high success rates (Schlan and Unna, 1949; Dixon *et al.*, 1950). However a few years later, carefully controlled trials showed that it was no better than a placebo (Block, 1953; Hampson *et al.*, 1954; Wolf and Pinsky, 1954). Originating from mephenesin, *meprobamate* (Equanil), which a few years ago was hailed as the drug of choice in these conditions (Borrus, 1955; Selling, 1955; Rickels *et al.*, 1959) has also decreased in popularity recently. In a critical review of the literature, Laties and Weiss (1958) point out the hollowness of many of the claims which so boosted its sales, particularly in the U.S.A. Though some carefully controlled trials demonstrated no advantage over placebo (Koteen, 1957) others, using similar doses, claim that it is of benefit in mild states of tension and anxiety (West and Da Fonseca, 1956; Hinton, 1958) probably because of its hypnotic effect which has been demonstrated by Borrus (1955) and Lasagna (1959). Certainly it has addictive properties, similar to those of the barbiturates (Ewing and Haizlip, 1958).

Other drugs which have been claimed to benefit states of anxiety and tension are *methylpentynol* (Oblivon) and its carbamate (Bourne, 1954; Gusterson, 1955); *hydroxyzine* (Atarax) (Farah, 1956; Robinson *et al.*, 1956), *phenaglycodol* (Ultran) (Kurtz, 1958) and *benactyzine* (Suavitil) (Davies, 1956; Hargreaves *et al.*, 1958). The last is also said to have some antidepressant properties (Alexander, 1956, 1958). However, the few controlled trials which have been carried out have not, on the whole, upheld these claims (Raymond and Lucas, 1956; Raymond *et al.*, 1957; Middlefell and Edwards, 1959). A possible exception is methylpentynol (Bockner, 1957) though, here again, its beneficial action may be due to its hypnotic effect (Simpson, 1954). It is perhaps significant that barbiturates are still widely used for the relief of anxiety and tension (Sargant, 1958). *Chlordiazepoxide* (Librium) has recently been introduced into this field and a well controlled study by Jenner *et al.* (1961) demonstrated a significant advantage over either placebo or amylobarbitone.

ANTIDEPRESSANTS

In the treatment of depression, stimulant drugs have a limited value. Apart from their having little effect in other than very mild depressive states with symptoms mainly of fatigue, their action is short lasting and may be followed by an even deeper depression. For this reason they are of most use when the depression is limited to one part of the day, e.g. early morning, or perhaps to counteract the occasional depressing effect of the major tranquillizers. *Amphetamine* is the best known of this type of drug. Recently its addictive properties have become more widely recognized and the identity of an amphetamine psychosis is now well established (Connell, 1958). *Phenmetrazine* (Preludin) (Evans, 1959) and *pipradol* (Meratran) (Begg and Reid, 1956) are likewise only of benefit in very mild depressions. Cases of addiction and toxic psychosis are well established with phenmetrazine (Evans, 1959) and hallucinations have been described following pipradol (Schou, 1956).

Methylphenidate (Ritalin) (Ferguson *et al.*, 1956; Ehrmantraut *et al.*, 1957; Robin and Wiseberg, 1958) also appears to be effective only in fatigue states and in very mild depressions. To our knowledge, toxic psychoses and states of addiction have not been described though the absence of addiction, in contrast to the older stimulants, may be due more to the difficulty in obtaining the drug than to its innate properties.

The most clearly defined group of drugs in the treatment of depression are the *amine oxidase inhibitors* (see also p. 57). Although there is no evidence to suggest that the depressive illnesses seen in clinical practice are due to a deficiency of brain 5-hydroxytryptamine (5-HT) or catechol amines, it is generally accepted that amine oxidase inhibitors afford symptomatic relief to many patients (Sargant, 1960). With the drugs and dosages used in clinical practice, improvement only starts after one or two weeks; if no benefit is apparent after a month, some other treatment is indicated. The earlier the beneficial change, the better the final outcome and *vice versa*, and the smaller the effective dose the better the result. It is a matter of controversy whether the type of patient most likely to respond to these drugs can be differentiated clinically (West and Dally, 1957; Alexander and Berkeley, 1959; Pare and Sandler, 1959). Perhaps of most interest is the question whether amine oxidase inhibitors are general euphoriants or whether they act only on those patients whose depression is due to a specific metabolic abnormality which has yet to be identified; the striking response noted in some patients compared with the apparent ineffectiveness in others suggests that the latter view may be true.

Depressive illnesses tend to improve spontaneously and so the generally quoted 60% improvement is largely meaningless, especially as many patients were only mildly depressed (Symposium, 1958). The 43% improvement in the placebo-controlled trial conducted by Kiloh *et al.*

(1960) may be a more realistic overall figure. Even when improvement occurs it is by no means a cure but rather a relief of symptoms. For this reason a maintenance dose must be continued until a natural remission occurs.

Iproniazid (Marsilid) on which most of the work has been done, has largely dropped out of use because of the incidence and severity of its side effects. These are described on p. 67. The newer inhibitors *phenelzine* (Nardil), *isocarboxazid* (Marplan) and *nialamide* (Niamid), like iproniazid, are hydrazine derivatives and their side effects are similar, though less common and severe. A possible exception is *pheniprazine* which seems to have a greater tendency than the other new amine oxidase inhibitors to produce jaundice (Holdsworth *et al.*, 1961) and may cause red-green colour blindness. It has now been withdrawn. A recent addition to this group of drugs is *tranylcypromine* (Parnate). This is not a hydrazine and claims have been made that it is relatively free from these side effects. However, one author stopped a therapeutic trial of the drug because of the occurrence, in three patients, of a state of collapse, associated with hypertension and symptoms of meningismus (Clarke, 1961).

With the possible exception of nialamide, which may be less useful, all these drugs are equally effective when given in adequate doses (Holt *et al.*, 1960; Crisp *et al.*, 1961; Dally and Rohde, 1961). Patients who are unresponsive to one drug seldom respond more than partially to another. Recently a competitive inhibitor of amine oxidase, *etryptamine* (Monase) has been introduced, but reports are too few for a proper assessment (Robie, 1961).

Although the amine oxidase inhibitors are now established as useful in the treatment of depression, it is still not proven that they owe their therapeutic properties to their action on amine oxidase. Attempts to correlate changes in mental state with amine oxidase inhibition (Feldstein *et al.*, 1960; Resnick *et al.*, 1960; Dewhurst and Pare, 1961) are largely invalidated by the inability, at present, to assess brain amine oxidase activity in man. It is known that the degree of inhibition of amine oxidase in brain does not always follow that of liver (Horita, 1961). Furthermore, it is the changes in concentrations of brain amines which are thought to be important in the antidepressant action of these drugs and these changes do not bear a straightforward relationship to the degree of amine oxidase inhibition (Gey and Pletscher, 1961). On another track, Pare and Sandler (1959) tried to reproduce the effects of iproniazid by giving 5-hydroxytryptophan and 3,4-dihydroxyphenylalanine, precursors of 5-hydroxytryptamine and the catecholamines respectively, to depressed patients who had previously been shown to improve as a direct result of treatment with iproniazid. In no instance was any improvement noted clinically.

The evidence in favour of the therapeutic properties being due to their inhibitory action on amine oxidase, has been summarized by Pletscher (1959). The main points are firstly, that there is a rough correlation between the inhibitory action on monoamine oxidase and the clinical effectiveness of the drug. Secondly, with the small doses used in man, there is only a slow development of amine oxidase inhibition and this is associated with a similarly delayed clinical effect. Thirdly, when the drug is stopped, amine oxidase activity only returns slowly and clinical relapse is also delayed.

The other major antidepressant drug is *imipramine* (Tofranil). Since its introduction in 1957 by Kuhn, it has become established as an effective antidepressant agent (Lehmann *et al.*, 1958; Blair, 1960) and although little has been learned about the mechanism of its therapeutic action, there is a suggestion that the more typical retarded endogenous depressions respond more favourably than the agitated and atypical ones (Crisp *et al.*, 1961; Dally and Rohde, 1961). Certainly the side effects are poorly tolerated in the anxious, tense patient. The overall incidence of improvement is probably similar to that obtained with the amine oxidase inhibitors and in a well controlled trial by Ball and Kiloh (1959), 66% of patients showed a good response compared with 21% treated with placebo. Dosage should be built up over a period of a week to a maximum of 150–300 mg./day. Symptom relief occurs within the first two weeks, but, as with the amine oxidase inhibitors, a maintenance dose of the drug must be continued until a natural remission occurs. In some chronic depressions, treatment may have to be continued indefinitely.

The side effects have been well reviewed by Brookfield (1960). Atropine-like side effects are common at the beginning of treatment but tend to disappear as it continues. In descending order of frequency they comprise, dryness of the mouth, tachycardia, and disturbances of accommodation. Sweating may also occur. A fine tremor is sometimes present though this may be manifested only in the form of an inner restlessness. More uncommonly there may be giddiness and postural hypotension, especially in the elderly (Delay and Deniker, 1959) who may also develop confusional and hallucinatory episodes at night (Delay and Deniker, 1959; Post, 1959; Blair, 1960). Convulsions occur in about 2% of patients and Delay and Deniker (1959) have described E.E.G. changes of an 'irritative' nature. Less in the nature of a side effect is a tendency to produce a state of hypomania and this may also occur when amine oxidase inhibitors are used. The state is due to an overdosage with the antidepressant and is particularly likely to occur in those manic-depressive illnesses when the patient was previously subject to mood swings. *Amytriptyline* (Tryptizol) is structurally and pharmacologically similar to imipramine; its clinical value is still uncertain.

A new drug, *chlorprothixene* (Taractan) is of interest as, although published reports are few (Geller, 1960; Ravn, 1960), it is claimed to combine the antidepressant properties of imipramine with those of a major tranquillizer.

In psychiatric practice the antidepressant drugs must bear comparison with electroconvulsive therapy (ECT) which, in favourable cases, affords a complete cure. On the one hand relief from symptoms with the antidepressant drugs may not be complete and treatment must be continued, perhaps for many months, until a natural remission occurs. Furthermore, in severely depressed or suicidal patients, the latent period before any improvement can be expected may be dangerous. On the other hand, the patient may be spared the unpleasantness and theoretical brain damage which may be associated with ECT. In general, the antidepressant drugs are of most use in the mild to moderately depressed patients who are suitable for treatment at home or in the outpatients' department, ECT being reserved for intractable patients or those in whom an effect is required quickly.

POLYPHARMACY

Finally, in a chapter of this kind, the common practice of using several drugs in combination should be discussed. The proponents of polypharmacy, such as Barsa (1960), point out that the drugs used in psychiatry are aimed at symptomatic relief rather than for the cure of a disease. They argue that since a particular drug will only affect certain 'target' symptoms, a battery of different drugs may be necessary to relieve all the symptoms in a particular patient. Certainly, it is common to use a major tranquillizer with a hypnotic side effect in restless senile patients and this is not far removed from the use of two drugs, one a tranquillizer and the other a hypnotic. On the other hand, it is a fact that when the diagnosis is clear, most psychiatrists will use only one drug, e.g. trifluoperazine for a classical schizophrenia with hallucinations and delusions. Similarly in a classical depression ECT alone, or perhaps one of the antidepressants by itself, will be used regardless of whether the patient is deluded, agitated, or, on the contrary, retarded. Polypharmacy is much more common in atypical cases, in outpatients and when the psychiatrist is not confident of his diagnosis. To the extent that polypharmacy is an admission of ignorance it is bad and in itself obscures the picture. If the psychiatrist is unable to arrive at a full assessment of the patient by the ordinary methods of history and examination, much valuable information can be gained by observing the response of the patient to drugs, provided these are given singly and on a logical basis. Even in those cases where a combination of drugs is justified, the doses of the various drugs should be prescribed separately

to suit the individual patient. There is no advantage, other than con-
venience, in prescribing a mixture, put out by a pharmaceutical firm,
where the ingredients are rigidly standardized regardless of the individual
patient's symptoms.

EXPERIMENTAL METHODS IN PSYCHOPHARMACOLOGY

In recent years there has been intense research activity concerned with
drugs which have psychological effects and which might therefore be of
use in psychiatry for treating mentally ill patients. Many new drugs,
especially 'tranquillizers' and 'antidepressants', have been introduced
and found valuable clinically, and this has also led to renewed attempts
to unravel the mode of action of older drugs like barbiturates and
amphetamine. The whole subject has now become known by the name
'psychopharmacology'.

This section is about general principles which underly the evaluation
of 'psycho-active' drugs by means of experiments on animals and man.
Since the main therapeutic function of these drugs is to change people's
feelings and behaviour, the most direct and the most widely used
approaches are those which seek to reproduce and measure such changes
in the laboratory. Increasingly it is now also possible to study concomitant physiological and biochemical changes in the nervous system,
and this is beginning to lead to a more basic understanding of the mode
of action of these drugs. Direct investigation of psychological changes is,
however, by definition crucial for meaningful evaluation, and it is with
the assessment of these changes that what follows is largely concerned.

Although studying the psychological changes produced by these drugs
is thus a direct way of evaluating their actions, the choice of methods
for doing this and even more so the interpretation of their results is
rarely straightforward. To measure psychological changes in an objective and quantitative way is intrinsically complex and difficult, especially
where feelings and other subtle characteristics are involved. For practical
reasons most of the work with drugs must be done on animals, mainly
rats and mice, whose brains and behaviour differ much more from
those of man than do for example their circulatory systems. Laboratory
experiments on man can only be done in a limited way, and large or
repeated doses of drugs and unpleasant or prolonged procedures cannot
easily be used: and in any case it is never certain how far the results of
laboratory experiments, whether the subjects be 'normal' volunteers or
psychiatric patients, can be generalized to actual clinical applications.
The only decisive evidence about the therapeutic value of drugs comes
from clinical trials on the kinds of patients for whom the drugs are
ultimately intended; but such trials are only justified after much
preliminary work in the laboratory, and the results moreover do not by

themselves tell one much about the mode of action of the drugs tested (see also pp. 68–76).

Because of all this, the evaluation of psycho-active drugs poses special problems and requires varied and flexible skills. There is an extensive literature on the techniques available and on what can and cannot be found out by means of them. Recently a number of reviews have been published which are specially relevant to the study of drugs (e.g. Craver, 1956; Dews and Skinner, 1956; Riley and Spinks, 1958; Cole and Gerard, 1959; Steinberg, 1959; Miller and Barry, 1960; Uhr and Miller, 1960; Ross and Cole, 1960; Dews and Morse, 1961; Hunt, 1961; Irwin, 1962).

How techniques are chosen and applied in a particular investigation largely depends on its main purpose: this may be (i) screening—the discovery and testing of new substances of potential value in the treatment of mental illness, or (ii) analytical investigation which aims at elucidating drug-behaviour relations in a more fundamental way. Such differences in aim can lead to important differences in procedure, though in practice there is often a good deal of overlap.

SCREENING

Because there is such tremendous interest in the discovery of new psycho-active drugs, a large proportion of research in psychopharmacology is concerned with screening. Screening tests must be reasonably sensitive and specific if they are not to miss promising compounds and if they are to exclude unpromising ones; and the tests must be quick and cheap to carry out so that large numbers of compounds can be screened. So far no single animal test has been found which will discriminate reliably between drugs which have different kinds of psychological effects in man, except for relatively crude differences in effect like predominantly stimulant or predominantly depressant actions. Such crude differences can be determined by administering large doses and observing gross changes in behaviour, e.g. sleep or convulsions; or by devices like activity cages which yield quantitative though arbitrary records of changes in the amount of movement animals make during a given period. Sometimes differences of this kind can be detected more readily if use is made of antagonistic or potentiating actions of drugs. For example, compounds with central stimulant actions can often be identified by finding out if they awaken anaesthetized animals; and conversely, animals can first be made hyperactive by amphetamine or other drugs, and new compounds can then be screened for their ability to depress this induced hyperactivity. Another kind of test for drugs with central depressant actions involves pre-treating animals with the new compound, usually in doses which by themselves do not produce sleep, and then putting the animal to sleep with a standard hypnotic like hexobarbitone. Nearly all drugs which have some depressant action on the central nervous system will prolong the sleeping time when tested in this way, and this sort of test has now become a routine procedure for screening tranquillizing drugs since promising compounds are unlikely to be missed. But a great variety of other drugs, e.g. adrenaline, histamine, lysergic acid diethylamide, some antidepressants (see p. 65), and 5-hydroxytryptamine, have also been shown capable of prolonging such sleeping times, and so the test is not specific.

Sometimes it is possible to detect slighter and more diverse effects of drugs on the behaviour of animals in the course of making preliminary observations, especially if observers are experienced and make use of aids like rating scales (Irwin, 1959; Norton, 1957). One way of constructing such rating scales is first to select and define a broad pattern of behaviour which is expected to be affected by the drug, e.g. 'excitement'; next a number of components of this pattern are distinguished which are thought to be characteristic of it and which are relatively easily observed, e.g. walking, running, rearing on hindlegs, sniffing, tail movements. A system of marks or scores is then devised for rating the frequency or intensity with which each component behaviour occurs in a given 'time sample', and animals are observed with and without drugs and the results are compared. Rating scales can be incorporated as useful adjuncts in almost any test methods which depend on observations of animal or of human behaviour.

In order to follow up preliminary observations of the effects of new compounds in a more objective and precise fashion, and particularly in order to detect subtle effects which are not obvious to inspection, a great variety of more specialized test methods has become widely used. Versions of two main kinds of approach are commonly adopted, based on either *'criterion behaviour'* or on *'criterion drugs'* (Russell, 1960; Report, 1961).

(a) Screening in terms of *'criterion behaviour'* ideally depends on the following steps: 1. Select a form of human abnormal behaviour which it is desired to modify, e.g. anxiety neurosis, and determine its basic characteristics. 2. Induce in animals a form of behaviour which as far as possible has similar characteristics. 3. Search for new drugs which modify this animal behaviour in relatively low doses. 4. Test these drugs in man—if possible in comparable laboratory experiments with normal volunteers (in practice this is seldom possible with new drugs), and finally in patients who show the abnormal behaviour originally selected.

As one would expect, among the animal tests which are most used for this type of screening are those which involve disrupting an animal's normal behaviour in some way, for example by subjecting it to noxious stimuli like electric shocks or to a 'conflict' situation where a hungry animal cannot both obtain food and avoid some sort of punishment. The disturbances of behaviour which may result from such treatment vary and largely depend on the particular experimental conditions: an animal's previously learnt habits may disintegrate, it may become unable to learn new ones, it may refuse to eat, may become aggressive, hyperactive or inactive, may show physiological reactions like altered respiration and heart rate and loss of weight, and it may make unusual, inappropriate or repetitive movements. Human subjects too can be exposed to mild forms of stress in the laboratory, and psychological and physiological reactions can be demonstrated and measured. How far the behaviour disturbances induced by such techniques in animals, or in human subjects, do in fact resemble real-life abnormal behaviour in psychiatric patients is at present difficult to say; the factors involved are complex and by no means fully understood, but if the experimental situations are carefully contrived the results can provide an approximate guide to clinical effectiveness (Russell, 1951). As for drugs, various substances can indeed reduce the effects of disrupting stimuli and so 'normalize' behaviour in some of these laboratory experiments; but they include drugs which clinically have other kinds of uses, e.g. alcohol, barbiturates, hyoscine and morphine, and in addition much depends, once again, on the details of the experimental situation. These kinds of test methods are intrinsically interesting and attractive, but for practical purposes they are not sufficiently specific or exact to be more than a fairly coarse screen. Many attempts have been made to refine them, both by making the experimental situations more precise and by using more than one test. For example, the aim may be to narrow the basis of screening by selecting only those compounds which modify animal behaviour based on fear, e.g. avoiding an electric shock at a signal, but which leave other kinds of learnt behaviour, e.g. pressing a button in order to obtain food, unimpaired; appropriate additional tests may then yield relevant information, but to demonstrate such selective actions of drugs, even approximately, requires complex analytical procedures which are beyond the scope of most screening programmes. Some kinds of differential effects can, however, be investigated fairly readily by using additional tests, for example whether behaviour is 'normalized' at doses which do not also produce gross disturbances of movement. There is evidence that drug-induced disturbances of movements in man, e.g. 'ataxia', can to some extent be predicted from tests of movements in animals, and it is possible that this may also be true of the extra-pyramidal symptoms which can result from treating patients with drugs like phenothiazines; correlations have been reported between the doses of different compounds which are liable to produce extra-pyramidal symptoms in patients and the doses of the same compounds which are active in tests of 'catalepsy' in animals ('Triangle', 1960). But while effects of drugs on movements may be important 'side effects', they are not usually the kinds of effect for which psycho-active drugs are primarily being screened.

(b) Screening in terms of '*criterion drugs*' usually proceeds as follows: 1. Choose a drug the clinical value of which is already established but on some aspects of which it is desired to improve, e.g. amylobarbitone, chlorpromazine, amphetamine. 2. Determine the effects of this drug in animals by means of a wide variety of tests. 3. Then use selected tests, e.g. the most sensitive or those which for other reasons seem especially diagnostic, to screen new compounds. 4. Test the new drugs which have been identified by this procedure in man. The third step in this sequence is probably the most difficult. Thus a given animal test may be very sensitive to the 'criterion drug' in the sense that it detects the presence of smaller doses of it than other tests do, but it does not follow automatically that the effect measured by this sensitive test has anything to do with the desirable clinical actions of the criterion drug, for which the new compounds are being screened. The variety of animal tests which has been used for this kind of screening is enormous, and many of them seem in fact extremely remote from any possible clinical relevance. The usual basis for selecting tests is in practice largely empirical; so long as tests are quick, simple, repeatable and relatively sensitive to the criterion drugs they may be thought worth using for screening in a trial-and-error fashion, and the results are evaluated mainly by statistical kinds of reasoning.

An example of such an approach is illustrated in Fig. 9 on which are plotted 'profiles' of drug actions based on data obtained by Janssen (1961). Along the vertical axis is a log scale representing ED50's (median effective doses), that is doses at which 50 % of animals tested showed the effect a test was designed to detect. Results for three different drugs are illustrated, pentobarbitone, chlorpromazine and haloperidol (p. 51). The large rectangles indicate the median lethal doses for each drug, and the numbered rectangles represent nine different tests which were performed on different groups of rats; the upper and lower edges of each rectangle are drawn in the positions of the 95 % fiducial limits for each test, which means roughly that 95 % of ED50's for the test would be expected to lie between these limits if the test were repeated indefinitely. The figure thus enables one to read off and compare the doses at which the different tests become sensitive to the effects of the three drugs for which the results have been plotted. The tests themselves were of many kinds: the first four depended on the ability of each of the three drugs to antagonize effects of another drug; test no. 5 was a test for 'catalepsy' which meant that each animal was placed in a standard unusual position and the test was 'positive' if the animal failed to correct this position in a fixed time; test no. 6 depended on the reduction by the drug of the animal's normal food intake by 50 %; no. 7 was a test for the loss of the righting reflex, and nos. 8 and 9 were tests for slight and deep hypothermia respectively. Inspection of the three 'profiles' suggests a number of conclusions. For example, the margin between the LD50 and the ED50's for nearly all the tests is much greater for chlorpromazine and haloperidol than for the barbiturate, and this is consistent with other evidence that the

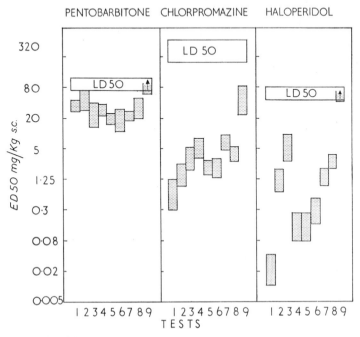

FIG. 9. 'Activity profiles' of three drugs. Along the vertical axis are log ED50's, and the rectangles represent nine different tests which were given to rats and which are described in the text. The upper and lower edges of each rectangle are drawn in the position of the 95% fiducial limits for that test. The diagram thus enables the doses to be read off at which the different tests become sensitive to each drug.

therapeutic indices of these newer drugs are apt to be high compared with barbiturates. Another feature of the profiles is that nearly all the tests for which results are given are affected by all three drugs, but for the barbiturate the ED50's are all very similar whereas for the other two drugs, and especially with haloperidol, they are spread out over a wide range. This suggests that all three drugs can have many similar effects, but that it is easier with the newer drugs to obtain selective effects, that is, some effects can be obtained with low doses which leave other kinds of behaviour unaffected. Evidence has been accumulating that such differences in dose margins are apt to be characteristic of many tranquillizing drugs as compared with barbiturates, and it is possible that this partly accounts for differences in their clinical efficacy.

Laboratory experiments in man also have suggested that, although barbiturates and some tranquillizing drugs can produce qualitatively similar effects, the dose margins seem to be different: thus it has been reported that a barbiturate produced 'elation' and other effects on people's moods only in relatively high doses which also produced drowsiness and impaired efficiency, but with two different tranquillizing drugs effects on mood became manifest at lower doses than those which produced drowsiness and inefficiency (Klerman *et al.*, 1960).

In a general way profiles of the kind illustrated can be used to describe similarities and differences between compounds, and in particular to identify compounds with new profiles and therefore possibly new patterns of action. How far generalizations made from such profiles can be applied to clinical effects largely depends on knowing more about the meaning of the tests themselves. Some of the tests referred to in the figure are relatively easy to interpret, e.g. those for the loss of the righting reflex (no. 7), for hypothermia (nos. 8 and 9), and perhaps also the test for 'catalepsy' (no. 5). The production of hypothermia is a well-known effect of chlorpromazine, and this is clearly illustrated in the figure; the possible significance of tests of 'catalepsy' for predicting extra-pyramidal side-effects in man has already been discussed, and if this is so then it might be useful to look for new compounds which have a relatively higher ED50 for tests like no. 5. With other kinds of tests the interpretation is far from obvious; for example test no. 1 is based on the inhibition of chewing movements induced by a very large dose of amphetamine, and it is difficult to understand on the basis of our present knowledge why this test should be the most sensitive of all the nine tests for both chlorpromazine and haloperidol. But until much more information about such underlying factors becomes available, it is justifiable to use the information derived from such profiles in an empirical way; if many compounds are compared and it is found that drugs which have similar clinical effects consistently have similar profiles—and in practice this is often found—then the profiles can be used to discriminate between drugs for screening purposes. Furthermore, the results of such empirical procedures may themselves lead to new information about the tests. For example, if tests which are intended to measure similar sorts of behaviour consistently yield different ED50's, this suggests that the underlying processes tested must be different; conversely, if different tests produce similar ED50's it does not prove that they are measuring the same underlying process, though in practice it may make possible economies of procedure.

From what has been said it will be clear that the screening of psycho-active drugs is at present still being carried out against a background of many unsolved problems, and partly because of this it often involves a prodigious amount of work with no guarantee of success at the end;

further progress must largely depend on the results of analytical investigations which will now be discussed.

ANALYTICAL INVESTIGATIONS

Broadly speaking, the aim of analytical studies is to determine selective effects of drugs in a way which will throw light on their fundamental mode of action. This can be done at several levels.

A primarily behavioural approach is illustrated by recent work of Miller (1960, 1961) and his colleagues. In one series of experiments the aim was to find out whether the effects of amylobarbitone in various *animal experiments* could all be accounted for by assuming that the drug directly and specifically reduced fear, or whether it acted in some other way. The first step was to set up several experimental situations in which rats were taught to obtain food or water rewards by running from varying distances towards them or by pressing levers. When they had learnt this, the effect of amylobarbitone on these performances was tested, and it was found that animals treated with the drug ran somewhat less quickly or pressed the lever rather less often to get their rewards than control animals. Next, fear was induced by giving the rats occasional electric shocks near the places where they got the rewards, and the shocks were always stronger the longer the distance an animal had had to run or the louder a tone which was being sounded as a signal for the shock. Under these conditions the control animals now ran much less fast or pressed the lever much less often in order to get rewards than they had done before the electric shocks were introduced, but the performance of the animals treated with amylobarbitone was hardly affected; this suggested that the drug protected the animals from the effects of fear. The results were moreover much the same for all the different test situations used: it did not matter whether the rewards were food or water, whether the animals had to run or to press levers to obtain them or whether the cues associated with the electric shocks were primarily visual and kinaesthetic (distance which had been run) or auditory (loudness of tone); hence it seemed unlikely that the effects of the drug were dependent merely on the peculiarities of a particular test situation. The ingredients of the experimental situations were then analysed still further. For example, in all the experiments described the procedure had involved first teaching animals to do something—to run or to press levers to get rewards—and only then were the shocks, and thus the behaviour based on fear, superimposed; therefore the drug might merely have modified the most recently acquired and presumably least well established habits, and not specifically habits based on fear. This possibility was studied by further tests where the effects of the drug on habits which had been established in different orders were determined; the results suggested that the selective effects on fear persisted, and that the drug did not act merely by weakening the most recently established habits most. In other tests the rats' ability to discriminate between different kinds of perceptual cue was tested. This was done in order to make sure that the drug did not produce its effects in the fear-tests merely by impairing sense perception and so making the rats less able to recognize the environments in which they got electric shocks; the results of these tests were complex and inconclusive and will have to be followed up by further experiments. Other experiments involving a similar approach but different drugs, especially alcohol and chlor-promazine, have recently been reported (Grossman and Miller, 1961).

The effects of drugs on *human behaviour* can be analysed in many ways. A large proportion of investigations has been concerned with ways in which drugs can alter the efficiency of various performances, and particularly with discovering the characteristics which determine to what extent different kinds of performance are selectively susceptible to the effects of drugs.

For example, the aim may be to find out how the performance of skills involving complex hand-eye co-ordination breaks down under the influence of alcohol. One method of studying this is to make subjects carry out a complicated and continuous task, for example a task which resembles driving a car along a track, which has been so arranged that different components like speed, various types of error, smoothness of movements and so forth can be recorded and analysed separately, and the effects of different doses of alcohol on these components can then be determined and compared quantitatively (Drew *et al.*, 1959). Comparisons can similarly be made not only between different components of the same task, but also between different tasks involving various kinds of performances, like reasoning and memory as well as sense perception or motor skill. By means of performance tests it is often possible to detect impairments of efficiency long before there are any clinical signs of intoxication. As a general rule relatively complex kinds of performance for which sustained attention is required are apt to be impaired to a greater extent and by smaller doses of central depressant drugs than simpler performances (Steinberg, 1954).

Recently there has been renewed interest in trying to improve efficiency by means of drugs, and the conditions under which drugs like amphetamine can bring about improvements have been much studied. Usually the most striking effects can be demonstrated if tasks are relatively simple, repetitive and prolonged, like doing easy mental arithmetic, tapping a morse key as fast as possible, or monitoring a radar-type screen to detect small irregularly spaced signals. With such tasks, amphetamine and similar drugs can often postpone the deterioration in performance which occurs as time goes on and which is usually attributed to 'fatigue', and this has led to the question of how far these

4

drugs have a direct effect on the *ability* to perform and how far they act in other ways, for example by counteracting boredom and so improving the subject's inclination to work. It has often been shown that these drugs make people feel interested, confident and energetic, but it is difficult to devise experiments which will solve this kind of problem conclusively (Plotnikoff *et al.*, 1960). Relevant evidence comes from a number of different lines of approach, and one kind of evidence is obtained from experiments in which the incentives that are given to subjects are varied. This can be done in various ways, for example incentives are high if subjects are made to compete with one another and so are working near the limits of their capacity; under such conditions drugs are not usually able to produce much further improvement in performance (Hauty and Payne, 1958; Steinberg, 1961), and this suggests that it is not the actual capacity to perform which is increased by drugs. There are exceptions, however, and the whole subject of improvements in performance due to drugs needs further study.

A large and growing number of investigations has been concerned with analysing possible *sites of action* of drugs in the brain by neurophysiological and other techniques and with relating them to behavioural effects. Technically this kind of work is often very difficult and complicated. In recent years the part played by the 'reticular activating system' has been particularly studied; it is now generally accepted that this system is closely involved in the regulation of sleep and wakefulness and possibly in the control of many other kinds of behaviour as well, and it also seems to be specially sensitive to the effects of some drugs (French, Verzeano and Magoun, 1953; Magoun, 1958; Feldberg, 1959).

Bradley and Key (1958) have studied the effects of drugs on thresholds for arousing sleeping animals. Cats were specially prepared (encéphale isolé preparations), and they could be stimulated in two ways; electrically through an electrode whose tip was fixed in the reticular formation, and by auditory stimuli which were standard noises whose loudness could be varied. Two criteria of 'arousal' were used: E.E.G. arousal, that is, changes in the animal's E.E.G. which typically occur when animals wake up, and waking up itself ('behavioural arousal') which depended on responses like the opening of eyes and the contraction of the nictitating membrane; thresholds were determined by the voltage of electrical stimulation or the loudness of noise needed to produce arousal. The effects of various drugs were analysed in this way and differential effects could be demonstrated. For example, amphetamine lowered thresholds to both kinds of stimulation and a barbiturate raised thresholds to both kinds of stimulation, but chlorpromazine had more selective effects: doses which caused only slight rises in the threshold to electrical stimulation of the reticular formation blocked responses to auditory stimulation completely. In other words,

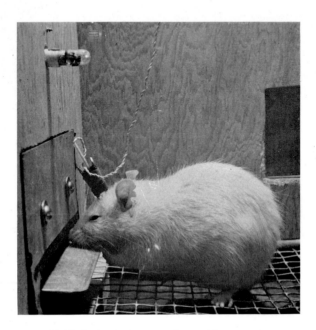

PLATE II 'Self-stimulation' experiment. The rat steps on a pedal which completes a circuit so that a small electric shock is delivered through the electrode implanted in its brain. Widely different but relatively stable rates of self-stimulation are elicited if electrodes are implanted in different parts of the brain, and these rates can be selectively modified by drugs.

To face p. 87

chlorpromazine was especially potent in reducing the effects of sensory stimulation on arousal, and this suggested that its main effects were not directly on the reticular formation, as is probably the case with barbiturates, but were 'more related to the influence of afferent signals impinging on the reticular formation via collaterals from sensory pathways'. This interpretation was consistent with the apparent indifference to sensory stimuli which has often been reported with chlorpromazine in intact animals and in man, and also with most other available neurophysiological evidence concerning the action of this drug (Bradley, 1962).

Another way of studying actions of drugs in the brain is by means of 'self-stimulation' techniques which were introduced some years ago (Olds and Milner, 1954). Stimulating electrodes are permanently implanted in different parts of the brain of rats and the circuit is so arranged that the rats can give their brains small electric shocks by stepping on a pedal (Plate II). Rats soon learn to stimulate themselves in this way and the frequency of stimulation largely depends on the position of the electrodes; specially 'rewarding' places in the brain have been identified, and also 'punishing' places where stimulation is avoided. In some places, especially in parts of the hypothalamus and in the septal region, very high self-stimulation rates of several thousand per hour can be obtained, and these contain among them areas which other kinds of experiment have also shown to be involved in various forms of emotional behaviour. Drugs can modify rates of self-stimulation differentially. For example, in the posterior hypothalamus self-stimulation rates of up to 5,000 per hour can normally occur, and in the anterior hypothalamus normal rates range from 400–1,100. With a small dose of chlorpromazine, however, self-stimulation of the posterior hypothalamus may be severely depressed, but in the anterior hypothalamus there may barely be any effect. It seems therefore that the drug produces some important change in the activity of the posterior hypothalamus (Olds, 1960).

The distribution and roles of substances which occur naturally in the brain have been much analysed by pharmacological and biochemical methods, and they are discussed elsewhere (Chapter 1). A special stimulus for this kind of work has been the hope that it might eventually lead to the discovery of biochemical factors involved in mental illnesses like schizophrenia, the causes of which are, as yet, poorly understood (Kety, 1959).

REFERENCES

* Denotes review

AGRANOFF, B. W., BRADLEY, R. M. and AXELROD, J. (1957). *Proc. Soc. exp. Biol.* (*N.Y.*), **96**, 261

ALEXANDER, L. (1956). *J. Amer. med. Ass.* **162**, 966

ALEXANDER, L. (1958). *J. Amer. med. Ass.* **166**, 1019

ALEXANDER, L. and BERKELEY, A. W. (1959). *Ann. N.Y. Acad. Sci.* **80**, 669

ALLGÉN, L. G., JÖNSSON, B. J., NAICKOFF, B., ANDEREN, M. L., HUUS, I. and
    NIELSEN, I. M. (1960). *Experientia*, **16,** 325
ANNALS OF THE NEW YORK ACADEMY OF SCIENCES (1957), **67,** 671
ANNOTATION (1958). *Brit. med. J.* **2,** 1586
AXELROD, J., HERTTING, G. and PATRICK, R. W. (1961). *J. Pharmacol. exp. Ther.*
    134, 325
AYD, F. J. (1960). *J. med. Soc. N.J.* **57,** 4
BALL, J. R. B. and KILOH, L. G. (1959). *Brit. med. J.* **2,** 1052.
BALZER, H. and HOLTZ, P. (1956). *Arch. exp. Path. Pharmak.* **227,** 547
BARRACLOUGH, C. A. and SAWYER, C. H. (1959). *Endocrinology*, **65,** 563
BARSA, G. A. (1960). *Amer. J. Psychiat.* **117,** 448
BARTHOLOMEW, A. A., BOURNE, G. L. and MARLEY, E. (1958). *Clin. Sci.* **17,** 629
BARTHOLOMEW, L. G., CAIN, J. C., FRAZIER, S. H., PETERSEN, M. C., FOULK, W. T.,
    SOULE, E. H., FLEISCHER, G. A. and OWEN, C. A. (1958). *Gastroenterology*,
    34, 1096
BARTHOLOMEW, A. A., CHAPPELL, P., MARLEY, E. and CHAMBERS, J. S. W. (1958).
    Lancet, **1,** 346
BEECHER, H. K. (1959). 'Measurement of Subjective Responses.' Oxford University
    Press
BEGG, W. G. A. and REID, A. A. (1956). *Brit. med. J.* **1,** 946
*BEIN, H. J. (1956). *Pharmacol. Rev.* **8,** 435
BENACK, R. T. (1961). *New England J. Med.* **264,** 294
BERGER, F. M. (1956). *Int. Rec. Med.* **169,** 184
BLAIR, D. (1960). *J. ment. Sci.* **106,** 891
*BLASCHKO, H. (1952). *Pharmacol. Rev.* **4,** 415
BLOCK, S. L. (1953). *Arch. Neurol. Psychiat. (Chicago)*, **69,** 727
BLOHM, T. R., SUMMERS, L. L. and GREENWOOD, R. L. (1954). *Fed. Proc.* **13,** 337
BOCKNER, S. (1957). *J. ment. Sci.* **103,** 218
BORRUS, J. C. (1955). *J. Amer. med. Ass.* **157,** 1596
BOURNE, G. (1954). *Lancet,* **2,** 522
*BRADLEY, P. B. (1962). In 'Physiological Pharmacology', Vol. 1. Ed. Root, W. S.
    and Hofmann, F. G. London: Academic Press. In press
BRADLEY, P. B. and KEY, B. J. (1958). *Electroenceph. clin. Neurophysiol.* **10,** 97
BRAMWELL, C., CAMPBELL, M. and EVANS, W. (1933). *Lancet,* **2,** 69
BRILL, H. (1959). 'Trifluoperazine'. London: Kimpton
BRILL, H. and PATTON, R. E. (1957). *Amer. J. Psychiat.* **114,** 509
BRILL, H. and PATTON, R. E. (1959). *Amer. J. Psychiat.* **116,** 495
*BRODIE, B. B., SPECTOR, S. and SHORE, P. A. (1959). *Pharmacol. Rev.* **11,** 548
BROOKFIELD, R. W. (1960). In the 'British Encyclopaedia of Medical Practice,
    Medical Progress.' London. p. 343
BROWN, B. B. and WERNER, H. W. (1954). *J. Pharmacol. exp. Ther.* **110,** 180
BROWN, B. G. and HEY, P. (1956). *Brit. J. Pharmacol.* **11,** 58
*CARLO, P. E. (1957). 'Psychotropic Drugs', p. 392. Ed. Garattini, S. and Ghetti, V.
    Amsterdam: Elsevier
CLARK, M. L. and JOHNSON, P. C. (1960). *J. clin. Endocr.* **20,** 641
CLARKE, J. A. (1961). *Lancet,* **1,** 618
COHN, V. H. and SHORE, P. A. (1960). *Fed. Proc.* **19,** 283
COLE, J. and GLEES, P. (1956). *Lancet,* **1,** 338
*COLE, J. O. and GERARD, R. W. (1959). 'Psychopharmacology. Problems in
    Evaluation.' Washington: Nat. Acad. Sci.
CONNELL, P. H. (1958). 'Amphetamine Psychosis.' London: Chapman and Hall
CORNE, S. J. and GRAHAM, J. D. P. (1957). *J. Physiol.* **135,** 339
COSTA, E., PSCHEIDT, G. R., VAN METER, W. G. and HIMWICH, H. (1961). *J. Phar-
    macol. exp. Ther.* **130,** 81
*CRAVER, B. N. (1956). *Ann. N.Y. Acad. Sci.* **64,** 463
CRISP, A. H., HAYS, P. and CARTER, A. (1961). *Lancet,* **1,** 17
DALLY, P. J. and ROHDE, P. (1961). *Lancet,* **1,** 8
DAVIES, E. B. (1956). *Brit. med. J.* **1,** 480

*DAVISON, A. N. (1958). *Physiol. Rev.* **38,** 729

DELAY, J. (1959). In 'Neuropsychopharmacology'. Ed. Bradley, P. B., Deniker, P., Radouco-Thomas, C. Amsterdam: Elsevier

DELAY, J. and DENIKER, P. (1959). *Canad. Psychiat. Ass. J.* **4** (suppl.), 100

*DELAY, J., DENIKER, P. and ROPERT, R. (1959). 'Psychopharmacology Frontiers.' London: Churchill

DELAY, J., DENIKER, P., ROPERT, R., BECK, H., BARANDE, R. and EURIEULT, M. (1959). *Presse méd.* **67,** 201

DELAY, J., DENIKER, P. and TARDIEU, Y. (1953). *Presse méd.* **61,** 1165

DELAY, J., PICHOT, P., LEMPERIÉRE, T. and ELISSALDE, B. (1960). *Acta neurol. psychiat. belg.* **60,** 21

DE MAAR, E. W. J., MARTIN, W. R. and UNNA, K. R. (1958). *J. Pharmacol. exp. Ther.* **124,** 77

DENBER, H. C. B. and BIRD, E. G. (1957). *Amer. J. Psychiat.* **113,** 972

DENHAM, J. and CARRICK, D. J. E. L. (1961). *J. ment. Sci.* **107,** 326

DESHAIES, G., RICHARDEAU, N., and DECHOSAL, F. (1957). *Ann. méd-psychol.* **115,** 417

DEWAR, H. A., HORLER, A. R. and NEWALL, D. J. (1959). *Brit. Heart J.* **21,** 315

DEWHURST, W. G. and PARE, C. M. B. (1961). *J. ment. Sci.* **107,** 239, 244

*DEWS, P. B. and MORSE, W. H. (1961). *Annu. Rev. Pharmacol.* **1,** 145

*DEWS, P. B. and SKINNER, B. F. (1956). *Ann. N.Y. Acad. Sci.* **65,** 247

DICKER, S. E. and STEINBERG, H. (1957). *Brit. J. Pharmacol.* **12,** 479

DICKER, S. E., STEINBERG, H. and WATSON, R. H. J. (1957). *J. Physiol. (Lond.),* **137,** 88P

DISEASES OF THE NERVOUS SYSTEM (1960). **21,** No. 2 supplement

DISEASES OF THE NERVOUS SYSTEM (1960). **21,** No. 3 supplement

DIVRY, P., BOBON, J. and COLLARD, J. (1960). *Acta neurol. psychiat. belg.* **60,** 7

DIXON, H. H., DICKEL, H. A., COEN, R. A. and HAUGUN, J. B. (1950). *Amer. J. med. Sci.* **220,** 23

DOMENJOZ, R. and THEOBALD, W. (1959). *Arch. int. Pharmacodyn.* **120,** 450

DOUGHTY, R. B. (1955). In 'Chlorpromazine in Mental Health'. London

DRASSDO, A. and SCHMIDT, M. (1954). *Med. Mschr.* **8,** 366

DREW, G. C., COLQUHOUN, W. P. and LONG, H. A. (1959). *MRC Memorandum No. 38*

EDISEN, C. B. and SAMUELS, A. S. (1958). *Arch. Neurol. Psychiat. (Chicago),* **80,** 481

EHRMANTRAUT, W. R., SHEA, J. G., TICKTIN, H. E. and FAZEKAS, J. F. (1957). *Arch. intern. Med.* **100,** 66

EISON, S. B., SABSHIN, M. and HEATH, H. (1959). *J. nerv. ment. Dis.* **128,** 256

ELTHERINGTON, L. G. and HORITA, A. (1960). *J. Pharmacol. exp. Ther.* **128,** 7

EVANS, J. (1959). *Lancet,* **2,** 152

EWING, J. A. and HAIZLIP, T. M. (1958). *Amer. J. Psychiat.* **114,** 835

FABING, H. D. (1955). *Science,* **21,** 208

FARAH, L. (1956). *Int. Rec. Med. Gen. Prac. Clin.* **169,** 379

*FELDBERG, W. (1959). *Brit. med. J.* **2,** 771

FELDMAN, P. E. (1956). *Amer. J. Psychiat.* **113,** 52

FELDSTEIN, A., HOAGLAND, H., RIVERA, M. R., FREEMAN, H. (1960). *J. Neuropsychiat.* **2,** 12

FERGUSON, J. T., LINN, F. V. Z., SHEETS, J. A., NICKELS, M. M. (1956). *J. Amer. med. Ass.* **162,** 1303

FOULDS, G. A. (1958). *J. ment. Sci.* **104,** 259

FOUTS, J. R. and BRODIE, B. B. (1956). *J. Pharmacol. exp. Ther.* **116,** 480

FRENCH, J. D., VERZEANO, M. and MAGOUN, H. W. (1953). *Arch. Neurol. Psychiat. (Chicago),* **69,** 505

FREYHAN, F. A. (1959). *Amer. J. Psychiat.* **115,** 577

FRIEND, D. G. (1960). *Clin. Pharmacol. Ther.* **1,** 5

FURCHGOTT, R. F., WEINSTEIN, P., HENBLE, H., BOZORGMEHRI, P. and MENSENDICK, R. (1955). *Fed. Proc.* **14,** 342

GADDUM, J. H. and KWIATKOWSKI, H. (1938). *J. Physiol. (Lond.),* **94,** 87

GELLER, W. (1960). *Med. Klin.* **55,** 554

GERTNER, S. B. (1961). *J. Pharmacol.* **131,** 223

GEY, K. F. and PLETSCHER, A. (1961). *J. Neurochem.* **6,** 239

GILLETE, J. R., DINGELL, J. V., SULSER, F., KUNTZMAN, R. and BRODIE, B. B. (1961). *Experientia,* **17,** 417

GLAZKO, A. J., DILL, W. A., WOLF, L. M. and KADENKO, A. (1956). *J. Pharmacol. exp. Ther.* **118,** 377

GOLDBERG, L. I. and SJOERDSMA, A. (1959). *J. Pharmacol. exp. Ther.* **127,** 212

GOLDMAN, D. (1958). *Amer. J. med. Sci.* **235,** 67

GRAY, S. and FORREST, A. D. (1958). *Brit. med. J.* **1,** 374

GREEN, A. L. and HAUGHTON (1961). *Biochem. J.* **78,** 172

GREEN, H. and ERICKSON, R. W. (1960). *J. Pharmacol. exp. Ther.* **129,** 237

GREIG, M. E., WALK, R. A. and GIBBONS, A. J. (1959). *J. Pharmacol. exp. Ther.* **127,** 110

GROSSMAN, S. P. and MILLER, N. E. (1961). *Psychopharmacologia,* **2,** 342

GUSTERSON, F. R. (1955). *Lancet,* **1,** 940

HALPERN, B. N. (1956). *C. R. Soc. Biol. (Paris),* **150,** 1152

HAMPSON, J. L., ROSENTHAL, D. and FRANK, J. D. (1954). *Bull. Johns Hopk. Hosp.* **95,** 170

HARGREAVES, G. R., HAMILTON, M. and ROBERTS, J. M. (1958). *J. ment. Sci.* **104,** 1056

HAUTY, G. T. and PAYNE, R. B. (1958). *Amer. J. publ. Health,* **48,** 571

HELMER, O. M. (1957). *J. Lab. Clin. Med.* **50,** 737

HERRMANN, B. and PULVER, R. (1960). *Arch. int. Pharmacodyn.* **126,** 454

HESS, S. M., SHORE, P. A. and BRODIE, B. B. (1956). *J. Pharmacol. exp. Ther.* **118,** 84

HESS, S., WEISSBACH, H., REDFIELD, B. G. and UDENFRIEND, S. (1958). *J. Pharmacol. exp. Ther.* **124,** 189

HIGH, J. P., HASSERT, G. L., RUBIN, B., PIALA, J. J., BURKE, J. C. and CRAVER, B. N. (1960). *Toxicol. appl. Pharmacol.* **2,** 540

HIMWICH, R. E. (1958). *Science,* **127,** 59

HINTON, J. M. (1958). *J. Neurol. Psychiat.* **21,** 301

HINTON, J. M. (1959). *J. ment. Sci.* **105,** 872

HOFFET, H. and CORNU, F. (1960). *Schweiz. med. Wschr.* **90,** 602

HOLDSWORTH, C. D., ATKINSON, M. and GOLDIE, W. (1961). *Lancet,* **2,** 621

HOLLISTER, L. E. (1958). *Calif. Med.* **89,** 1

HOLLISTER, L. E., ERICKSON, G. V., MOTZENBECKER, P. (1960). *J. clin. exp. Psychopath.* **21,** 15

HOLT, J. P., WRIGHT, E. R. and HECKER, A. O. (1960). *Amer. J. Psychiat.* **171,** 533

HOLTEN, C. H. and SONNE, E. (1955). *Acta pharmacol. (Kbh.)* **11,** 148

HOLZER, G. and HORNYKIEWICZ, O. (1959). *Arch. exp. Path. Pharmak.* **237,** 27

HORITA, A. (1958). *J. Pharmacol. exp. Ther.* **122,** 176

HORITA, A. (1961). *Toxicol. appl. Pharmacol.* **3,** 474

HORNYKIEWICZ, O. (1958). *Brit. J. Pharmacol.* **13,** 91

HUCKER, H. B. and PORTER, C. C. (1961). *Fed. Proc.* **20,** 172

*HUNT, H. F. (1961). *Annu. Rev. Pharmacol.* **1,** 125

IRWIN, S. (1959). In 'Research Conference on the Therapeutic Community'. Ed. Denber, H. C. B. Springfield, Ill.: Thomas

IRWIN, S. (1962). *Science,* **136,** 123

JANSSEN, P. A. J. (1961). *Arzneimittel-Forschung,* **11,** 819, 932

JANSSEN, P. A. J., DE WESTERINGH, C. V., JAGENEAU, A. H., DEMOEN, P. J. A., HERMANS, B. K. F., DAELE, G. H. P. V., SCHELLEKENS, H. L., DER EYKEN, C. A. M. V. and NIEMEGEERS, C. J. E. (1959). *J. Medicinal Pharmaceutical Chem.* **1,** 281

JANSSEN, P. A. J., JAGENEAU, A. H. and NIEMEGEERSE, J. E. (1960). *J. Pharmacol. exp. Ther.* **129,** 471

JENNER, F. A., KERRY, R. J. and PARKIN, D. (1961). *J. ment. Sci.* **107,** 575, 583

J. AMER. MED. ASS. (1958). **166,** 1040

KAHN, M. and PAREZ, V. (1958). *Am. J. Med.* **25,** 898

*KETY, S. S. (1959). *Science,* **129,** 1528, 1590

KILOH, L. G., CHILD, J. P. and LATNER, G. (1960). *J. ment. Sci.* **106,** 1139

KINROSS-WRIGHT, J. (1959). *J. Amer. med. Ass.* **170,** 1283

KINROSS-WRIGHT, J. (1959). *Ann. N.Y. Acad. Sci.* **80,** 840

KLERMAN, G. L., DiMASCIO, A., HAVENS, L. L. and SNELL, J. E. (1960). *Arch. gen. Psychiat.* **3,** 4

KLINE, N. S. (1954). *Ann. N.Y. Acad. Sci.* **59,** 107

KLINE, N. S. (1958). *J. clin. exp. Psychopath.* **19,** suppl. 1, 72

KLINE, N. S. (1958). *Ass. Res. nerv. Dis. Proc.* **37,** 218

KOECHLIN, B. and ILIEV, V. (1959). *Ann. N.Y. Acad. Sci.* **80,** 804

KOELLE, G. B. (1946). *J. Pharmacol. exp. Ther.* **88,** 232

KOTEEN, H. (1957). *Ann. int. Med.* **47,** 978

KRIVOY, W. (1957). *Proc. Soc. exp. Biol. (N.Y.)* **96,** 18

KUHN, R. (1957). *Schweiz. med. Wschr. vol.* **35/36,** 1135

KURTZ, P. L. (1958). *Canad. med. Ass. J.* **78,** 209

LAROCHE, M-J. and BRODIE, B. B. (1960). *J. Pharmacol. exp. Ther.* **130,** 134

LASAGNA, L. (1959). *Res. Publ. Ass. nerv. ment. Dis.* **37,** 325

LATIES, V. G. and WEISS, B. (1958). *J. chron. Dis.* **7,** 500

LEHMANN, H. E., CAHN, C. H. and DE VERTEUIL, R. L. (1958). *Canad. psychiat. Ass. J.* **3,** 155

LEMIEUX, G., DAVIGNON, A. and GENEST, J. (1956). *Canad. med. Ass. J.* **74,** 522

LEWIS, A. (1959). In 'Neuropsychopharmacology'. Ed. Bradley, P. B., Deniker, P. and Radouco-Thomas, C. Amsterdam: Elsevier

LOMAS, J., BOARDMAN, R. H. and MARKOWE, M. (1955). *Lancet,* **1,** 1144

MAAS, A. R. and NIMMO, M. J. (1959). *Nature (Lond.),* **184,** 547

*MAGOUN, H. W. (1958). 'The Waking Brain.' Springfield, Ill.: Thomas

MALAMUD, W., BARTON, W. E., FLEMING, A. M., MIDDLETON, P. H. K., FRIEDMAN, T. T. and SCHLIFER, M. J. (1957). *Amer. J. Psychiat.* **114,** 193

MARGOLINS, S., PERLMAN, P. L., VILLANI, F. and McGAVACK, T. H. (1951). *Science,* **114,** 384

MARLEY, E. (1959). *Brit. J. Pharmacol.* **14,** 284

MARLEY, E. and CHAMBERS, J. S. W. (1956). *Brit. med. J.* **2,** 1467

MARLEY, E. and VANE, J. R. (1958). *Brit. J. Pharmacol.* **13,** 364

MARSHALL, E. F., STIRLING, G. S., TAIT, A. C. and TODRICK, A. (1960). *Brit. J. Pharmacol.* **15,** 35

MEIER, R., GROSS, F. and TRIPOD, J. (1954). *Klin. Wschr.* **32,** 445

MIDDLEFELL, R. and EDWARDS, K. C. S. (1959). *J. ment. Sci.* **105,** 792

MIELKE, F. A. (1957). *Amer. J. Psychiat.* **114,** 134

*MILLER, N. E. (1961). *Amer. Psychologist,* **16,** 12

*MILLER, N. E. and BARRY, H. (1960). *Psychopharmacologia,* **1,** 169

MILLER, R. E., MURPHY, J. V. and MIRSKY, J. A. (1957). *J. Pharmacol. exp. Ther.* **120,** 379

MORAN, N. C. and BUTLER, W. M. (1956). *J. Pharmacol. exp. Ther.* **118,** 328

MULLER, O. F., GOODMAN, N. and BELLET, S. (1961). *Clin. Pharmacol. Ther.* **2,** 300

NIEMEGEERS, C. J. E. and JANSSEN, P. A. J. (1960). *J. Pharmacy Pharmacol.* **12,** 744

NND (1961). *New and Non-official Drugs,* p. 472

NORTON, S. (1957). In 'Psychotropic Drugs'. Ed. Garattini, S. and Ghetti, V. Amsterdam: Elsevier

OLDS, J. (1960). In 'Electrical Studies on the Unanesthetized Brain'. Ed. Ramey, E. R. and O'Doherty, D. S. New York: Hoeber-Harper

OLDS, J. and MILNER, P. (1954). *J. comp. physiol. Psychol.* **47,** 419

PALMER, H. (1960). *Brit. med. J.* **2,** 944

PAPATHEODOROU, C. A., KRIEGER, H. P. and WAGMAN, I. H. (1958). *J. Mt. Sinai Hosp.* **25,** 427

PARE, C. M. B. and SANDLER, M. (1959). *Lancet,* **1,** 282

PARE, C. M. B. and SANDLER, M. (1959). *J. Neurol. Psychiat.* **22,** 247

PELLMONT, B., SIEMER, F. A., BESENDORF, H., BÄCHTOLD, H. P. and LÄUPPI, E. (1960). *Helv. physiol. pharmacol. Acta,* **18,** 241

PIALA, J. J., HIGH, J. P., HASSERT, G. L., BURKE, J. C., and CRAVER, B. N. (1959). *J. Pharmacol. exp. Ther.* **127,** 55
PLETSCHER, A. (1959). *Ann. N.Y. Acad. Sci.* **80,** 1039
PLETSCHER, A. (1961). *Dtsch. med. Wschr.* **86,** 647
PLETSCHER, A. and BERNSTEIN, A. (1958). *Nature (Lond.),* **181,** 1133
PLETSCHER, A. and BESENDORF, H. (1959). *Experientia,* **15,** 25
PLETSCHER, A. and PELLMONT, B. (1958). *J. clin. exp. Psychopath.* **19** (suppl.), 163
*PLOTNIKOFF, N., BIRZIS, L., MITOMA, C., OTIS, L., WEISS, B. and LATIES, V. (1960). 'Drug Enhancement of Performance.' Menlo Park, Calif.: Stanford Research Institute
PLUMMER, A. J., MAXWELL, R. A. and EARL, A. E. (1957). *Schweiz. med. Wschr.* **87,** 370
PLUMMER, A. J., SHEPPARD, H. and SCHULERT, A. R. (1957). 'Psychotropic Drugs.' Ed. Garattini, S. and Ghetti, V. Amsterdam: Elsevier
POST, F. (1959). *Brit. med. J.* **2,** 1252
PROCKOP, D. J., SHORE, P. A. and BRODIE, B. B. (1959). *Ann. N.Y. Acad. Sci.* **80,** 643
QUINN, G. P., SHORE, P. A. and BRODIE, B. B. (1959). *J. Pharmacol. exp. Ther.* **127,** 103
RANDALL, L. O., SCHALLEK, W., HEISE, G. A., KEITH, E. F. and BAGDON, R. E. (1960). *J. Pharmacol. exp. Ther.* **129,** 163
RATHOD, N. H. (1958). *Lancet,* **1,** 611
RAVN, J. (1960). *Wien. klin. Wschr.* **72,** 192
RAYMOND, M. J. and LUCAS, C. J. (1956). *Brit. med. J.* **1,** 952
RAYMOND, M. J., LUCAS, C. J., BEESLEY, M. L., O'CONNELL, B. A. and ROBERTS, J. A. F. (1957). *Brit. med. J.* **2,** 63
REES, W. L. (1960). *Brit. med. J.* **2,** 522
REES, W. L. and LAMBERT, C. (1955). *J. ment. Sci.* **101,** 834
*REPORT (1961): 'Behavioral research in preclinical psychopharmacology'. *Psychopharmacol. Serv. Center Bull.* Sept. p. 1
RESNICK, O., HAGOPIAN, M., HOAGLAND, H. and FREEMAN, H. (1960). *Arch. gen. Psychiat.* **2,** 459
RICHTER, D. and TINGEY, A. H. (1939). *J. Physiol. (Lond.),* **97,** 265
RICKELS, K., CLARK, T. W., EWING, J. H., KLINGENSMITH, W. C., MORRIS, H. M. and SMOCK, C. D. (1959). *J. Amer. med. Ass.* **171,** 1649
*RILEY, H. and SPINKS, A. (1958). *J. Pharmacol.,* **10,** 657, 721
ROBIE, T. R. (1961). *J. Neuropsychiat.* **2** (suppl. I), 531
ROBIN, A. A. and WISEBERG, S. (1958). *J. Neurol. Psychiat.* **21,** 55
ROBINSON, H. M., ROBINSON, R. C. B. and STRAHAN, J. F. (1956). *J. Amer. med. Ass.* **161,** 604
ROBISON, M. M., LUCAS, R. A., MacPHILLAMY, H. B., BARRETT, W. and PLUMMER, A. J. (1961). *Experientia,* **17,** 14
ROBSON, J. M. and KEELE, C. A. (1950 and 1956). 'Recent Advances in Pharmacology.' London: Churchill
ROIZIN, L., TRUE, C. and KNIGHT, M. (1959). *Res. Publ. Ass. nerv. ment. Dis.* **37,** 285
*ROSS, S. and COLE, J. O. (1960). *Annu. Rev. Psychol.* **11,** 415
*RUSSELL, R. W. (1951). 'The Comparative Study of Behaviour.' London: Lewis
*RUSSELL, R. W. (1960). *Psychopharmacol. Serv. Center Bull.* Dec. p. 1
SARGANT, W. (1958). *Brit. med. J.* **2,** 1031
SARGANT, W. (1960). *Psychosomatics,* **1,** 74
SCHAYER, R. W., WU, K. Y. T., SMILEY, R. L. and KOBAYASKI, Y. (1954). *J. biol. Chem.* **210,** 259
SCHERBEL, A. L. (1961). *Arch. Int. Med.* **107,** 37
SCHLAN, L. S. and UNNA, K. R. (1949). *J. Amer. med. Ass.* **140,** 672
SCHNEIDER, J. A. and EARL, A. E. (1954). *Fed. Proc.* **13,** 150
SCHOU, M. (1956). *Brit. med. J.* **1,** 1236
SCHWARTZ, M. A. (1960). *J. Pharmacol. exp. Ther.* **130,** 157
SELLING, L. S. (1955). *J. Amer. med. Ass.* **157,** 1594

SHEE, J. C. (1960). *Brit. med. J.* **2**, 507

SHEPHERD, M. (1957). 'A Study of the Major Psychoses in an English County.' Maudsley Monograph No. 3. London: Chapman and Hall

SHEPHERD, M. (1961). 'Neuropsychopharmacology.' Ed. Rothlin, E. Vol. 2. Amsterdam: Elsevier

SHEPHERD, M. and WATT, D. C. (1956). *J. Neurol. Psychiat.* **19**, 232

SHEPPARD, H., TSIEN, W. H., RODEGKER, W. and PLUMMER, A. J. (1960). *Toxicol. appl. Pharmacol.* **2**, 353

SICARD, J. A. (1921). *Rev. neurol. (Paris)* **53**, 672

SICARD, J. A. (1923). *Presse méd.* **23**, 265

SIMPSON, R. G. (1954). *Lancet*, **1**, 883

SJOERDSMA, A., GILLESPIE, L., Jr. and UDENFRIEND, S. (1958). *Lancet*, **2**, 159

SJOERDSMA, A., OATES, J. A. and GILLESPIE, L. (1960). *Proc. Soc. Exp. Biol. Med.* **103**, 485

SJOERDSMA, A., OATES, J. A., ZALTZMAN, P. and UDENFRIEND, S. (1959). *J. Pharmacol. exp. Ther.* **126**, 217

SNOW, P. J. D. and ANDERSON, D. E. (1959). *Brit. Heart J.* **21**, 323

SPENCER, J. N., PORTER, M., FROEHLICH, H. L. and WENDEL, H. (1960). *Fed. Proc.* **19**, 277

STEINBERG, H. (1954). *Quart. J. exp. Psychol.* **6**, 170

*STEINBERG, H. (1959). In 'Quantitative Methods in Human Pharmacology and Therapeutics'. Ed. Laurence, D. R. London: Pergamon

*STEINBERG, H. (1961). *Rev. Psychol. appl.* **11**, 361

STERNBACH and REEDER. (See Randall *et al.*, 1960)

STONE, C. A. (1961). Memorandum of the Merck Institute

*SYMPOSIUM on 'Brain Mechanisms and Drug Action' (1957). Ed. Fields, W. S. Springfield: Thomas

*SYMPOSIUM (1958). 'The Biochemical and Clinical Aspects of Marsilid and other Monoamine Oxidase Inhibitors.' *J. clin. exp. Psychopath.* **19** (suppl. 1)

SYMPOSIUM (1959). *Ann N.Y. Acad. Sci.* **80**, 551

TABOR, C. W., TABOR, H., ROSENTHAL, S. M. and BAUER, H. (1954). *J. Pharmacol. exp. Ther.* **110**, 48

TAESCHLER, M. and CERLETTI, A. (1959). *Nature (Lond.)*, **184**, 823

TAYLOR, J. D., WYKES, A. A., GLADISH, Y. C. and MARTIN, W. B. (1960). *Nature (Lond.)*, **187**, 941

'TRIANGLE' (1960). *The Sandoz Journal of Medical Science*, **4**, 205

TURNER, W. J., CARL, A., MERLIS, S. and WILCOXON, F. (1958). *Arch. Neurol. Psychiat.* **79**, 597

UDENFRIEND, S., WEISSBACH, H. and BOGDANSKI, D. F. (1957). *Ann. N.Y. Acad. Sci.* **66**, 602

UDENFRIEND, S., WITKOP, B., REDFIELD, B. G. and WEISSBACH, H. (1958). *Biochem. Pharmacol.* **1**, 160

*UHR, L. and MILLER, J. G. (1960). 'Drugs and Behavior.' New York: Wiley

VELARDO, J. T. (1958). *Fertil. and Steril.* **9**, 60

VERNIER, V. G. (1961). *Dis. Nerv. Syst.* **22**, 7 (suppl.)

WAITZKIN, L. (1958). *Ann. intern. Med.* **49**, 607

WALKENSTEIN, S. S., KNEBEL, E. M., MACMULLEN, J. A. and SEIFTER, J. (1958). *J. Pharmacol. exp. Ther.* **123**, 254

WECKOWICZ, T. E. and WARD, T. F. (1960). *J. ment. Sci.* **106**, 1008

WEISKRANTZ, L. (1957). 'Psychotropic Drugs'. Ed. Garattini, S. and Ghetti, V. Amsterdam: Elsevier

WEISKRANTZ, L. and WILSON, W. A. (1955). *Ann. N.Y. Acad. Sci.* **61**, 36

WERNER, G. (1959). *Amer. J. med. Sci.* **237**, 123

WEST, E. D. and DA FONSECA, A. F. (1956). *Brit. med. J.* **2**, 1206

WEST, E. D. and DALLY, P. J. (1957). *Brit. med. J.* **1**, 1491

WING, L. (1956). *J. ment. Sci.* **102**, 530

WOLF, S. and PINSKY, R. H. (1954). *J. Amer. med. Ass.* **155**, 339

ZBINDEN, G., RANDALL, L. O. and MOE, R. A. (1960). *Dis. Nerv. Syst.* **21** (2), 89

ZELLER, E. A., BARSKY, J. and BERMAN, E. R. (1955). *J. biol. Chem.* **214,** 267

ZELLER, E. A., BARSKY, J., FOUTS, J. R., KIRCHEIMER, W. F. and VAN ORDEN, L. S. (1952). *Experientia,* **8,** 349

ZELLER, E. A., BLANKSMA, L. A., BURKARD, W. P., PACHA, W. L. and LAZANAS, J. C. (1959). *Ann. N.Y. Acad. Sci.* **80,** 583

ZELLER, E. A., PACHA, W. L. and SARKAR, S. (1960). *Biochem. J.* **76,** 45P

CHAPTER 3
CATECHOL AMINES

If a pair of twins could maintain the fiction that there was really only one of them for the first 45 years of their life, it would cause considerable confusion to their friends; this confusion would resolve when the dual nature was discovered. However, their activities would then be regarded with a certain amount of suspicion and if, on their 55th birthday, they announced that there was a third, but less active brother, it would not be much of a shock. This is a fair analogy to the story of the catechol amines and of the part they play in the body. Injections of extracts of suprarenal gland were shown by Oliver and Schäfer (1895) to cause a rise in blood pressure and by Lewandowsky (1899) to produce effects very similar to those produced by stimulating sympathetic nerves; Langley (1901) confirmed and extended these observations. Both Takamine (1901) and Abel (1902) concentrated the active principle of the suprarenal medulla and Abel named this epinephrine: purified extracts soon became available commercially as adrenaline.

The idea that adrenaline might be the chemical transmitter at sympathetic nerve endings was first proposed by Elliott in 1904. In spite of intensive work on adrenaline and on what Dale was to call other 'sympathomimetic' amines (Elliott, 1905; Barger and Dale, 1910), Elliott's idea was not confirmed experimentally until Loewi (1921) showed that stimulation of the sympathetic nerve of the frog's heart did in fact release a chemical which he called 'acceleransstoff'. In the same year Cannon and Uridil (1921) showed that stimulation of the hepatic nerves also caused a discharge of a substance which behaved like adrenaline; many others confirmed these findings. But there was something wrong; the effects of sympathetic nerve stimulation did not always correspond exactly to the effects of injected adrenaline (Barger and Dale, 1910). For many years, various theories were canvassed to explain the inexactness; for instance, Cannon and Rosenblueth (1933) suggested that the adrenaline liberated at sympathetic nerve endings combined with something in the receptive substances to form sympathin E (excitatory) or sympathin I (inhibitory) (for review see Rosenblueth, 1950).

Bacq (1933) first suggested that there might be a twin lurking in the background, that sympathetic nerve stimulation might cause a liberation of noradrenaline. This suggestion received some confirmation from the work of Stehle and Ellsworth (1937) and of Greer et al. (1938) who showed that stimulation of the hepatic nerves in cats liberated a substance which behaved very much more like noradrenaline than like adrenaline.

It was not until 1946, however, that the second twin (noradrenaline) was shown to occur naturally in the body (von Euler, 1946) in organs rich in adrenergic nerves.

It became possible to separate the twins by chemical means and to show that stimulation of adrenergic nerves released not adrenaline but noradrenaline (Gaddum and Goodwin, 1947; Peart, 1949; Folkow and Uvnäs, 1948). It was also found that the adrenal medulla contained noradrenaline as well as adrenaline; indeed, tumours of the adrenal glands might contain mostly noradrenaline (Holton, 1949).

With the recognition of adrenaline and noradrenaline as individual naturally occurring substances, the confusion was resolving. More recently, however, it has been shown that a third pharmacologically active amine, albeit less potent, occurs in tissues. Schümann (1956) extracted and identified dopamine (hydroxytyramine, 3:4 dihydroxy-phenylethylamine) from sympathetic nerves and ganglia; Carlsson *et al.* (1958) also found dopamine in brain. In some organs such as the lung, liver, jejunum and colon, the catechol amine content consists almost entirely of dopamine and this seems to be stored in granules of non-nervous cells (von Euler and Lishajko, 1957; Schümann, 1959). In other organs, about half of the catechol amines is dopamine, probably associated with nerve fibres (von Euler and Lishajko, 1958); in the adrenal medulla, only 2% of the total catechol amine is dopamine. In the brain, both dopamine and noradrenaline are present, but in different sites (Bertler and Rosengren, 1959*a*, *b*). Recently, Axelrod (1960*a*) has discovered yet another catechol amine, N-methyl adrenaline, as a small proportion (2%) of the total catechol amines in the adrenal glands of various mammals.

Isopropylnoradrenaline was also said to account for 2% of the adrenal catechol amines (Lockett, 1954), and to be released on stimulation of bronchial nerves (Lockett, 1957): it is now believed that this substance is not isopropylnoradrenaline, but an active metabolite of noradrenaline (Eakins and Lockett, 1961).

To summarize, four catechol amines have been positively identified in the body. Adrenaline acts mainly as a hormone. Noradrenaline acts as a hormone, as a transmitter of nerve impulses and as an intermediate in adrenaline formation. The role of dopamine is established as a precursor of noradrenaline and adrenaline, but it is not yet clear whether it has a separate physiological function of its own. The role of N-methyl adrenaline, if any, is not known.

ESTIMATION OF CATECHOL AMINES IN BIOLOGICAL FLUIDS
AND TISSUE EXTRACTS

The separation and identification of the extremely small quantities of adrenaline, noradrenaline and dopamine that normally occur in tissue extracts depends upon chemical and biological methods that distinguish between three such closely related compounds. To add to the difficulties, other active substances may be extracted at the same time, such as histamine and 5-hydroxytryptamine. Various methods for the estimation of noradrenaline and adrenaline have been described (see reviews by Gaddum, 1950; von Euler, 1950; Pekkarinen, 1954; von Euler, 1956). Methods for estimating dopamine have been described by Carlsson and Waldeck (1958); Weil-Malherbe (1960) and Schümann (1956).

The estimation of adrenaline and noradrenaline in the suprarenal glands is relatively easy because there is so much amine present. In urine of patients with a phaeochromocytoma there may also be enough present to estimate them fairly simply by measuring the blood pressure rise after intravenous injection into a cat (von Euler, 1952), or by their action on the rabbit intestine *in vitro* (Mann, 1953). In all other tissues and fluids the amounts of adrenaline, noradrenaline and dopamine are so small that very special procedures have to be used for their collection, extraction and estimation. For instance, to measure accurately the concentrations of free adrenaline or noradrenaline in blood one has to avoid damage to the platelets which store not only 5-HT, but may also contain adrenaline and noradrenaline (Born, Hornykiewicz and Stafford, 1958). This means that the blood has to be collected and kept in cooled siliconed vessels to avoid clotting.

The catechol amines are usually separated from each other and from other substances either by absorption on to aluminium oxide or by paper partition chromotography (Goldenberg *et al.*, 1949; Crawford and Outschoorn, 1950; Vogt, 1954. Sometimes there is sufficient catechol amine present for it to be identified and estimated on the paper chromatogram itself, following oxidation to give a coloured product (Hökfelt, 1951); but more usually the amines are eluted from the paper and estimated either chemically or biologically. Although chemical methods are becoming more sensitive (see Symposium on catechol amines, 1959) they are still 50–100 fold less sensitive than biological methods. For instance, in a rat which has been pithed (Shipley and Tilden, 1947) or received urethane and hexamethonium (Vogt, 1952), as little as 1 ng. noradrenaline gives a measurable rise in blood pressure. Adrenaline can be estimated by its inhibitory effect on contractions of the rat's uterus induced by carbachol (de Jalon, Bayo and de Jalon, 1945; Gaddum, Peart and Vogt, 1949). When results are required rapidly and when it is known that adrenaline or noradrenaline are released into the blood stream, their concentrations can be estimated directly by a combination of isolated organ and whole animal technique in which a continuous stream of blood is made to bathe or superfuse the isolated test organs (Vane, 1958). By a suitable choice of test organs the proportions of adrenaline and noradrenaline can be determined.

Several chemical methods have been developed for the determination of adrenaline or noradrenaline. Early methods depended upon the estimation of a coloured product of the catechol amine (Whitehorn, 1935) but with these the concentrations of adrenaline in the blood were unbelievably high (Ghosh *et al.*, 1951).

Most of the chemical methods now in use depend upon measuring the fluorescence either of trihydroxyindoles, which the catechol amines form when oxidized with suitable reagents (Ehrlén, 1948; Lund, 1949*a*, *b*, *c*; von Euler and Floding, 1955), or of their condensation products with ethylenediamine (Weil-Malherbe and Bone, 1952). The use of the spectrophotofluorometer (Bowman, Caulfield and Udenfriend, 1955) has helped to make fluorescent methods more specific. Both biological and chemical methods for assaying catechol amines are surveyed in Section I of the Symposium on catechol amines (1959). Because dopamine has less biological activity than adrenaline or noradrenaline, it is usually determined by modifications of the above chemical methods (Carlsson and Waldeck, 1958; Carlsson, 1959; Weil-Malherbe, 1960).

The availability of labelled catechol amines and their precursors has also made it possible to estimate them by radioactive measurements, but in such determinations, as in the chemical methods, care has to be taken to exclude metabolic products from the estimation.

THE FORMATION OF CATECHOL AMINES IN THE BODY

The use of labelled chemicals has increased enormously our knowledge of the way in which adrenaline and noradrenaline are synthesized in the body. The steps in the synthesis shown in Fig. 10 were first proposed by Blaschko (1939) and by Holtz (1939) but many years elapsed

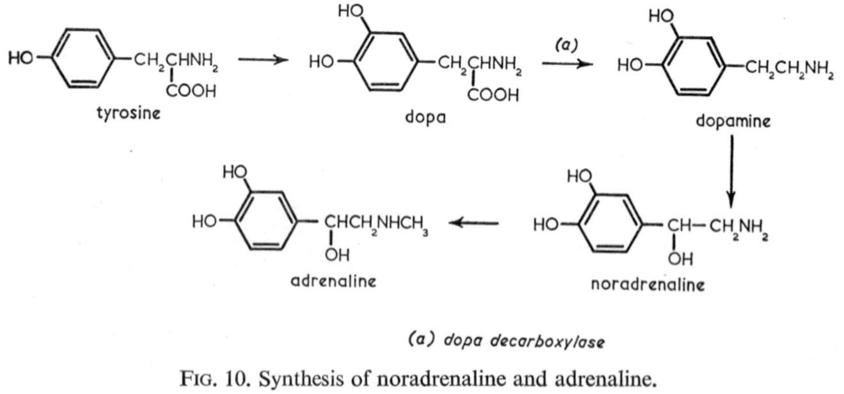

(a) dopa decarboxylase

FIG. 10. Synthesis of noradrenaline and adrenaline.

before definitive evidence for the sequence was obtained. First, it was shown that the adrenal medulla could convert noradrenaline to adrenaline (Bülbring, 1949; Bülbring and Burn, 1949). Then, Demis *et al.*

(1955, 1956) incubated labelled dopa with homogenates of bovine adrenal medulla and identified small amounts of labelled dopamine and labelled noradrenaline. It had been shown earlier that the enzyme L-dopa decarboxylase (Holtz *et al.*, 1938), which converts L-dopa to dopamine, is present in the suprarenal medulla (Langemann, 1951; Holtz and Bachmann, 1952; Westermann, 1957); so are small amounts of dopamine itself (Goodall, 1951; Sheppard and West, 1953; Dengler, 1957). With these individual steps confirmed, the sequence was demonstrated as a whole; for *in vivo* and *in vitro*, medullary tissue converts labelled L-tyrosine or L-dopa into the correspondingly labelled amines, dopamine, noradrenaline and adrenaline (Hagen, 1956; Pellerin and D'Iorio, 1957; Kirshner and Goodall, 1956; Goodall and Kirshner, 1957; Masuoka *et al.*, 1956; Leeper and Udenfriend, 1956; Udenfriend and Wyngaarden, 1956).

The key enzyme in the synthesis, L-dopa decarboxylase, has been found also in sympathetic nervous tissue and in different parts of the brain (Holtz and Westermann, 1956); the same reactions were demonstrated in homogenates of sympathetic nerves and ganglia incubated with labelled L-tyrosine or L-dopa (Goodall and Kirshner, 1958) with the important difference that the synthesis went no further than noradrenaline.

Each step in the formation of adrenaline must be catalysed by enzymes but apart from L-dopa decarboxylase, remarkably little is known about any of them. Thus, although Kaufman (1959) has studied the conversion of phenylalanine to tyrosine, the enzyme which converts L-tyrosine to L-dopa has not received much attention. This enzyme must have a special and selective function, for the following reason: there appears to be no biochemical distinction between L-dopa decarboxylase and 5-hydroxy-L-tryptophan decarboxylase. In other words, it is thought that the same enzyme serves to decarboxylate L-dopa to dopamine and 5-hydroxy-L-tryptophan to 5-hydroxytryptamine (Holtz and Westermann, 1957; Westermann *et al.*, 1958; Bertler and Rosengren, 1959*b*). Thus, cells of the adrenal medulla, which selectively store catechol amines contain the decarboxylating enzyme, as do enterochromaffin cells, which selectively store 5-HT. The selection of the right substrate must therefore take place at the stage before the decarboxylating enzyme. Possibly, cells which store catechol amines have an enzyme which converts L-tyrosine to L-dopa, whereas cells which store 5-HT have an enzyme which converts L-tryptophan to 5-hydroxy-L-tryptophan.

In summary, the cells which synthesize catechol amines receive from the blood L-tyrosine and convert it into L-dopa. This is changed to dopamine by L-dopa decarboxylase in the cytoplasm (Schümann, 1958). The dopamine is stored in cytoplasmic granules, or converted into noradrenaline by the enzyme dopamine β-oxidase (Demis *et al.*, 1956; Goodall and Kirshner, 1958; Udenfriend and Wyngaarden, 1956) which is present in the granules. The noradrenaline may be stored in granules or, in some cells, changed to adrenaline by a methylating enzyme in the cytoplasm (Kirshner and Goodall, 1957). In these cells the adrenaline must then go back into granules for storage. Cells which store dopamine may possibly release it as a transmitter; but it seems more likely, especially in nerve cells, that excitation leads to rapid synthesis and release of noradrenaline. It is known that nervous excitation increases the rate of synthesis of noradrenaline and adrenaline, for prolonged stimulation does not alter the noradrenaline content of nerves (Luco and Goni, 1948) or of ganglia (Vogt, 1954). Similarly, although prolonged splanchnic stimulation brings about the release of considerable amounts of catechol amine from the adrenal medulla, the concentration in the medulla decreases little (Elliott, 1912; Hökfelt and McLean, 1950; Holland and Schümann, 1956). On the other hand, if the adrenal glands are depleted with reserpine it takes a week for the catechol amine content to recover (Butterworth and Mann, 1957) and even longer if the gland is denervated (Kroneberg and Schümann, 1959).

THE DISTRIBUTION OF CATECHOL AMINES

If the adrenal medulla is exposed to potassium bichromate or chromic acid the cells stain brown (Henle, 1865). Kohn (1898, 1903) suggested that cells which undergo this reaction should be called chromaffin cells. This name is used for them almost universally, although other suggestions have been made, such as phäochrome, phaeochrome, pleochrome and fuscogenic cells. Chromic acid, bichromate and other oxidizing agents induce coloration by oxidizing the catechol amines; the oxidized products condense to form insoluble coloured polymers which resemble melanin (Gérard *et al.*, 1930). Because the catechol amines are reducing agents, chromaffin cells react also with ammoniacal silver solution to give deposits of metallic silver. Using the bichromate reaction, chromaffin cells can be easily identified in the adrenal medulla and in other parts of the body.

As well as dopamine, noradrenaline and adrenaline, 5-hydroxytryptamine will also bring about the chromaffin reaction in cells in which it is stored; thus the Kultschitzky cells or enterochromaffin cells of Erspamer are also truly chromaffin. Boyd (1960) has pointed out that the distinction between chromaffin cells containing adrenaline and those containing 5-HT on simply histochemical grounds is not always convincing.

THE ADRENAL MEDULLA

The adrenal medullae of mammals contain two types of cell, one of which stores adrenaline and the other noradrenaline (for references see

Eränkö, 1960). These two cell types probably have different physiological functions, for insulin causes almost total loss of the adrenaline from the medulla but does not diminish its content of noradrenaline (Eränkö, 1952, 1954; Hillarp and Hökfelt, 1954; Vogt, 1954; Coupland, 1958); on the other hand, small doses of reserpine cause a selective loss of noradrenaline (Eränkö and Hopsu, 1958; Camanni and Molinatti, 1958). Although these conclusions depend upon histochemical evidence, there is also physiological evidence that different types of nerve stimuli may cause preferential secretion of either adrenaline or noradrenaline from the adrenal medulla (Brücke *et al.*, 1952; Redgate and Gellhorn, 1953; Folkow and von Euler, 1954).

The proportions of adrenaline and noradrenaline in the adrenal medulla vary greatly in different species and under different conditions (von Euler, 1956). Of the total catechol amine in the adrenal medulla, average values for noradrenaline are 4·5% in the rabbit, 11% in the guinea pig, 45% in the cat, 70% in the hen, and about 20% in man (Goldenberg, 1951; von Euler, 1951, 1954, 1956).

OTHER SPECIALIZED CELLS CONTAINING CATECHOL AMINES

Chromaffin cells are found also in the organs of Zuckerkandl, in the carotid body, in paraganglia situated near the first part and arch of the aorta and in the pelvic plexuses and gonads (see Boyd, 1960). Little is known about the function of these cells, but it has been suggested that, because noradrenaline is in the carotid body, it has a humoral role there (Lever *et al.*, 1959). Much interest has been shown in a diffuse system of chromaffin cells described by Adams-Ray *et al.* (1958) and Niebauer and Wiedmann (1958). These cells are scattered throughout the body; they are most concentrated in the walls of the blood vessels of the cutis but they are present also in lung, liver, uterus, urinary bladder, heart, nerves, and striated muscle. In fact the only tissue in which Adams-Ray *et al.* could not find such cells was the placenta. Histochemical reactions suggest that the cells contain either adrenaline or noradrenaline. The cells are always closely related to non-medullated autonomic nerve fibres.

SYMPATHETIC NERVES

It is now thought that the main catechol amine released by sympathetic nerves is noradrenaline. However, it must be remembered that some organs also contain high concentrations of dopamine (see p. 2) and that a variable but small amount of adrenaline is released together with noradrenaline when some sympathetic nerves are stimulated (Peart, 1949; Mann and West, 1951; Outschoorn, 1952; Mirkin and Bonny-castle, 1954). The adrenaline may, however, come from chromaffin cells (von Euler, 1956). It is very difficult by pharmacological or physiological means to tell whether a catechol amine is stored in nerve endings or in chromaffin cells associated with nerve endings. One method, pointed out by von Euler (1960*a*), is to cut postganglionic sympathetic nerves; when the fibres degenerate the concentration of noradrenaline in the tissue declines whereas that of adrenaline does not. This suggests that noradrenaline is associated with sympathetic nerve endings and adrenaline with some other structures, possibly the chromaffin cells.

THE STORAGE OF CATECHOL AMINES

In the adrenal medulla, pressor amines are largely stored within intracellular particles or granules (Blaschko and Welch, 1953; Hillarp and Nilson, 1953; Hillarp *et al.*, 1953). The particles can be separated from cell debris, nuclei and microsomes by differential centrifugation. Moreover, by centrifuging through layers of sucrose of increasing density the particles can be separated from mitochondria (Blaschko *et al.*, 1956; Blaschko, Hagen and Hagen, 1957; Hillarp, 1958). The granules that are rich in catechol amines are rich also in adenine nucleotides and contain the enzyme which converts dopamine into noradrenaline. They lack the enzymes characteristic of mitochondria, succinic dehydrogenase, fumarase and amine oxidase; only negligible amounts of catechol amines are present in the mitochondrial fraction.

Electron micrographs of adrenal medullary cells show numerous, densely osmiophilic, granules up to 100 mμ in diameter, lying between the endoplasmic reticulum; these are, in fact, the granules which store the catechol amines (Hagen and Barrnett, 1960). The chemical composition of the chromaffin granules is most unusual. They consist of 68% water, 6·7% catechol amines, 4·5% adenosine phosphates, 11·5% proteins and 7% lipids (Hillarp, 1959). In other words, 21% of their dry weight is made up of amines, 15% of adenosine phosphates, 35% of protein and 22% of lipids. There are strong reasons for believing that the acidic phosphate groups of the adenosine phosphates combine with and neutralize the basic groups of the catechol amines; this is probably the fundamental storage mechanism (Hillarp, Högberg and Nilson, 1955; Blaschko *et al.*, 1956). Although the principal nucleotide present is adenosine triphosphate (ATP), adenosine diphosphate (ADP) and adenylic acid (AMP) are also present; their relative amounts vary from species to species. In the normal resting gland, the total number of negative charges on the adenine nucleotides is balanced by the total number of positive charges on the catechol amines (Blaschko *et al.*, 1956; Hillarp, 1958).

In sympathetic nerve fibres about half of the noradrenaline is also stored in granules about 20–100 mμ in diameter (Schümann, 1958; von Euler, 1958) and the ATP content of these granules is similarly equivalent to the amine content (Schümann, 1958). The rest of the noradrenaline and the dopamine is in the cytoplasm (Schümann, 1960;

von Euler, 1960*b*). In brain (see p. 10) the catechol amines are found in granules (Chrusćiel, 1960) which are very much smaller than those in nerve and adrenal medulla and resemble more the vesicles which contain acetylcholine (Whittaker, 1959).

The association of catechol amines with adenine nucleotides in specialized granules makes one wonder how the catechol amines are released from the cell. It could be, for example, that release of the amines follows passively the utilization of the high energy phosphate of the ATP.

THE INACTIVATION OF CATECHOL AMINES

There are three routes of inactivation for adrenaline and noradrenaline; one depends on the enzyme amine oxidase, the second on the

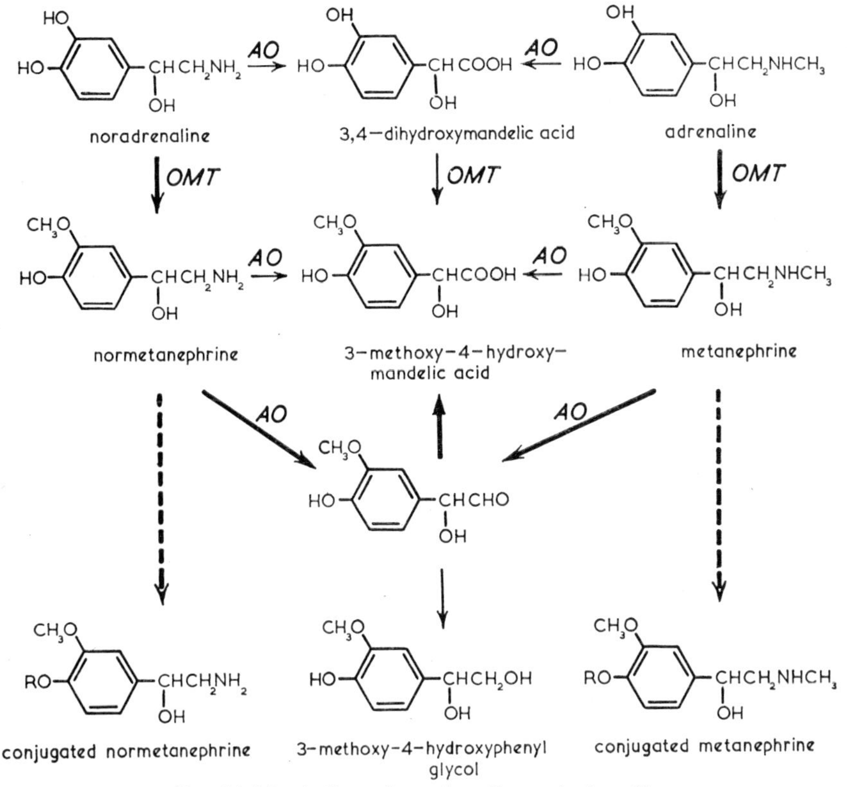

noradrenaline   3,4–dihydroxymandelic acid   adrenaline

normetanephrine   3–methoxy–4–hydroxy–mandelic acid   metanephrine

conjugated normetanephrine   3–methoxy–4–hydroxyphenyl glycol   conjugated metanephrine

FIG. 11. Metabolism of noradrenaline and adrenaline.
AO—amine oxidase; OMT—O-methyl transferase

enzyme catechol O-methyl transferase and the third on the uptake of amines by tissues. The enzyme amine oxidase is found in almost every tissue in the body (see Blaschko, 1952). It is easy to show *in vitro* that the enzyme oxidizes the side chain of many amines, such as adrenaline, noradrenaline, tyramine, phenylethylamine, tryptamine and 5-HT, and for some time it was held that amine oxidase was mainly responsible for inactivation of catechol amines in the body. However, if inhibitors of amine oxidase are administered to an animal, the effects of adrenaline, noradrenaline and 5-HT are not potentiated (Griesemer *et al.*, 1953; Corne and Graham, 1957; Vane, 1959), although those of tryptamine and tyramine are (Vane, 1959). The idea that amine oxidase is of importance in the physiological inactivation of catechol amines began, therefore, to be treated with reserve.

Recent work has shown this caution to be justified, for another enzyme, catechol O-methyl transferase has been found. The discovery of derivatives of adrenaline and noradrenaline methylated in the 3-hydroxy position of the phenyl ring (Armstrong *et al.*, 1957; Axelrod, 1957; Axelrod *et al.*, 1959) led to a detailed study of the fate of adrenaline and noradrenaline in man and of the methylating enzyme. Labelled adrenaline was administered intravenously and its metabolites were isolated from the urine; this showed that approximately 68% of administered adrenaline is O-methylated to metanephrine; 23% is deaminated, oxidized or reduced before O-methylation and the remainder is excreted conjugated or unchanged. Noradrenaline is metabolized in essentially the same manner as adrenaline. The methylated compounds normetanephrine and metanephrine are either conjugated, or attacked by amine oxidase to form 3-methoxy-4-hydroxy mandelic acid. The various routes of inactivation are shown in Fig. 11. The major role of amine oxidase is therefore secondary to O-methyl transferase and the failure of amine oxidase inhibitors to potentiate the effects of catechol amines is understandable. Whether or not amine oxidase is important for the inactivation of brain catechol amines is discussed in Chapter 11.

The discovery of O-methyl transferase was followed by a search for specific inhibitors of the enzyme. Over 20 years ago it was shown that catechol, pyrogallol, quercitin and similar compounds would potentiate the biological effects of adrenaline and noradrenaline (Bacq, 1936; Lavollay, 1941): on re-investigation, they were all found to be inhibitors of catechol-O-methyl transferase (Bacq *et al.*, 1959; Axelrod and Laroche, 1959; Axelrod and Tomchick, 1959). This was additional evidence for the role of O-methyl transferase as the primary step in the inactivation of adrenaline and noradrenaline.

When catechol amines are injected intravenously into mice they disappear from the tissues in two distinct phases. There is a rapid fall in concentration in the first five minutes during which about 55% of adrenaline and 40% of noradrenaline are O-methylated. This is followed by a much slower decline in concentration; $1\frac{1}{2}$ hours later for adrenaline and 6 hours later for noradrenaline, 20% of the administered catechol amine is still retained as such by the tissues (Axelrod, 1960*b*).

Endogenous noradrenaline is also bound to tissues. When the splenic nerve is stimulated noradrenaline appears in the splenic venous blood; the amount that appears depends on the state of the tissue. About 12 hours after central denervation, which might be expected to starve the tissue of noradrenaline, very little of the noradrenaline released by nerve stimulation appears in the blood stream; almost all of it is retained in the spleen. If phenoxybenzamine is given, which blocks receptors for noradrenaline, very much more transmitter appears in the blood stream; similarly, after a burst of rapid stimulation which might be expected to load the tissues with transmitter, more noradrenaline appears in the blood during a subsequent period of stimulation. As it takes at least 12 hours for the tissues to lose their noradrenaline there must be a firm binding of noradrenaline at sites other than the nerve endings themselves (Brown and Gillespie, 1957; Brown, Davies and Gillespie, 1958; Brown, Davies and Ferry, 1959; Brown, 1960). Because these take-up sites are blocked by phenoxybenzamine the word 'receptor' has been used to describe them, but there is, as yet, no proof that these sites are the same spots on the cell membranes with which noradrenaline normally combines to produce its biological effect. Phenoxybenzamine may block not only these 'active receptors' but also some other uptake sites for catechol amines. Another possibility is that liberated noradrenaline may be taken back into the nerve ending (Paton, 1960).

Whatever the mechanism, there is no doubt that noradrenaline and, to a lesser extent, adrenaline can be taken up by tissues, held in an inactive form and kept there out of the circulation for several hours. Consequently, this process must be important in the inactivation of catechol amines. It may also be related to the process by which cocaine and many other basic drugs potentiate the actions of catechol amines. For many years, it has been known that receptors for catechol amines become supersensitive a few days after cutting the sympathetic nerve supply to an organ. After injections of ganglion blocking agents, bretylium, guanethidine or cocaine, the effects of catechol amines are also potentiated. This similarity between the effects of denervation and the effects of 'pharmacological denervation' has led to the supposition that the processes involved are similar (see Emmelin, 1961). There are, however, objections to this idea as applied to the effects of catechol amines: for instance, the potentiation which follows the injection of bretylium occurs almost instantaneously whereas it takes an hour or more for the nerves to be blocked. The potentiation induced by hexamethonium may outlast the blocking effect of hexamethonium on the ganglia.

The potentiation of the effects of catechol amines by cocaine is accompanied by higher blood levels of the catechol amines, for a longer time (Trendelenburg, 1959; Muscholl, 1961). By different methods, Axelrod (1960*b*) has also shown that substances such as reserpine, chlorpromazine, imipramine and amphetamine interfere with the tissue binding of catechol amines, as does phenoxybenzamine (see above). Vane (unpublished) has found that after substances such as hexamethonium and bretylium, the blood levels of injected noradrenaline are also sufficiently higher to account for the increased effects. Furthermore, although there is no evidence for the release of catechol amine into the bloodstream by tyramine in normal animals (Vane, 1960), traces can be detected if the animal has been pre-treated with hexamethonium. These results suggested that hexamethonium was in some way interfering with the take up of catechol amine by the tissues, without affecting the combination of catechol amine with the receptors. It was therefore proposed (Vane, unpublished) that drugs such as ganglion blocking agents, bretylium, guanethidine and possibly cocaine, all being basic in nature, will combine with non-specific acidic radicals in the tissues, but not with the specific receptors for catechol amines. When these agents are absent, noradrenaline will combine both with the specific sites and with the non-specific sites. The combination with the non-specific sites would be sufficient to reduce the amount of noradrenaline available for combination with receptors. When the non-specific sites are blocked by other basic compounds, more noradrenaline would be free for receptor combination, and the effect obtained would be greater. The conception of non-specific take up sites, or 'sites of loss' has been reviewed in general terms by Veldstra (1956) and has been applied by Cavallito (1957) in connection with neuro-muscular blocking agents.

The fate of catechol amines therefore depends upon at least three simultaneous processes of inactivation, which reduce the concentration of amine in the circulation greatly within 2 minutes. These separate but parallel inactivation processes can be affected by a variety of agents. Many inhibitors of amine oxidase are known (see p. 57). Catechol-O-methyl transferase is inhibited by pyragallol and similar compounds and tissue binding may be reduced by several compounds.

Work on catechol-O-methyl transferase is still in its early stages but it is already helping the clinician. The estimation of 3-methoxy-4-hydroxy mandelic acid in the urine is used in the diagnosis of phaeochromocytoma. The substance is extracted by absorption on to an ion exchange resin; after elution it is converted into vanillin which is estimated colorimetrically (Sandler and Ruthven, 1959*a, b*, 1960). Other methods have also been described (Armstrong and MacMillan, 1959; Kraupp *et al.*, 1959; La Brosse *et al.*, 1958; Robinson *et al.*, 1959; Gitlow *et al.*, 1960). In normal adults, urinary excretion of 3-methoxy-4-hydroxy mandelic acid in 24 hours is from 4 to 8 mg.; in cases of proved phaeochromocytoma the excretion is between 10–50 mg.

RECEPTORS FOR CATECHOL AMINES

Catechol amines have many and varied actions in the body; they stimulate the heart, contract vascular smooth muscle, dilate the bronchi, inhibit intestinal smooth muscle and affect metabolism in various ways. The range and pattern of effects is characteristic for each individual catechol amine.

Most of the excitatory or stimulatory effects are blocked by specific antagonists such as ergotoxine and phenoxybenzamine; the inhibitory effects, the metabolic effects, and the stimulant action on the heart are not. This separation into effects which are antagonized by blocking agents and effects which are not has led to the idea that there are two types of receptor (Ahlquist, 1948): receptors blocked by ergotoxine, dibenamine, phenoxybenzamine, etc. are called α receptors and those which are not blocked are called β receptors. More recently, compounds have been discovered which selectively block the β receptors (Powell and Slater, 1958; Mayer and Moran, 1960; Ariëns, 1960); these are similar in structure to the catechol amines, except that the ring hydroxyl groups have been replaced by chloro groups. Because the inhibitory effects of catechol amines on intestinal smooth muscle were not completely blocked by either type of antagonist, another receptor (the δ receptor) was proposed (Furchgott, 1959). However, a combination of both types of antagonist gives complete block, suggesting that the inhibitory effects of catechol amines on intestinal smooth muscle are produced by a mixture of α and β receptors (Ahlquist and Levy, 1959; Furchgott, 1960).

Noradrenaline acts mainly on α receptors, isopropylnoradrenaline mainly on β receptors, and adrenaline acts on both. By using the two types of antagonist and by comparing the activity of noradrenaline with isoprenaline, the distribution of α and β receptors has been plotted throughout the body.

Although the receptors for catechol amines have had these names for many years we are only just beginning to learn something about their fundamental nature. Important advances have been made using chemical, biochemical and electrophysiological techniques and it is fascinating to see how a general picture of the receptor is emerging from these different approaches. The primary action of catechol amines (see also p. 201) on many tissues is to promote the formation from ATP of a cyclic nucleotide, adenosine-3',5'-phosphate (Sutherland and Rall, 1960). The enzyme which converts ATP to cyclic adenylate requires a bivalant metal such as magnesium; Belleau (1960) suggested that the hydroxyl groups of the catechol nucleus combine with a bivalant metal ion attached to the enzyme. The cyclic adenylate stimulates the formation of active phosphorylase which accelerates glycogenolysis (Fig. 12). It is interesting to note that ATP is thus intimately connected with catechol amines not only in their storage but also in their effects on metabolism.

It is possible that this cyclase system is the actual β-receptor; this idea is supported by the fact that isoprenaline is the most effective of the catechol amines upon the system and adrenaline is generally more effective than noradrenaline. The cyclase system may be in the cell membrane, or inside the cell (Sutherland, 1960).

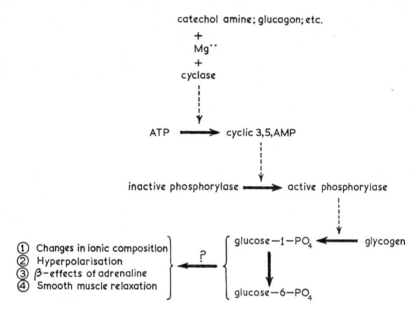

FIG. 12. The role of cyclic 3,5-adenosine monophosphate in glycogenolysis (modified from Sutherland and Rall, 1960).

Using electrophysiological techniques, Bülbring (1960) has shown that on intestinal smooth muscle, adrenaline can have two actions which may be linked respectively with the α and β effects. One is a direct action on the membrane, leading to an increase in permeability of the membrane to one or several ions. This makes the membrane less stable and more excitable and might even cause depolarization. The other action is metabolic and can be measured as an increase in phosphorylase activity, presumably following the formation of cyclic adenylate. Bülbring suggests that this affects the functional state of the cell by making more energy available, which can be used either to bring about a contraction or to hyperpolarize the cell membrane through active ion transport, thereby making the membrane less excitable. The hypothesis implies that in smooth muscle catechol amines induce both α and β effects simultaneously and that the effect that is observed is the resultant of two opposing actions. When contraction is produced the direct action on membrane permeability predominates; when relaxation is produced the metabolic effect predominates. Under the influence of adrenaline, the active extrusion of sodium from the cell is approximately doubled and the uptake of sodium is lessened (Goodford and Hermansen, 1960). This action on the 'sodium pump' may be the final membrane-stabilizing stage of a chain of metabolic events initiated by the action of adrenaline on the formation of cyclic adenylate.

When adrenaline stimulates glycogenolysis more lactic acid is produced. Lundholm and Mohme-Lundholm (1960) think that the inhibitory effects of adrenaline are caused by the direct action of this lactic acid. Whichever hypothesis is true, it certainly seems that the inhibitory effects of adrenaline are linked with a stimulation of a chain of metabolic events, initiated by the formation of cyclic adenylate. Although the excitatory effects are thought to be due to depolarization of the muscle membrane, Schild (1960) has shown that when smooth muscle is completely depolarized by immersion in potassium methyl sulphate Ringer, adrenaline can still produce contraction or relaxation.

The synergism between the results of Sutherland, Bülbring and Belleau is very striking and should lead, before long, to the identification for the first time, of an actual adrenaline receptor.

THE ACTIONS OF CATECHOL AMINES IN THE BODY

These actions both in animals and in man have been extensively reviewed (Goodman and Gilman, 1955; Drill, 1958; Ginsburg and Cobbold, 1960) and only a brief account will be given here. Intravenous infusions of noradrenaline in man bring about bradycardia of reflex origin, an increase in total peripheral resistance and a rise in blood pressure. With adrenaline, the heart rate increases, the peripheral resistance falls and the mean blood pressure remains almost unchanged. Isoprenaline is the most potent of the amines in increasing the heart rate and reducing the peripheral resistance; the mean blood pressure falls. All three amines increase the depth of respiration by some mechanism other than a direct action on the respiratory centre (Coles *et al.*, 1956; Young, 1957).

The cardiovascular effects in man agree well with the idea that noradrenaline acts mainly on α receptors, isoprenaline on β receptors and adrenaline on both. Thus, the action of noradrenaline on skeletal muscle blood vessels is constrictor; after phenoxybenzamine, the effect is abolished but no dilator component is seen. However, the constrictor effect of intra-arterial infusions of adrenaline is reversed by phenoxybenzamine to dilatation, showing that both types of receptor are involved (Ginsburg and Cobbold, 1960).

THE RELEASE OF CATECHOL AMINES

The Release of Catechol Amines from Nerve Endings

The classical idea of transmission in an adrenergic neurone is of a nerve impulse liberating noradrenaline from the nerve endings, close to the site of action. The noradrenaline diffuses to the site of action and combines with the receptors. Recently, evidence has been presented that another, less direct mechanism exists. Reserpine depletes adrenergic neurones of their noradrenaline, thereby reducing their effectiveness when the nerves are stimulated. Following an infusion of noradrenaline the nerve becomes effective once more (Burn, 1960), suggesting that noradrenaline has been taken up out of the circulation into the stores associated with the nerve endings. Even in normal cats, the effects of sympathetic stimulation are increased after an infusion of noradrenaline. It is well known that in the presence of atropine, acetylcholine produces many effects that are 'adrenergic' rather than 'cholinergic'; for example, acceleration and increase in force of heart muscle, constriction of vessels, erection of hair tufts and contraction of the spleen. These adrenergic effects of acetylcholine are indirect for they are reduced or abolished after depletion by means of reserpine, of the stores of noradrenaline. Furthermore, in animals which have received reserpine, stimulation of adrenergic nerves such as those going to the spleen, produces apparently cholinergic effects, which are potentiated by eserine and reduced by atropine. This evidence suggested to Burn and Rand that in sympathetic nerves, there was an unknown proportion of cholinergic fibres which first released acetylcholine; the acetylcholine in turn released catechol amine either from stores in the nerve endings themselves or from closely associated chromaffin cells. From the pattern of distribution of acetyl-cholinesterase in adrenergic nerves, Koelle (1961) has also concluded that acetylcholine may play a part in the transmission process in a proportion of sympathetic nerve endings.

Basing his argument upon the actions of bretylium and hemicholinium, Burn (1961) has now extended the idea of an underlying cholinergic mechanism to include *all* postganglionic sympathetic fibres. From its chemical structure, he adduces that bretylium is more likely to act in relation to acetylcholine than to noradrenaline. Concentrations of bretylium which blocked the release of catechol amine by sympathetic nerve stimulation also blocked the release of catechol amine by injected acetylcholine, but not by tyramine (Hukovic, 1960; Burn, 1961). Burn therefore suggests that just as acetylcholine is specifically blocked by atropine at the receptors associated with para-sympathetic nerve endings, by tubocurarine at the neuro-muscular junction and by hexamethonium at ganglia, so it is blocked at the terminations of postganglionic sympathetic fibres by bretylium. Since all postganglionic sympathetic nerves are blocked by bretylium, they must all be mediated by a primary release of acetylcholine.

Hemicholinium interferes with the synthesis of acetylcholine (MacIntosh *et al.*, 1956) by preventing the access of choline to choline acetylase (Gardiner, 1961). The fact that hemicholinium blocks transmission in some isolated sympathetic nerve-smooth muscle preparations (Chang and Rand, 1960) has been taken as further evidence that these nerves are cholinergic in nature.

General acceptance of this new hypothesis will depend to a large extent upon further research on the specificity of both bretylium and hemicholinium and anatomical work on the nerve endings themselves. Against the idea that all sympathetic nerves have an underlying cholinergic mechanism are the experiments of Gardiner and Thompson (1961). Even with high doses of hemicholinium they were unable to affect transmission in the postganglionic sympathetic supply to the isolated nictitating membrane of the cat. Thompson (1960) could find no evidence for cholinergic fibres in the postganglionic supply to the nictitating membrane. Hellmann and Thompson (1961), using a histochemical staining technique, found cholinesterase only in the Harderian gland; there was none in the smooth muscle cells of the membrane nor in the great majority of the nerve fibres supplying the muscle.

Substances which block release from nerve endings

Substances such as phenoxybenzamine block the α-effects of catechol amines in the body, by preventing their combination with the receptors. The use of these substances in clinical medicine is limited because, with the receptors blocked, noradrenaline cannot be used to restore the blood pressure should the dose of antagonist prove too large. Of great interest, therefore, was a compound which prevented the release of noradrenaline from sympathetic nerve endings. This compound was xylocholine (see also p. 310) or choline 2, 6-xylyl ethyl bromide (TM10). Although it had many other actions its primary one was to reduce or abolish for long periods the responses to stimulation of adrenergic nerves (Willey, 1957; Exley, 1956, 1957). It was first thought that this block of adrenergic nerves was linked with the powerful local anaesthetic action of the drug (Hey and Willey, 1953, 1954) but it was later found that analogues of the compound, although powerful anaesthetics, failed to block the release of transmitter from the postganglionic sympathetic supply to the nictitating membrane. Moreover, xylocholine did not affect parasympathetic nerve stimulation. When adrenergic nerves were blocked by xylocholine, the postganglionic action potentials were unimpaired (Exley, 1960). Xylocholine has no action on L-dopa-decarboxylase but the effects of xylocholine on isolated preparations such as the nerve-smooth muscle preparation of the intestine (Finkleman, 1930) could easily be reversed by adding dopamine. This led to the hypothesis that xylocholine was acting by preventing the conversion of dopamine to noradrenaline, the last stage in its synthesis (Bain and Fielden, 1957). The suggestion was supported by work with suspensions of adrenal medullary tumour cells which had been exposed to radioactive dopamine. The presence of xylocholine diminished the formation of noradrenaline from radioactive dopamine (Bain, 1960).

The ability of xylocholine selectively to block the sympathetic nervous system by preventing release of noradrenaline led to a search for compounds with similar action but with fewer side effects. So far, two have become of clinical importance, bretylium (Boura, Copp and Green, 1959) and guanethidine (Maxwell, Mull and Plummer, 1959). These substances are further discussed on p. 311. Although bretylium is similar to xylocholine it is said to have quite a different mode of action. Measurement of the distribution of radioactive bretylium in animals shows it to be concentrated apparently selectively, in sympathetic ganglia and postganglionic sympathetic nerve trunks (Boura et al., 1960). Up to 500 times the concentration of bretylium is found in sympathetic nerves as compared with parasympathetic nerves. This selective concentration in adrenergic nerves together with a strong local anaesthetic action (Boura and Green, 1959) has led to the hypothesis that bretylium acts as a local anaesthetic selectively on sympathetic nerves because it is concentrated in them. If this is so, the local anaesthetic action must be limited to the fine nerve terminals, for Exley (1960) showed that under the influence of bretylium the postganglionic distal portion of the cat's splanchnic nerves still responds to stimulation by a burst of action potentials. Although structurally dissimilar, guanethidine, [2-(octahydro-l′-azocinyl)-ethyl] -guanidine sulphate has an effect similar to that of bretylium, but more prolonged. It is unlikely that guanethidine acts through its local anaesthetic action on postganglionic nerves (Bein, 1960) for even after high doses postganglionic action potentials are normal (Maxwell et al., 1960).

All three drugs have some initial sympathomimetic activity; xylocholine releases catechol amines from tissues (Coupland and Exley, 1957) but the amounts liberated are not sufficient to account for the block of the nerve ending and the release is very slow. Large doses of bretylium have to be used to produce sympathomimetic effects (Boura and Green, 1959). Sheppard and Zimmermann (1959, 1960) showed that guanethidine reduces the concentration of catechol amines in the spleen, the heart and arteries, but not in the brain or the adrenal medulla; and Jaques (1960) found that it lowers the concentration of 5-hydroxytryptamine in the small intestine of mice and rabbits. It is possible that the depletion of catechol amines is important as far as the actions of guanethidine are concerned. If so, then guanethidine could be regarded as having some peripheral actions similar to reserpine and some similar to bretylium (Burn, 1961).

Because the effects of these three agents are on the nerve terminal, the actions of circulating adrenaline and noradrenaline on their receptors are not reduced; indeed they are potentiated (see earlier). None of these substances reduces the output of catechol amines from the adrenal glands.

Theoretically, agents which will effectively and selectively block the sympathetic nervous system should be beneficial in some types of hypertension. They do not prevent the actions of noradrenaline should the blood pressure require to be raised after an overdosage, nor do they block the parasympathetic system, as do the ganglion-blocking drugs. Bretylium and guanethidine have been much used in the treatment of hypertension and this is discussed on p. 311.

The release of catechol amines from the adrenal gland

Acetylcholine, histamine and 5-hydroxytryptamine all bring about the release of catechol amines in a short burst from the adrenal gland. Reserpine, on the other hand, brings about their slow but prolonged release. A single dose of reserpine reduces the concentration of catechol amines in nervous tissue and in chromaffin cells to very low levels within 24 hours. Small doses of reserpine are said to deplete the adrenal medulla selectively of noradrenaline (Eränkö and Hopsu, 1958; Camanni and Molinatti, 1958). As the depletion by reserpine is a slow process, pharmacological effects of the released catechol amines are usually only seen after the administration of amine oxidase inhibitors (Eltherington and Horita, 1960) or cocaine (Horita, 1958), although Muscholl and Vogt (1957) have shown that within the first hour after administration of reserpine to rabbits, the concentrations of catechol amines increase in the blood. Gillis and Lewis (1956) have shown that reserpine antagonizes the actions of catechol amines, so the circulating reserpine may not only cause the slow liberation of catechol amines but may also prevent their reaction with the receptors. How amine oxidase inhibitors bring out the pharmacological effects of the circulating noradrenaline is not clearly understood.

Substances which block release from the adrenal medulla

Ganglion blocking drugs in general are less active on the adrenal medulla than on ganglion cells although they block both. For instance, the medulla is blocked by a series of methonium compounds of which the most potent is hexamethonium, just as it is on ganglia (Marley and Paton, 1961). Recently a new compound, N, N-diisopropyl-N'-isoamyl-N'-diethylaminoethyl urea (Gardier *et al.*, 1960) has been said to block the adrenal medulla selectively and to prevent the release of catechol amines but not to block ganglia.

Release of catechol amines from other stores

Injections of reserpine lead to the loss of catechol amines and 5-hydroxytryptamine from almost all tissues in the body, including the adrenal glands (Pletscher *et al.*, 1955; Shore *et al.*, 1955; Holzbauer and Vogt, 1956; Muscholl and Vogt, 1958; Carlsson and Hillarp, 1956; Paasonen and Krayer, 1957), the heart (Bertler *et al.*, 1956), the aorta of rabbit and dog, the spleen, iris and tail skin of the cat and the ear skin of the rabbit (Burn and Rand, 1957; Burn and Rand, 1958*a*, 1959; Burn *et al.*, 1959).

It has been known for many years that reactions of some sympathomimetic amines, such as tyramine, are different from those of adrenaline although the chemical structure is similar. For instance, the pressor action of tyramine is abolished by cocaine (Tainter and Chang, 1927), whereas that of adrenaline is increased (Fröhlich and Loewi, 1910). About a week after sympathetic denervation of an organ the actions of tyramine are also reduced or abolished (Meltzer, 1904; Burn, 1932; Fleckenstein and Stöckle, 1955). The observation of Carlsson *et al.* (1957) that tyramine had no pressor action in a cat pretreated with reserpine suggested to Burn and Rand that the lack of action of tyramine in such animals was due to the absence of noradrenaline and that the normal pressor action of tyramine depended on the release of noradrenaline. The hypothesis suggests therefore, that tyramine acts *indirectly*, through a release of noradrenaline from tissue stores. This also explains the lack of action of tyramine after sympathetic denervation because noradrenaline disappears from the denervated tissues (Goodall, 1951; von Euler and Purkhold, 1951). Furthermore, in cats pretreated with reserpine, infusions of noradrenaline restored the pressor action of tyramine suggesting that noradrenaline had been taken up into the empty tissue stores (Burn and Rand, 1960*a*). Infusions of dopa or dopamine, but not of adrenaline, also restored the pressor effects of tyramine. Even in normal cats the actions of tyramine were increased after an infusion of noradrenaline (Burn and Rand, 1960*b*). Corresponding experiments on the isolated colon taken from rabbits pretreated with reserpine, show that sympathetic stimulation has little effect; after bathing the organ in noradrenaline sympathetic stimulation has a much greater effect (Gillespie and Mackenna, 1959). In atria isolated from untreated rabbits, adding noradrenaline to the bathing fluid greatly increases the subsequent effect of nicotine or tyramine, despite frequent changes of bathing fluid between the drugs (Azarnoff and Burn, 1961).

That the action of tyramine may be mediated by a release of noradrenaline from stores in tissues poses at least two problems; the first is whether other sympathomimetic amines act in the same way; and the second is whether released noradrenaline circulates in the blood stream. Burn and Rand (1958b) have shown that if an animal is treated with reserpine many compounds with structures similar to tyramine have no action, but that it is restored after infusions of noradrenaline. These compounds include phenylethylamine, amphetamine, phenylethanolamine, and several others in which the phenyl ring has only one hydroxyl group or no substituents at all. Vane (unpublished) has also shown that several methoxyphenylethylamines have no action in cats pretreated with reserpine. If many sympathomimetic amines act on smooth muscle indirectly through the release of noradrenaline, the accepted structure-action relationships need substantial re-interpretation. Only the catechol compounds, which act directly, should be used for arguing structure-action relationships with respect to receptors for adrenaline and noradrenaline in smooth muscle, for if the action of substances such as tyramine and amphetamine is indirect, they cannot combine with the same receptor as does noradrenaline.

Attempts to demonstrate the possibility that noradrenaline is released into the blood stream by tyramine and similar substances have been made in two ways; Vane (1960) used the blood-bathed organ technique to monitor continuously the arterial blood from an animal for increase of concentration of catechol amines. Intravenous injections of as little as 0·1 μg. adrenaline or noradrenaline relax the test organ (a rat stomach strip) when the circulating amine reaches it, showing that the method is sensitive to very low blood concentrations of catechol amines. To make the test with tyramine, a stomach strip was taken from a rat pretreated with reserpine, so that the local stores of catechol amine were depleted. An intravenous injection of 1 mg. or more tyramine into the cat caused no relaxation of the rat stomach strip although there was a substantial pressor response; the concentration of catecholamine in the blood must have been less than 1 ng./ml. Such low concentrations cannot produce profound cardiovascular effects. If, however, a normal rat stomach strip is bathed in blood from the cat, it will relax almost immediately to tyramine injected directly into the blood bathing the strip. Thus, the strip reacts to tyramine without any catechol amine reaching it in the blood; the local stores of noradrenaline in the muscle, when released, are sufficient to cause a typical relaxation of the same muscle. The cats used in these experiments were anaesthetized with chloralose and their adrenal glands were in the circulation. Lockett and Eakins (1960a, b) claim that after intravenous tyramine in adrenalectomized cats which had received both atropine and hexamethonium as well as an anaesthetic, they can detect up to 15 μg. of catechol amine per 100 ml. plasma in aortic blood although none in carotid blood. Such high concentrations should be easily detectable by other methods. The pretreatment with hexamethonium may be important in this respect (see page 106).

Burn and Rand suggested that what is released by tyramine is noradrenaline; but there is some evidence that it may be adrenaline. West (1960) showed that during an infusion of small quantities of noradrenaline the actions of single injections of noradrenaline itself were suppressed whereas those of tyramine and of adrenaline were potentiated.

EFFECTS OF SUBSTANCES WHICH BLOCK RELEASE OF CATECHOL AMINES

The prior administration of cocaine prevents the pressor effects of tyramine and of similar drugs but potentiates the pressor effects of catechol amines. This has led to the suggestion that cocaine prevents the release of noradrenaline from storage sites (Burn and Rand, 1959; Macmillan, 1959). Bretylium and guanethidine do not block the pressor effects of tyramine.

OTHER ACTIONS OF SYMPATHOMIMETIC AMINES

If the sympathomimetic effects of tyramine and similar agents are indirect, they cannot combine to any great extent with receptors for catechol amines. Thus, on isolated smooth muscle, many of the non-catechol 'sympathomimetic' amines do not produce an adrenaline-like effect. They do, however, have actions on tryptamine receptors in preparations such as the rat stomach strip, the guinea pig ileum and the isolated rabbit duodenum (Vane, 1960). Contractions of these tissues produced by amphetamine, mescaline, 5-HT and tryptamine are all selectively antagonized by antagonists for 5-HT, such as brom LSD. The combination of phenylethylamines with tryptamine receptors has also been shown on the isolated clam heart (Greenberg, 1960). In lightly anaesthetized cats, amphetamine and other phenylethylamines cause a chemoreceptor reflex similar to that produced by 5-HT (Vane, 1960). Amphetamine has also been shown to depolarize ganglion cells (Reinert, 1960).

Work in the last few years has resolved many of the anomalies connected with the metabolism and actions of sympathomimetic amines. To a large extent, this is due to the use of new drugs as tools for research. Just as receptors have been characterized by the use of specific antagonists, so the storage and release mechanisms have been characterized by drugs like reserpine, xylocholine and bretylium. Similarly, our knowledge of the synthesis and inactivation of catechol amines depends upon the use of labelled chemicals, enzyme antagonists and refinements in biochemical techniques.

REFERENCES

* Denotes review

References to 'Adrenergic Mechanisms' are to the Ciba Foundation *Symposium on Adrenergic Mechanisms, edited by Vane, J. R., Wolstenholme, G. E. W., and O'Connor, M. London: Churchill (1960).

ABEL, J. J. (1902). *Johns Hopk. Hosp. Bull.* **13,** 29
ADAMS-RAY, J., NORDENSTAM, H. and RHODIN, J. (1958). *Acta neuroveg. (Wien).* **18,** 304
AHLQUIST, R. P. (1948). *Amer. J. Physiol.* **153,** 586
AHLQUIST, R. P. and LEVY, B. (1959). *J. Pharmacol. exp. Ther.* **127,** 146
ARIËNS, E. J. (1960). In Adrenergic Mechanisms, p. 264
ARMSTRONG, M. D., MCMILLAN, A. and SHAW, K. N. F. (1957). *Biochim. Biophys. Acta,* **25,** 442
*ARMSTRONG, M. D. and MCMILLAN, A. (1959). *Pharmacol. Rev.* **11,** 394
AXELROD, J. (1957). *Science,* **126,** 400
AXELROD, J. (1960a). *Biochim. Biophys. Acta,* **45,** 614
AXELROD, J. (1960b). In Adrenergic Mechanisms, p. 28
AXELROD, J., KOPIN, I. J. and MANN, J. D. (1959). *Biochim. Biophys. Acta,* **36,** 576
AXELROD, J. and LAROCHE, M. J. (1959). *Science,* **130,** 800
AXELROD, J. and TOMCHICK, R. (1959). *Nature (Lond.),* **184,** 2027
AZARNOFF, D. L. and BURN, J. H. (1961). *Brit. J. Pharmacol.* **16,** 335
BACQ, Z. M. (1933). *Arch. int. Physiol.* **36,** 167
BACQ, Z. M. (1936). *Arch. int. Physiol.* **42,** 340
BACQ, Z. M., GOSSELIN, L., DRESSE, A. and RENSON, J. (1959). *Science,* **130,** 453
BAIN, W. A. (1960). In Adrenergic Mechanisms, p. 131
BAIN, W. A. and FIELDEN, R. (1957). *Lancet,* **2,** 472
BARGER, G. and DALE, H. H. (1910). *J. Physiol.* **41,** 19
BEIN, H. J. (1960). In Adrenergic Mechanisms, p. 162
BELLEAU, B. (1960). In Adrenergic Mechanisms, p. 223
BERTLER, A., CARLSSON, A. and ROSENGREN, E. (1956). *Naturwissenschaften,* **43,** 521
BERTLER, A. and ROSENGREN, E. (1959a). *Experientia,* **15,** 10
BERTLER, A. and ROSENGREN, E. (1959b). *Experientia,* **15,** 382
BLASCHKO, H. (1939). *J. Physiol.* **96,** 50P
*BLASCHKO, H. (1952). *Pharmacol. Rev.* **4,** 415
BLASCHKO, H., BORN, G. V. R., D'IORIO, A. and EADE, N. R. (1956). *J. Physiol.* **133,** 544
BLASCHKO, H., HAGEN, J. M. and HAGEN, P. (1957). *J. Physiol.* **139,** 316
BLASCHKO, H. and WELCH, A. D. (1953). *Arch. exp. Path. Pharmak.* **219,** 17
BORN, G. V. R., HORNYKIEWICZ, O. and STAFFORD, A. (1958). *Brit. J. Pharmacol.* **13,** 411
BOURA, A. L. A., COPP, F. C., DUNCOMBE, W. G., GREEN, A. F. and McCOUBREY, A. (1960). *Brit. J. Pharmacol.* **15,** 265
BOURA, A. L. A., COPP, F. C. and GREEN, A. F. (1959). *Nature (Lond.),* **184,** BA70
BOURA, A. L. A. and GREEN, A. F. (1959). *Brit. J. Pharmacol.* **14,** 536
BOWMAN, R. L., CAULFIELD, P. A. and UDENFRIEND, S. (1955). *Science,* **122,** 32
BOYD, J. D. (1960). In Adrenergic Mechanisms, p. 63
BROWN, G. L. (1960). In Adrenergic Mechanisms, p. 116
BROWN, G. L., DAVIES, B. N. and FERRY, C. B. (1959). *J. Physiol.* **147,** 13P
BROWN, G. L., DAVIES, B. N. and GILLESPIE, J. S. (1958). *J. Physiol.* **143,** 41
BROWN, G. L. and GILLESPIE, J. S. (1957). *J. Physiol.* **138,** 81
BRÜCKE, F., KAINDL, F. and MAYER, H. (1952). *Arch. int. Pharmacodyn.* **88,** 407
BÜLBRING, E. (1949). *Brit. J. Pharmacol.* **4,** 234
BÜLBRING, E. (1960). In Adrenergic Mechanisms, p. 275
BÜLBRING, E. and BURN, J. H. (1949). *Brit. J. Pharmacol.* **4,** 202
BURN, J. H. (1932). *J. Pharmacol. exp. Ther.* **46,** 75
BURN, J. H. (1960). In Adrenergic Mechanisms, p. 326
BURN, J. H. (1961). *Brit. med. J.* **1,** 1623

BURN, J. H., LEACH, E. H., RAND, M. J. and THOMPSON, J. W. (1959). *J. Physiol.* **148**, 332
BURN, J. H. and RAND, M. J. (1957). *Lancet*, **2**, 1097
BURN, J. H. and RAND, M. J. (1958a). *Brit. med. J.* **1**, 903
BURN, J. H. and RAND, M. J. (1958b). *J. Physiol.* **144**, 314
BURN, J. H. and RAND, M. J. (1959). *J. Physiol.* **147**, 135
BURN, J. H. and RAND, M. J. (1960a). *Brit. J. Pharmacol.* **15**, 47
BURN, J. H. and RAND, M. J. (1960b). *J. Physiol.* **150**, 295
BUTTERWORTH, K. R. and MANN, M. (1957). *Brit. J. Pharmacol.* **12**, 415
CAMANNI, F. and MOLINATTI, G. M. (1958). *Acta endocr. (Kbh.)* **29**, 369
CANNON, W. B. and ROSENBLUETH, A. (1933). *Amer. J. Physiol.* **104**, 557
CANNON, W. B. and URIDIL, J. E. (1921). *Amer. J. Physiol.* **58**, 353
*CARLSSON, A. (1959). *Pharmacol. Rev.* **11**, 300
CARLSSON, A. and HILLARP, N. Å. (1956). *Kungl. fysiogr. Sällsk Förhandl.* **26**, No. 8
CARLSSON, A., LINDQUIST, M., MAGNUSSEN, T. and WALDECK, B. (1958). *Science*, **127**, 471
CARLSSON, A., ROSENGREN, E., BERTLER, A. and NILSSON, J. (1957). In 'Psychotropic Drugs', p. 363. Ed. Garattini, S. and Chetti, V. Amsterdam: Elsevier
CARLSSON, A. and WALDECK, B. (1958). *Acta physiol. scand.* **44**, 293
CAVALLITO, C. J. (1957). Curare and Curare-like agents, p. 288. Amsterdam: Elsevier
CHANG, V. and RAND, M. J. (1960). *Brit. J. Pharmacol.* **15**, 388
CHRUSĆIEL, T. L. (1960). In Adrenergic Mechanisms, p. 539
COLES, D. R., DUFF, F., SHEPHERD, W. H. T. and WHELAN, R. F. (1956). *Brit. J. Pharmacol.* **11**, 346
CORNE, S. J. and GRAHAM, J. D. P. (1957). *J. Physiol.* **135**, 339
COUPLAND, R. E. (1958). *J. Endocrin.* **17**, 191
COUPLAND, R. E. and EXLEY, K. A. (1957). *Brit. J. Pharmacol.* **12**, 306
CRAWFÓRD, T. B. B. and OUTSCHOORN, A. S. (1950). *Brit. J. Pharmacol.* **6**, 8
DEMIS, D. J., BLASCHKO, H. and WELCH, A. D. (1955). *J. Pharmacol. exp. Ther.* **113**, 14
DEMIS, D. J., BLASCHKO, H. and WELCH, A. D. (1956). *J. Pharmacol. exp. Ther.* **117**, 208
DENGLER, H. (1957). *Arch. exp. Path. Pharmak.* **231**, 373
*DRILL, V. A. (1958). Pharmacology in Medicine. New York: McGraw Hill
EAKINS, K. E. and LOCKETT, M. F. (1961). *Brit. J. Pharmacol.* **16**, 108
EHRLÉN, I. (1948). *Farm. Revy.* **47**, 242
ELLIOTT, T. R. (1904). *J. Physiol.* **31**, Proc. XX
ELLIOTT, T. R. (1905). *J. Physiol.* **32**, 401
ELLIOTT, T. R. (1912). *J. Physiol.* **44**, 374
ELTHERINGTON, L. G. and HORITA, A. (1960). *J. Pharmacol. exp. Ther.* **128**, 7
*EMMELIN, N. (1961). *Pharmacol. Rev.* **13**, 17
ERÄNKÖ, O. (1952). *Acta anat.* **16**, suppl. 17
ERÄNKÖ, O. (1954). *Acta path. microbiol. scand.* **36**, 219
ERÄNKÖ, O. (1960). In Adrenergic Mechanisms, p. 103
ERÄNKÖ, O. and HOPSU, V. (1958). *Endocrinology*, **62**, 15
EULER, U. S. VON. (1946). *Acta physiol. scand.* **12**, 73
*EULER, U. S. VON. (1950). In 'Methods in Medical Research', in Chicago: Year Book Publishers, **3**, 116
*EULER, U. S. VON. (1951). *Pharmacol. Rev.* **3**, 247
EULER, U. S. VON. (1952). *Scand. J. clin. Lab. Invest.* **4**, 254
*EULER, U. S. VON. (1954). *Pharmacol. Rev.* **6**, 15
*EULER, U. S. VON. (1956). 'Noradrenaline'. Springfield: Thomas
EULER, U. S. VON. (1958). *Acta physiol. scand.* **43**, 155
EULER, U. S. VON. (1960a). In Adrenergic Mechanisms, p. 509
EULER, U. S. VON. (1960b). In Adrenergic Mechanisms, p. 493
EULER, U. S. VON and FLODING, I. (1955). *Acta physiol. scand.* **33**, suppl. 118, 57

EULER, U. S. VON and LISHAJKO, F. (1957). *Acta physiol. pharmacol. neerl.* **6**, 295
EULER, U. S. VON. and LISHAJKO, F. (1958). *Acta physiol. scand.* **42**, 333
EULER, U. S. VON. and PURKHOLD, H. (1951). *Acta physiol. scand.* **24**, 218
EXLEY, K. A. (1956). *J. Physiol.* **133**, 70P
EXLEY, K. A. (1957). *Brit. J. Pharmacol.* **12**, 297
EXLEY, K. A. (1960). In Adrenergic Mechanisms, p. 158
FINKLEMAN, B. (1930). *J. Physiol.* **70**, 145
FLECKENSTEIN, A. and STÖCKLE, D. (1955). *Arch. exp. Path. Pharmaka.* **224**, 401
FOLKOW, B. and EULER, U. S. VON. (1954). *Circulat. Res.* **2**, 191
FOLKOW, B. and UVNÄS, B. (1948). *Acta physiol. scand.* **15**, 365
FRÖHLICH, A. and LOEWI, O. (1910). *Arch. exp. Path. Pharmak.* **62**, 160
*FURCHGOTT, R. F. (1959). *Pharmacol. Rev.* **11**, 429
FURCHGOTT, R. F. (1960). In Adrenergic Mechanisms, p. 246
*GADDUM, J. H. (1950). In 'Methods in Medical Research'. Chicago: Year Book Publishers, **3**, 116
GADDUM, J. H. and GOODWIN, L. G. (1947). *J. Physiol.* **105**, 357
GADDUM, J. H., PEART, W. S. and VOGT, M. (1949). *J. Physiol.* **108**, 476
GARDIER, R. W., ABREU, B. E., RICHARDS, A. B. and HERRLICH, H. C. (1960). *J. Pharmacol. exp. Ther.* **130**, 340
GARDINER, J. E. (1961). *Biochem. J.* **81**, 297
GARDINER, J. E. and THOMPSON, J. W. (1961). *Nature (Lond.)*, **191**, 86
GÉRARD, P., CORDIER, R. and LISON, L. (1930). *Bull. Histol. Tech. micr.* **7**, 133
GHOSH, N. C., DEB, C. and BANERJEE, S. (1951). *J. biol. Chem.* **192**, 867
GILLESPIE, J. S. and MACKENNA, B. R. (1959). *J. Physiol.* **147**, 31P
GILLIS, C. N. and LEWIS, J. J. (1956). *J. Pharm (Lond.)*, **8**, 606
GINSBURG, J. and COBBOLD, A. F. (1960). In Adrenergic Mechanisms, p. 173
GITLOW, S. E., MENDLOWITZ, M., KHASSIS, S., COHEN, G. and SHA, J. (1960). *J. clin. Invest.* **39**, 221
GOLDENBERG, M. (1951). *Amer. J. Med.* **10**, 627
GOLDENBERG, M. APGAR, V., DETERLING, R. and PINES, K. L. (1949). *J. Amer. med. Ass.* **140**, 776
GOODALL, MC. C. (1951). *Acta physiol. scand.* **24**, suppl. 85
GOODALL, MC. C. and KIRSHNER, N. (1957). *J. biol. Chem.* **226**, 213
GOODALL, MC. C. and KIRSHNER, N. (1958). *Circulation*, **17**, 366
GOODFORD, P. J. and HERMANSEN, K. (1960). *J. Physiol.* **153**, 29P
*GOODMAN, L. S. and GILMAN, A. (1955). The Pharmacological basis of therapeutics. New York: Macmillan
GREENBERG, M. J. (1960). *Brit. J. Pharmacol.* **15**, 365
GREER, C. M., PINKSTON, J. O., BAXTER, J. H. and BRANNON, E. S. (1938). *J. Pharmacol. exp. Ther.* **62**, 189
GRIESEMER, E. C., BARSKY, J., DRAGSTEDT, C. A., WELLS, J. A. and ZELLER, E. A. (1953). *Proc. Soc. exp. Biol. (N.Y.)* **84**, 699
HAGEN, P. (1956). *J. Pharmacol. exp. Ther.* **116**, 26
HAGEN, P. and BARRNETT, R. J. (1960). In Adrenergic Mechanisms, p. 83
HENLE, J. (1865). *Z. rat. Med.* **24**, 142
HEY, P. and WILLEY, G. L. (1953). *J. Physiol.* **122**, 75P
HEY, P. and WILLEY, G. L. (1954). *Brit. J. Pharmacol.* **9**, 471
HELLMAN, K. and THOMPSON, J. W. (1961). *J. Physiol.* **159**, 11P
HILLARP, N. Å. (1958). *Acta physiol. scand.* **43**, 82
HILLARP, N. Å. (1959). *Acta physiol. scand.* **47**, 271
HILLARP, N. Å. HÖGBERG, B. and NILSON, B. (1955). *Nature (Lond.)*, **176**, 1032
HILLARP, N. Å. and HÖKFELT, B. (1954). *Endocrinology*, **55**, 255
HILLARP, N. Å., LAGERSTEDT, S. and NILSON, B. (1953). *Acta physiol scand.* **29**, 251
HILLARP, N. Å. and NILSON, B. (1953). *Kungl. fysiogr. Sällsk. Förhandl.* **23**, No. 4
HÖKFELT, B. (1951). *Acta physiol. scand.* **25**, suppl. 89, p. 41
HÖKFELT, B. and MCLEAN, J. M. (1950). *Acta physiol. scand.* **21**, 258
HOLLAND, W. C. and SCHÜMANN, H. J. (1956). *Brit. J. Pharmacol.* **11**, 449
HOLTON, P. (1949). *J. Physiol.* **108**, 525

HOLTZ, P. (1939). *Naturwissenschaften,* **27,** 724
HOLTZ, P. and BACHMANN, F. (1952). *Naturwissenschaften,* **39,** 116
HOLTZ, P., HEISE, R. and LÜDTKE, K. (1938). *Arch. exp. Path. Pharmak.* **191,** 87
HOLTZ, P. and WESTERMANN, E. (1956). *Arch. exp. Path. Pharmak.* **227,** 538
HOLTZ, P. and WESTERMANN, E. (1957). *Arch. exp. Path. Pharmak.* **231,** 311
HOLZBAUER, M. and VOGT, M. (1954). *Brit. J. Pharmacol.* **9,** 249
HOLZBAUER, M. and VOGT, M. (1956). *J. Neurochem.* **1,** 8
HORITA, A. (1958). *J. Pharmacol. exp. Ther.* **122,** 474
HUKOVIĆ, S. (1960). *Brit. J. Pharmacol.* **15,** 117
JALON, P. G. DE, BAYO, J. B. and JALON, M. G. DE. (1945). *Farmacoterap. act.* **2,** 313
JAQUES, R. (1960). Quoted by Bein, H. J., in Adrenergic Mechanisms, p. 162
KAUFMAN, S. (1959). *J. biol. Chem.* **234,** 2677
KIRSHNER, N. and GOODALL, MC. C. (1956). *Fed. Proc.* **15,** 110
KIRSHNER, N. and GOODALL, MC. C. (1957). *Fed. Proc.* **16,** 73
KOELLE, G. (1961). *Nature (Lond.),* **190,** 208
KOHN, A. (1898). *Prag. med. Wschr.* **23,** 197
KOHN, A. (1903). *Arch. mikr. anat.* **62,** 263
KRAUPP, O., STORMANN, H., BERNHEIMER, H. and OBENAUS, H. (1959). *Klin. Wschr.* 37, 76
KRONEBERG, G. and SCHÜMANN, H. J. (1959). *Experientia,* **15,** 234
LA BROSSE, E. H., AXELROD, J. and SJOERDSMA, A. (1958). *Fed. Proc.* **17,** 386
LANGEMANN, H. (1951). *Brit. J. Pharmacol.* **6,** 318
LANGLEY, J. N. (1901). *J. Physiol.* **27,** 234
LAVOLLAY, J. (1941). *C. R. Soc. Biol. (Paris),* **135,** 1193
LEEPER, L. C. and UDENFRIEND, S. (1956). *Fed. Proc.* **15,** 298
LEVER, J. D., LEWIS, P. R. and BOYD, J. D. (1959). *J. Anat. (Lond.),* **93,** 478
LEWANDOWSKY, M. (1899). *Arch. Anat. Physiol. Lpz. (Physiol. Abt.)* 360
LOCKETT, M. F. (1954). *Brit. J. Pharmacol.* **9,** 498
LOCKETT, M. F. (1957). *Brit. J. Pharmacol.* **12,** 86
LOCKETT, M. F. and EAKINS, K. E. (1960a). *J. Pharm (Lond.),* **12,** 513
LOCKETT, M. F. and EAKINS, K. E. (1960b). *J. Pharm (Lond.),* **12,** 720
LOEWI, O. (1921). *Pflüg. Archiv,* **189,** 239
LUCO, J. V. and GONI, F. (1948). *J. Neurophysiol.* **11,** 497
LUND, A. (1949a). *Acta pharm. tox. (Kbh.)* **5,** 75
LUND, A. (1949b). *Acta pharm. tox. (Kbh.)* **5,** 121
LUND, A. (1949c). *Acta pharm. tox. (Kbh.)* **5,** 137
LUNDHOLM, L. and MOHME-LUNDHOLM, E. (1960). In Adrenergic Mechanisms, p. 305
MACINTOSH, F. C., BIRKS, R. I. and SASTRY, P. B. (1956). *Nature (Lond.),* **178,** 1181
MACMILLAN, W. H. (1959). *Brit. J. Pharmacol.* **14,** 385
MANN, M. (1953). *J. Pharm (Lond.),* **5,** 1024
MANN, M. and WEST, G. B. (1951). *Brit. J. Pharmacol.* **6,** 79
MARLEY, E. and PATON, W. D. M. (1961). *J. Physiol.* **155,** 1
MASUOKA, D. T., SCHOTT, H. F., AKAWIE, R. J. and CLARK, W. G. (1956). *Proc. Soc. exp. Biol. (N.Y.)* 93, 5
MAXWELL, R. A., MULL, R. P. and PLUMMER, A. J. (1959). *Experientia,* **15,** 267
MAXWELL, R. A., PLUMMER, A. J., SCHNEIDER, F., POVALSKI, H. and DANIEL, A. I. (1960). *Schweiz. med. Wschr.* **90,** 109
MAYER, S. E. and MORAN, N. C. (1960). *J. Pharmacol. exp. Therap.* **129,** 271
MELTZER, S. J. (1904). *Amer. J. Physiol.* **11,** 37
MIRKIN, B. L. and BONNYCASTLE, D. D. (1954). *Amer. J. Physiol.* **178,** 529
MUSCHOLL, E. (1961). *Brit. J. Pharmacol.* **16,** 353
MUSCHOLL, E. and VOGT, M. (1957). *Brit. J. Pharmacol.* **12,** 532
MUSCHOLL, E. and VOGT, M. (1958). *J. Physiol.* **141,** 132
NIEBAUER, G. and WIEDMANN, A. (1958). *Acta neuroveg. (Wien)* **18,** 280
OLIVER, G. and SCHÄFER, E. A. (1895). *J. Physiol.* **18,** 230
OUTSCHOORN, A. S. (1952). *Brit. J. Pharmacol.* **7,** 616
PAASONEN, M. K. and KRAYER, O. (1957). *Fed. Proc.* **16,** 326

PATON, W. D. M. (1960). In Adrenergic Mechanisms, p. 124
PEART, W. S. (1949). *J. Physiol.* **108**, 49
*PEKKARINEN, A. (1954). *Pharmacol. Rev.* **6**, 35
PELLERIN, J. and D'IORIO, A. (1957). *Canad. J. Biochem.* **35**. 151
PLETSCHER, A., SHORE, P. A. and BRODIE, B. B. (1955). *Science*, **122**, 374
POWELL, C. E. and SLATER, I. H. (1958). *J. Pharmacol. exp. Therap.* **122**, 480
REDGATE, E. S. and GELLHORN, E. (1953). *Amer. J. Physiol.* **174**, 475
REINERT, H. (1960). In Adrenergic Mechanisms, p. 373
ROBINSON, R. RATCLIFFE, J. and SMITH, P. (1959). *J. clin. Path* **12**, 541.
*ROSENBLUETH, A. (1950). The transmission of nerve impulses at neuro-effector junctions and peripheral synapses. Massachusetts Institute of Technology, New York Technology Press, Wiley, London, Chapman & Hall, Ltd
SANDLER, M. and RUTHVEN, C. R. J. (1959a). *Lancet*, **2**, 114
SANDLER, M. and RUTHVEN, C. R. J. (1959b). *Lancet*, **2**, 1034
SANDLER, M. and RUTHVEN, C. R. J. (1960). In Adrenergic Mechanisms, p. 40
SCHILD, H. O. (1960). In Adrenergic Mechanisms, p. 288
SCHÜMANN, H. J. (1956). *Arch. exp. Path. Pharmak.* **235**, 1
SCHÜMANN, H. J. (1958). *Arch. exp. Path. Pharmak.* **234**, 17
SCHÜMANN, H. J. (1959). *Arch. exp. Path. Pharmak.* **236**, 474
SCHÜMANN, H. J. (1960). In Adrenergic Mechanisms, p. 6
SHEPPARD, D. M. and WEST, G. B. (1953). *J. Physiol.* **120**, 15
SHEPPARD, H. and ZIMMERMANN, J. (1959). *Pharmacologist*, **1**, 69
SHEPPARD, H. and ZIMMERMANN, J. (1960). Quoted by Bein, H. J., in Adrenergic Mechanisms, p. 162
SHIPLEY, R. E. and TILDEN, J. H. (1947). *Proc. Soc. exp. Biol. N.Y.* **64**, 453
SHORE, P. A., SILVER, S. L. and BRODIE, B. B. (1955). *Science*, **122**, 284
STEHLE, R. L. and ELLSWORTH, H. C. (1937). *J. Pharmacol. exp. Therap.* **59**, 114
SUTHERLAND, E. W. (1960). In Adrenergic Mechanisms, p. 500
SUTHERLAND, E. W. and RALL, T. W. (1960). In Adrenergic Mechanisms, p. 295
*Symposium on Catecholamines (1959). *Pharmacol. Rev.* **11**, 241–300
TAINTER, M. L. and CHANG, D. K. (1927). *J. Pharmacol. exp. Ther.* **30**, 193
TAKAMINE, J. (1901). *Therap. Gaz.* **27**, 221
THOMPSON, J. W. (1960). *Ph. D. thesis*, University of London
TRENDELENBURG, U. (1959). *J. Pharmacol. exp. Ther.* **125**, 55
UDENFRIEND, S. and WYNGAARDEN, I. B. (1956). *Biochim. biophys. Acta*, **20**, 48
VANE, J. R. (1958). *J. Physiol.* **143**, 75P
VANE, J. R. (1959). *Brit. J. Pharmacol.* **14**, 87
VANE, J. R. (1960). In Adrenergic Mechanisms, p. 356
*VELDSTRA, H. (1956). *Pharmacol. Rev.* **8**, 339
VOGT, M. (1952). *Brit. J. Pharmacol.* **7**, 325
VOGT, M. (1954). *J. Physiol.* **123**, 451
WEIL-MALHERBE, H. (1960). In Adrenergic Mechanisms, p. 544
WEIL-MALHERBE, H. and BONE, A. D. (1952). *Biochem. J.* **51**, 311
WEST, G. B. (1960). In Adrenergic Mechanisms, p. 524
WESTERMANN, E. (1957). *Biochem. Z.* **328**, 405
WESTERMANN, E., BALZER, H. and KNELL, J. (1958). *Arch. exp. Path. Pharmak.* **234**, 194
WHITEHORN, J. C. (1935). *J. biol. Chem.* **108**, 633
WHITTAKER, V. P. (1959). *Biochem. J.* **73**, 37P
WILLEY, G. L. (1957). *Brit. J. Pharmacol.* **12**, 128
YOUNG, I. M. (1957). *J. Physiol.* **137**, 374

CHAPTER 4

5-HYDROXYTRYPTAMINE

(Serotonin, Enteramine)

The recent history of 5-hydroxytryptamine (5-HT) starts with the chemical identification of it in serum by Rapport in 1949. This was quickly followed by proof that enteramine, found by Erspamer in the alimentary tract of a great variety of vertebrates and invertebrates, is 5-hydroxytryptamine (Erspamer and Asero, 1952). Once the pure substance became available knowledge of its distribution and actions went ahead rapidly. No attempt will be made here to review the early history of our knowledge of this substance; an account of that will be found in the last edition of this book or, in more detail, in the reviews by Erspamer (1954) and Page (1954) and in the Symposium edited by Lewis (1958). Interest in 5-HT was very much stimulated by the discovery in 1953 of large amounts in the brain. This aspect is dealt with below but the reader is also referred to Chapter 1 (p. 10) where it is discussed in relation to other pharmacologically active substances in the brain.

IDENTIFICATION AND ESTIMATION

Knowledge of the normal and abnormal physiology of 5-HT has been much facilitated by the development of reliable methods of estimation. Early work depended mainly on bioassay but a sensitive and reliable fluorimetric method which enables large numbers of estimations to be carried through with considerable accuracy in a short time has now been developed and is more convenient. For the estimation of very small quantities however one of the very sensitive biological methods is still necessary.

BIOLOGICAL METHODS

Usually the tissue is extracted with acetone and the clear solution containing 5-HT separated by filtration or centrifugation and evaporated to dryness *in vacuo* at a temperature below 35° C. With high concentrations of acetone, polypeptides like oxytocin, vasopressin, bradykinin and substance P, which contract plain muscle, are not extracted. The following isolated organs are suitable for the assay:

(i) *Rat uterus* (Erspamer, 1953; Gaddum, 1953) or *rat colon* (Dalgleish *et al.*, 1953). The uterus is much more sensitive during oestrus than at other stages in the cycle and either a rat in oestrus, selected by vaginal smear, or one which has received an injection of an oestrogen

18 hours previously, is used. Neither of these preparations is sensitive to histamine and atropinization prevents interference by acetylcholine. Sensitivity: 4 to 10 ng./ml.

(ii) *Rat stomach* (Vane, 1957). This preparation is also insensitive to histamine and response to acetylcholine is abolished by hyoscine. Sensitivity: <1 ng./ml.

(iii) *Venus mercenaria heart* (Twarog and Page, 1953) or *Spisula solida heart* (Gaddum and Paasonen, 1955). The amplitude of the heart beat of these molluscs is increased by 5-HT whereas they are insensitive to adrenaline, histamine, substance P and adenosine compounds. The action of acetylcholine can be blocked by benzoquinonium. Sensitivity: 1 ng./ml.

PHOTOMETRIC AND FLUOROMETRIC METHODS (Udenfriend *et al.*, 1955a and *b*; Kuntzman *et al.*, 1961)

5-HT is extracted into n-butanol from a salt-saturated solution buffered to pH 10, and after washing with buffer at this pH, re-extracted into 3N HCl by the addition of heptane to the butanol solution. This procedure removes other indoles including tryptophan, 5-hydroxytryptophan and 5-hydroxyindoleacetic acid. The extracted 5-HT is then estimated either photometrically or fluorimetrically.

(i) *Photometric estimation.* 5-HT forms a chromophore with 1-nitroso-2-naphthol. At least 10 µg. 5-HT contained in 2 ml. extract is needed.

(ii) *Fluorimetric estimation.* In strong acid solution 5-HT, when activated by ultraviolet light, fluoresces with a yellow light. About 50 ng./ml. extract is needed for estimation; smaller amounts can be detected.

PAPER CHROMATOGRAPHY

The chromatographic separation and identification of indoles has been much developed in recent years. An account is given by Jepson (1958). The least amount of 5-HT for identification by staining on a paper chromatogram is about 0·5 µg.

DISTRIBUTION IN MAMMALS

The largest quantities of 5-HT are found in the *gastrointestinal tract* where it is confined to the mucosa. It is contained in the enterochromaffin cells which are pyramidal cells squeezed in between the cells of the mucosa with their bases on the basement membrane. They are distributed throughout the stomach and small and large intestine and have also been described in other organs (Feyerter, 1953), but whether or not they all contain 5-HT is not known. In the alimentary canal the largest amounts of 5-HT are found in the pyloric part of the stomach and the upper part of the small intestine (Feldberg and Toh, 1953), and the least in the colon. From the mucosa it is able to escape into the lumen of the intestine (Bülbring and Lin, 1958) and probably also into the blood stream (Erspamer and Testini, 1959).

There is evidence that the amount stored in the intestine is modified by changes in the intestinal flora. It has been found (Sullivan, 1960, 1961) that rats fed on a meat diet have larger amounts of 5-HT in the wall of the small intestine than rats fed on a mixed diet; and in these circumstances there is also an increase in intestinal aerobic bacteria. Further, the addition of certain antibiotics to the diet of mice and rats also increases the amount of 5-HT in the intestinal wall. Neither diet nor antibiotics, however, change the amount in the brain.

In the blood, 5-HT is contained in *platelets*; virtually none is found in platelet-free plasma if this has been prepared in such a way as to avoid platelet damage. Inappreciable amounts are found in leucocytes and none can be extracted from red cells. The reason for the large amount in platelets becomes clear when platelets are incubated with 5-HT; there is a rapid absorption and in 90 minutes human platelets become nearly saturated and then contain about 5 times as much as they did originally (Humphrey and Jaques, 1954; Hardisty and Stacey, 1955). The concentration in the platelets may be as much as 1000 times that in the surrounding liquid (Born and Gillson, 1959) and uptake is most rapid at body temperature. Cooling to $20°$ C. halts the uptake which can also be depressed by a rise in the pH of the suspending solution and by a number of drugs in low concentration (Stacey, 1961). Born, Ingram and Stacey (1958) found that the amount of 5-HT which platelets from different individuals contained when they are saturated varied with the amount of adenosine triphosphate (ATP) in them and suggested that it is bound to ATP, as catechol amines are bound in the suprarenal medulla, and Baker *et al.* (1959) have obtained further evidence of this by finding that when homogenized platelets are centrifuged, 5-HT and ATP separate in the same dense layer. Binding of 5-HT within platelets does not, of course, exclude the possibility of an active transport mechanism (Hughes and Brodie, 1959) on the surface of platelets and recent evidence on the competitive antagonism of tryptamine to the uptake of 5-HT tends to confirm the existence of such a mechanism (Stacey, 1961).

The amounts of 5-HT in platelets of different species varies enormously. In man 10^8 platelets, occupying a volume of about $1·3$ mm.[3] contain about 60 ng. 5-HT while in the same number of rabbit platelets, which are slightly smaller, there is about 15 times as much. Considerable amounts are also to be found in the *spleen*, and when the amounts in platelets and spleen of different species are compared the correspondence makes it seem likely that 5-HT in the spleen is derived from platelets. This is in agreement with the finding that the spleen is unable to make 5-HT from its precursor 5-hydroxytryptophan (v. *infra*).

In 1953 Twarog and Page found 5-HT in the *nervous system* and Amin, Crawford and Gaddum (1954) described its distribution. They noticed that it was contained in grey matter and not in medullated fibres and that its distribution corresponded closely with the distribution of noradrenaline. The cerebral cortex, cerebellum, spinal cord, dorsal and ventral roots and sympathetic ganglia contained little or none. The highest concentrations were found in certain subcortical nuclei and in the area postrema, a chemoreceptor area associated with the vomiting centre lying in the wall of the fourth ventricle. Recently Giarman and Friedman (1960) have found large amounts in the pineal gland of man, monkeys and ox; in fact the concentrations reported in some human and simian pineal glands are the highest found in any neural tissue. This is referred to below in the section on melatonin (p. 146). A more detailed account of 5-HT in the central nervous system is contained in Chapter 1 (p. 13) and the distribution of it and of enzymes synthesizing and inactivating it is given in Table 1 (p. 2).

The only other considerable source of 5-HT in mammals is in the *mast cells* of rats and mice (Benditt *et al.*, 1955; Parratt and West, 1957), and it is the mast cells which give the skin of these animals their high 5-HT content. The mast cells of man, cat, dog, rabbit, guinea pig and cow contain little or none.

Walaszek and Abood (1957) and Baker (1958, 1959) have investigated the *intracellular localization* of 5-HT in brain and intestine respectively. In both sites it was found to be largely contained in granules which sedimented with mitochondria in centrifuged homogenates but which could be shown to be heavier than mitochondria by means of a density gradient (p. 6) and to resemble in density the granules carrying histamine in mast cells and catechol amines in the adrenal medulla (p. 102). In the adrenal medulla and intestine, amines are associated with adenosine triphosphate (Prusoff, 1960) and it is possible that in both situations adenosine triphosphate is in ionic combination with stored amines.

The significance to be attached to the finding of a large or small amount of an amine stored in a certain situation is questionable. A small amount might indicate that it plays no important part in the tissue or that utilization and destruction is keeping pace with synthesis. The presence of an enzyme synthesizing the amine is probably a better guide to its functional importance in the area. The distribution of 5-HTP decarboxylase, the enzyme synthesizing 5-HT, is discussed in the next section.

SYNTHESIS AND METABOLISM

The biological synthesis of 5-HT has been worked out largely by Udenfriend (1957) and his colleagues and its course is indicated in the first part of Fig. 13. Synthesis starts from tryptophan but little is known of the sites at which this substance is hydroxylated to 5-hydroxytrypto-phan (5-HTP). Cooper and Melcer (1961) have synthesized 5-HTP from typtophan *in vitro* using homogenates of guinea pig intestinal mucosa in the presence of ascorbic acid and Cu^{++}. The activity was contained in

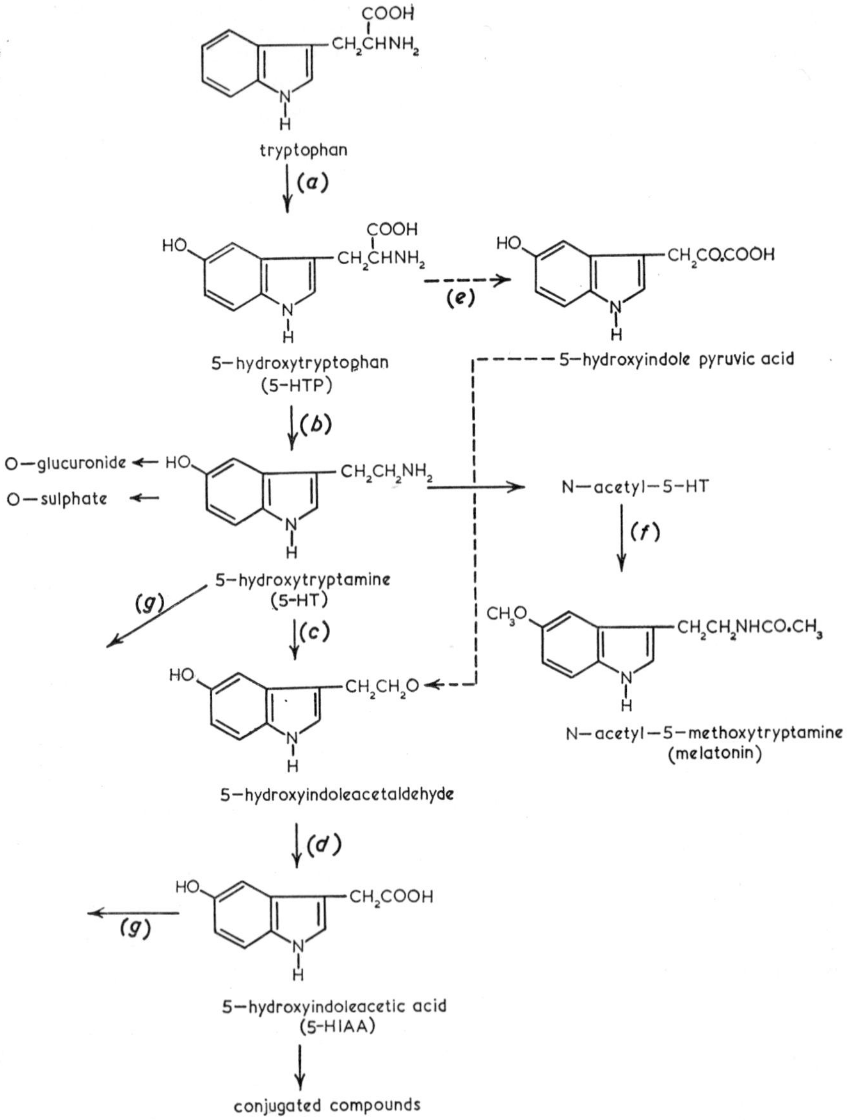

FIG. 13. Main pathways in the biosynthesis and metabolism of 5-hydroxytryptamine.
(a) *tryptophan hydroxylase*   (e) *amino-acid oxidase*
(b) *5-HTP decarboxylase*   (f) *indole O-methyl transferase*
(c) *amine oxidase*   (g) *coeruloplasmin*
(d) *aldehyde dehydrogenase*

particulate fractions of the cells and the soluble fraction contained an inhibitor. No activity could be detected in large intestine, liver, spleen or brain. There is good evidence that tryptophan is used *in vivo* in the synthesis of hydroxyindoles, for a patient with a malignant carcinoid tumour. when given ¹⁴C labelled tryptophan excreted ¹⁴C labelled 5-hydroxyindoles in his urine, and Eber and Lembeck (1957) and Zbinden and Pletscher (1958) found that the hydroxyindole metabolism of rats was depressed when they were on a low tryptophan diet. An active tryptophan hydroxylase has also been prepared from bacteria.

Table 8

5-hydroxytryptamine (μg./g. tissue) naturally present, and formed from added substrate

	Present		Formed	
	Guinea Pig	Rabbit	Guinea Pig	Rabbit
Kidney	—	0·03	200	45
Liver	—	0·4	25	15
Stomach	1·40	4·9	33	—
Spleen	1·06	19·6	3·3	4·65
Platelets	—	1·4	—	0
Bone marrow	—	0·33	0	0·65
Area postrema	0·21 (dog)		0 (ox)	
Sympathetic ganglia	0 (dog)		16·6 (dog)	

(Gaddum and Giarman, 1956)

The decarboxylating enzyme responsible for the formation of 5-HT from 5-HTP is widely distributed and its activity in many tissues is high. Since tryptophan hydroxylase cannot be found in many of them it must be presumed that supplies of 5-HTP come from the small intestine via the blood stream though none has been detected in the blood. The decarboxylation reaction must go on more rapidly than the preceding step for whereas tryptophan is found in the tissues, 5-HTP is not; presumably it is decarboxylated as fast as it is formed. For this, as for other decarboxylations, pyridoxal-5-phosphate is the co-enzyme and in pyridoxal deficiency 5-HT synthesis and its concentration in the brain and other tissues is depressed. The decarboxylase activity of various tissues is shown in Table 8. In general there is a similarity in the distribution of 5-HT and the enzyme which synthesizes it, but there are notable exceptions to this rule and the amounts of the two do not always run parallel. In the nervous system the area postrema contains much 5-HT and no decarboxylase, and sympathetic ganglia contain much decarboxylase and little 5-HT. Outside the nervous system only the intestine and kidney contain large amounts of decarboxylase, while the stomach and liver contain smaller amounts. Bone marrow and platelets have none; platelets, like the area postrema, must therefore acquire 5-HT ready made and we have already seen that they have a special mechanism for this. The mast cells of rats and mice, which store 5-HT, are able to synthesize it (Schindler *et al.*, 1959) but are unable to destroy it. There is now evidence (Wilson and Brodie, 1961) that the area postrema shares with the pineal gland and the pituitary an ability to absorb amines from the blood which the rest of the nervous system does not possess. Elsewhere the blood brain barrier prevents the brain from acquiring 5-HT from the blood (Bhargava and Borison, 1955) although it is permeable to 5-HTP. It is therefore probable that the 5-HT in the brain is synthesized by it.

A number of inhibitors of 5-HTP decarboxylase are known and the subject has been reviewed by Clark (1959). The most active inhibitors so far found are certain chalcones (Yuwiler *et al.*, 1959) and a group of phenylalanine derivatives investigated *in vitro* by Sourkes (1954). Smith (1960) has shown that the subcutaneous injection of mice with α-methyldihydroxyphenylalanine (α-methyldopa) depresses the concentration of 5-HT in brain and intestine, and causes sedation. In man α-methyldopa will reduce 5-HT synthesis in patients with the malignant carcinoid syndrome and lower the blood pressure of patients with hypertension (p. 316). The pharmacological effects of decarboxylase inhibitors cannot yet be interpreted with certainty as a number of other reactions may also be affected. Thus it is probable that tryptophan-, 5-HTP- and dopadecarboxylase are identical and the synthesis of tryptamine and of dopamine, the precursor of noradrenaline, is therefore likely to be affected by them. Further, histamine, tyramine and gamma-amino-butyric acid, to mention only four substances having powerful pharmacological actions, are also formed by decarboxylation.

5-HT is easily oxidized, first by amine oxidase to the aldehyde and then by aldehyde dehydrogenase to 5-hydroxyindoleacetic acid (5-HIAA) which is excreted in the urine. In man this substance accounts for about 30% of an injected dose of 5-HT. The other principal metabolite is N-acetyl-5-HT (McIsaac and Page, 1959) which may account for up to 25%. In addition small amounts of O-glucuronide (Weissbach *et al.*, 1961) and O-sulphate are excreted and traces of unchanged 5-HT (in man about 50 μg. 5-HT per day). The kidney contains much amine oxidase and this, no doubt, prevents more 5-HT reaching the urine. In the rabbit nearly all 5-HIAA formed is conjugated with glycine and excreted as 5-hydroxyindoleaceturic acid but this does not occur to any great extent in man. It is also known that 5-HT and 5-HIAA are oxidized by the coeruloplasmin of mammalian serum and the biological significance of this is discussed by Blaschko and Levine (1960).

The metabolism of 5-HT is complex and in spite of great advances in the last few years there is still a considerable fraction unaccounted for and it is important that this should be remembered when metabolic studies are interpreted.

The administration of amine oxidase inhibitors such as iproniazid, leads in some species to the accumulation of 5-HT, and to a lesser degree, of noradrenaline in the tissues where they are stored (Spector *et al.*, 1960), see Fig. 3 (p. 19). However, the interpretation of the pharmacological effects observed is complicated because there are several other naturally occurring amines (e.g. dopamine and tyramine), also oxidized by amine oxidase, and the concentration of these substances may also be affected. Other amine oxidase inhibitors which have been of value in investigations of this kind are β-phenylisopropylhydrazine and the harmala alkaloids but many others have been produced as a result of the discovery of their value in psychiatric treatment (see Chapter 1, p. 18 and Chapter 2, p. 57).

RATE OF TURNOVER OF 5-HT

By using ^{14}C labelled tryptophan and 5-HTP, Udenfriend and Weissbach (1958) have estimated the half life of 5-HT in platelets, spleen, stomach and intestine of rabbits. For platelets and spleen this was 33 hours, a figure which is similar to that obtained for the half life of platelets. This implies that 5-HT absorbed into a platelet remains there as long as the platelet circulates and is not exchanged or released. In the stomach and intestine the half life was 10 and 17 hours respectively. Because of the small amount of 5-HT contained in the brain compared with that in the blood in the brain, this method could not be used to estimate the half life of brain 5-HT. However by determining the rate of increase of brain 5-HT after administration of the quick-acting amine oxidase inhibitor harmaline, it was estimated that the half life must be a matter of minutes. If these estimations are confirmed they would show that the rate of synthesis of 5-HT is of the same order in the gastrointestinal tract as the brain of rabbits, even though the former tissue contains 25 to 50 times as much 5-HT as the latter.

PHARMACOLOGICAL ACTIONS

CARDIOVASCULAR SYSTEM

The changes in the circulation following the intravenous injection of 5-HT into experimental animals are complex and have only been incompletely analysed. Both a rise and a fall in blood pressure may be seen in the same animal and there are marked species differences in the responses. The subject has been reviewed in detail by Page (1957, 1958).

In dogs and rats three phases in the blood pressure response may be seen: a *transient fall* in pressure, accompanied by cardiac slowing, followed by a *small rise*, followed by a *prolonged fall*. The relative size and duration of these changes varies considerably from animal to animal, with the dose injected and with the initial blood pressure. Small doses and high pressures favour depressor effects and large doses and low pressures favour pressor effects (Outschoorn and Jacob, 1960). In cats and rabbits depressor effects predominate. The following factors appear to be concerned in these changes:

(i) *The initial transient fall in blood pressure and bradycardia.* This can, to a large extent, be eliminated by vagotomy or by the administration of atropine and appears to be due to a von Bezold-like reflex. A fall in blood pressure and bradycardia also follows the infusion of 5-HT into a coronary artery (Dawes and Comroe, 1954) and this is abolished by cooling the vagi (Kottegoda and Mott, 1955). In cats this chemoreflex response is like that caused by the injection of phenyldiguanide and both responses are reversibly inhibited by 2-naphthylguanidine (Fastier *et al.*, 1959).

(ii) *The small rise in pressure* is probably due to increased cardiac output and peripheral vasoconstriction. In dogs MacCannon and Horvath (1954) found that after the injection of 5-HT there was an increase in both pulmonary and systemic vascular resistances and this was followed by a rise in cardiac output.

(iii) *The prolonged fall in pressure* was attributed by Page and McCubbin (1956) to peripheral inhibition of neurogenic vasoconstriction because they found that in dogs it was eliminated by ganglion blocking drugs and by pithing. The site in the nervous system of this inhibition is not known. Ganglionic blockade seems unlikely, in view of Trendelenburg's (1957) observation that 5-HT increased the contraction of the nictitating membrane of the cat, in response to submaximal preganglionic stimulation, by facilitating transmission at the ganglion (see p. 135).

Infusion of 5-HT intra-arterially also causes very varied results. On the *pulmonary vessels* it is powerfully constrictor in the cat, dog and man; according to Ginzel and Kottegoda (1953) in the cat and dog it is more active than adrenaline and noradrenaline. It also reduces the blood flow through the *rabbit ear* and this has been used as a method of assay. Perfusion of the human *placenta* at constant minute volume inflow with added 5-HT causes an increase in perfusion pressure (Åström and Samelius, 1957). On the other hand infusion into the dog *fore limb* leads to the dilatation of small vessels and large arteries. The action on renal vessels is discussed below.

Le Messurier *et al.* (1959) found that in *man* intravenous infusions of 1 to 3 mg. 5-HT creatinine sulphate (0·4 to 1·3 mg. base) per minute caused sometimes a fall, sometimes a rise in arterial pressure but always an increase in pulse rate and an increase in forearm flow. This is in agreement with Page (1957) who found that cardiac output was doubled and peripheral resistance halved after a large infusion. Intravenous infusions also cause intense venous constriction, which may be very painful and may obstruct the infusion, and a flush. A flush in the hand was seen by Roddie *et al.* (1955) during infusion into the brachial artery. For the first 2 minutes the hand was bright red and there was a transient increase in blood flow through the limb but subsequently the limb became dusky blue and at the end of 10 minutes the fingers were deeply cyanosed. In some subjects small petechial haemorrhages appeared. The main effect on blood flow under these conditions was a decrease, but the volume of the limb increased. These changes might be due to constriction on the venous side of the capillaries but of this there is at present no proof. The human umbilical vein contracts to concentrations of 0·1 µg./ml. (Panigel and Mayer, 1959).

Feldberg and Smith (1953) have shown that 5-HT releases histamine from cat skin and this raises the question as to how much the vascular effects seen may be secondary to this. However, 5-HT is not a very powerful histamine releaser and rather high doses are needed.

RESPIRATORY SYSTEM

During intravenous infusion, hyperpnoeic and apnoeic responses may both be seen. The hyperpnoeic response with moderate doses is lost on section of the carotid sinus nerve and is due to stimulation of chemo-receptors. In this 5-HT resembles acetylcholine, nicotine and lobeline but differs from these substances in that the action is unaffected by hexamethonium (Ginzel and Kottegoda, 1954). Very large doses stimu-late respiration by a central action (McCubbin *et al.*, 1956).

The cause of the apnoeic responses has been less thoroughly investi-gated. According to Mott and Paintal (1953) stimulation of receptors between the great veins and the left atrium is partly responsible for the apnoea but a central action has also been suggested (Ginzel, 1957).

5-hydroxytryptamine is a powerful bronchoconstrictor. This has been shown by a number of authors in a variety of animals to be a direct action on the bronchial muscle. References are given by Konzett (1956) who found in cats that lysergic acid diethylamide and its 2-bromo-derivative specifically antagonize this action; atropine and antihista-mines have a much weaker action. Herxheimer (1955) showed that when guinea-pigs inhaled a 5-HT aerosol they developed a syndrome similar to that caused by anaphylaxis and by inhalation of histamine and acetylcholine aerosols, but unlike histamine it was rarely fatal. This he thought to be due to the development of tachyphylaxis.

KIDNEY

The antidiuretic action of 5-HT, first described by Erspamer (1953), has been confirmed by a number of observations on dog, rat and man. The mechanism by which it is brought about, however, is still a subject of dispute as is also Erspamer's suggestion that 5-HT is a true renal hormone. Abrahams and Pickford (1956) found that the injection of 10 to 20 μg./kg. into the cubital vein of conscious dogs caused anti-diuresis only on those occasions when the injection was followed by panting and a rise in aortic pressure. Antidiuresis was associated with a fall in both renal plasma flow and glomerular filtration rate, and they concluded that it was mainly caused by reflexes from receptors in the thorax. Spinazzola and Sherrod (1957), also using unaesthetized dogs, found that an infusion of 10 to 20 μg./kg./min. had an antidiuretic action and that this was accompanied by an increased renal plasma flow, an increase in the ratio of the concentration of inulin in the urine to that in the plasma and a decrease in the ratio of urine volume to inulin clearance. At the lower doses there was no decrease in glomerular filtration rate and they concluded that at this dose level 5-HT enhanced tubular reabsorption of water. Only at the higher doses was there a reduction in glomerular filtration rate, which might in part explain the greater antidiuretic effect of these doses.

Rats are more sensitive to the antidiuretic action of 5-HT and Del Greco, Masson and Corcoran (1956) found that 5 μg./kg./min. was effective and that the action was dependent on reduced glomerular filtration. A similar association of reduced glomerular filtration and anti-diuresis was found by Schneckloth et al. (1957) who infused 5-HT into normal human subjects.

Large and repeated injections of 5-HT into rats cause necrosis of the cortex of the kidney (Hedinger and Langemann, 1955; Page and Glendening, 1955) and the latter authors have suggested that the renal changes in women who have died more than 24 hours after premature separation of the placenta may be due to the liberation of 5-HT from platelets as a result of blood clotting.

PLAIN MUSCLE

Mammalian plain muscle in the alimentary tract, uterus, urinary bladder and ureters (Abrahams and Pickford, 1956), bronchial tract, pupil and nictitating membrane (Reid and Rand, 1952) is contracted by 5-HT and Evans and Schild (1953) have shown that it elicits powerful rhythmical contractions of the amniotic membrane of the 10 to 12 day incubated chick. This membrane is free from all nerve cells and fibres and contraction indicates that 5-HT has a direct effect on plain muscle. The bronchoconstrictor action has been discussed above in the section on respiration, the actions on the alimentary tract and uterus are discussed below.

ALIMENTARY TRACT

Doses of 10 to 100 ng. 5-HT/ml. cause a contraction of the longitu-dinal muscle of isolated segments of guniea-pig ileum. When larger doses are left in the bath the contraction gradually diminishes and the intestine is then found to be insensitive to further doses and to tryptamine but to have retained its sensitivity to acetylcholine, histamine and substance P. From this Gaddum (1953) concluded that there must be specific receptors for tryptamine compounds. Atropine and lysergic acid diethylamide both antagonize the action of 5-HT on the intestine but antagonism is incomplete even with large doses and increasing the dose finally fails to cause further antagonism. By the simultaneous application in pairs of drugs having an antagonistic action, Gaddum and Picarelli (1957) obtained results which could be explained if there are two kinds of receptors in intestine: D-receptors, blocked by phenoxybenzamine (dibenzyline) and lysergic acid diethylamide (LSD), and M-receptors, blocked by morphine, atropine and cocaine. D-receptors are blocked by drugs which are thought to have an effect on plain muscle and are therefore probably in the muscle itself. M-receptors are blocked by drugs which probably act on nervous tissue though the precise site of their action is unknown. Since phenoxybenzamine and LSD also block the action of 5-HT on the uterus and rabbit ear, the receptors in these organs are also classified as D-receptors.

The effect of 5-HT on the peristaltic activity of isolated loops of guinea-pig intestine has been investigated by Bülbring and Lin (1958). They devised a modification of Trendelenburg's preparation in which fluid ran at a constant rate into the proximal end of a horizontally placed piece of guinea-pig intestine immersed in Ringer in an organ bath and was collected as it was expelled from the distal end under the influence of peristalsis. They were able to record the intra-luminal pressure at which the reflex was elicited together with the rate of fluid transport. When 5-HT was added to the fluid traversing the lumen of the gut it stimulated peristalsis, lowered the threshold of pressure eliciting the reflex, increased the frequency of the contractions and increased the rate of transport of fluid. A similar result was obtained when 5-HTP was perfused through the lumen of the gut, and the addition of pyridoxal, the co-enzyme for decarboxylation, enhanced the effect of 5-HTP. These and the other observations led them to the conclusion that pressure receptors in the mucosa were responsible for the initiation of the peristaltic reflex and that these were sensitized by 5-HT. When 5-HT was added to the bath, so that it came in contact with the serosal surface of the gut, there was a transitory stimulation followed by paralysis of the reflex. After further analysis with the help of blocking agents, Bülbring and Crema (1958) concluded that 5-HT not only sensitizes pressure receptors but also sensitizes the muscles and ganglia to the transmitter acetylcholine, and that it is this action which is responsible for the transitory stimulation seen when it is applied to the outside of the intestine. Larger amounts lead to ganglionic block and paralysis.

Bülbring and Crema (1959) then did similar experiments on the intestine of an anaesthetized guinea-pig in which the circulation of the loop of intestine was still intact. They found that in this preparation the infusion of 5-HT into the lumen did not stimulate peristalsis but that the intra-arterial infusion of small quantities caused vigorous peristalsis at a lower intra-luminal pressure than previously. 5-HTP on the other hand was effective by both routes and caused an increased storage of 5-HT in the intestine. It appeared that *in vivo*, mechanisms for the removal of 5-HT prevented a suitable concentration being reached at the sensory receptors when it was given intra-luminally. Only when there was rapid synthesis from the precursor could the stimulant effect be obtained.

Evidence that 5-HT plays a normal physiological role in peristalsis was obtained when Bülbring and her co-workers found that 5-HT is released from the intestinal wall into the lumen of the gut, and that this release was related to the intra-luminal pressure both in the isolated intestine and in the living animal. During a burst of peristaltic activity, release was greater than during periods of quiescence. Using large intestine Lee (1960) has carried out experiments similar to those of Bülbring and concluded that 5-HT has here a similar effect on peristalsis and that it is released by distension but not by stimulation of extrinsic nerves.

The infusion of 5-HT or its precursor 5-HTP intravenously in man gives rise to intestinal colic and evacuation of the bowels. Colic and watery diarrhoea are present in nearly 90% of patients with malignant argentaffinomas. When all these points are taken together, although there is no proof that 5-HT plays an important part in normal peristalsis, there is strong circumstantial evidence that this is so.

The infusion of 5-HT into dogs has been found to increase mucus secretion. If given concurrently with an infusion of histamine, the volume and the acidity of the juice secreted in response to the histamine is reduced but this reduction does not occur after bilateral cervical vagotomy (Black *et al.*, 1958). In rats, very large doses of 5-HT cause haemorrhagic erosions of the glandular part of the gastric mucosa.

UTERUS

The isolated rat uterus contracts to 5-HT. Its sensitivity is greatest during oestrus and declines during dioestrus and after ovariectomy, but sensitivity is restored to the maximum 24 hours after the injection of oestradiol (Robson *et al.*, 1954). Human uterus *in vitro* is also stimulated by 5-HT (Garrett, 1958). Abrahams and Pickford (1956) found that the infusion of 1 µg. or more per kg. intravenously into conscious or anaesthetized dogs elicited uterine contractions but attempts to elicit contractions in the human uterus by intravenous infusion have met with little success. Probably the concentration in the blood reaching the uterus is too low because of rapid elimination. Poulson *et al.* (1960) gave large doses subcutaneously to mice in all stages of pregnancy. The pregnancies were interrupted and there were marked placental haemorrhages leading to death of the foetus (p. 287).

AUTONOMIC GANGLIA

Injection of 5-HT into the blood supply of the superior cervical ganglion of the cat augments both the response in the nictitating membrane and the action potentials in the postganglionic nerve, caused by stimulation of the preganglionic nerve by submaximal shocks. Histamine and pilocarpine have a similar effect in facilitating transmission through the ganglion, and the actions of all three are antagonized by small doses of morphine (Trendelenburg, 1957). The site of action is probably the ganglion cell and the receptors on it would thus appear to resemble the M-receptors of Gaddum and Picarelli (see p. 133). Transmission through the stellate ganglion of the rat is also facilitated by 5-HT (Hertzler, 1961).

CENTRAL NERVOUS SYSTEM

The effects of 5-HT on the brain are discussed on p. 17. They cannot easily be assessed by injection by the subcutaneous or intravenous routes because the amine passes the blood brain barrier with difficulty and the large doses needed produce powerful cardiovascular effects. Doses of 20 mg./kg. intraperitoneally have a sedative effect on mice and Feldberg and Sherwood (1954) found a somewhat similar effect in cats when the injection was made into a lateral cerebral ventricle through a cannula implanted in the skull. The animal became quiescent but appeared to be catatonic rather than drowsy for when put in an unnatural position it tended to remain in it rather than adopt a more normal one.

OTHER ACTIONS

Large doses of 5-HT have been shown by Steiner *et al.* (1957) to cause a thrombocytosis and Langendorff and Melching (1959) have found that a single dose of 20 mg./kg. will protect mice against whole body irradiation with X-rays.

INJECTION OF 5-HT IN MAN

The effect on the circulation has been described above (p. 130). Human subjects who have had 1 to 2 mg. intravenously have experienced nausea and dizziness, feelings of tightness across the chest with difficulty in breathing, a desire to empty the bowels and bladder and intestinal colic. Intravenous infusions of 1 to 3 mg./min. cause marked hyperpnoea; tidal air is always increased, respiratory rate sometimes (Parks *et al.*, 1960). These effects are of short duration (Spies and Stone, 1952; Page, 1954). Intradermal injections are painful and Armstrong, Dry and Keele (1953) have shown that when tested on the exposed base of a human skin blister, pain is caused by concentrations as low as 10^{-6} to 10^{-7}M. 5-hydroxytryptamine was much more potent in this respect than other tryptamine derivatives tested and than acetylcholine and histamine.

PHARMACOLOGICAL ACTIONS OF 5-HYDROXYTRYPTOPHAN

When 5-HTP is injected into dogs there is a rise in the amount of 5-HT in brain, liver, heart and blood. This is accompanied by tremors, ataxia, dilatation of the pupil, loss of light reflex, lachrymation, salivation, tachycardia and hyperpnoea. Small doses decrease activity while larger doses cause excitement and disorientation (Bogdanski *et al.*, 1958). These effects are due to its penetration into tissues and the formation of 5-HT from it. Both tissue concentrations of 5-HT and actions are accentuated by pretreatment with iproniazid which delays destruction of the 5-HT formed. In man the predominant effect of 5-HTP administration is stimulation of the gastrointestinal tract, and this prevents the giving of doses sufficiently large to cause central effects (Davidson *et al.*, 1957).

5-HYDROXYTRYPTAMINE IN DISEASE

Changes in hydroxyindole metabolism or in the concentration of 5-HT in the blood have been found in the malignant carcinoid syndrome, in some forms of mental deficiency and in some blood diseases.

MALIGNANT CARCINOID SYNDROME

Carcinoid tumours may develop anywhere along the gastrointestinal tract or in the appendages. Primary tumours are most common in the appendix and in the small and large intestine but also occur in the stomach and gall bladder and have been described recently in the bronchial tree (for refs. see Annotation, 1960). Their origin from argentaffin cells was first described by Gosset and Masson (1914). At first they were thought to be benign tumours but it is now known that they frequently become malignant and that this change is particularly common in those occurring in the small and large intestine. The syndrome associated with the development of malignancy was first described by Isler and Hedinger (1953) and by Thorson *et al.* (1954). It consists of watery diarrhoea, colic, flushing of the skin, attacks of bronchoconstriction resembling asthma and often oedema and ascites associated with valvular heart lesions and right heart failure. Attacks of flushing, abdominal pain and bronchoconstriction occur spontaneously but may sometimes be provoked and are reported to have been induced by: palpation of the tumour; anxiety; alcoholic drinks; meals, especially those containing much fat; intravenous injections of adrenaline or noradrenaline (Peart *et al.*, 1961). The flush varies very much in different individuals. It usually starts in the face, which becomes deep red in colour, and there is often a sensation of burning and fullness. The flush then spreads with a patchy distribution over the neck and trunk; neighbouring areas may be bright red, plum coloured or white. It usually disappears within a few minutes but patches may last much longer and in long-standing cases there is often permanent coarsening of the skin of the face and there may be telangiectases. There is no wheal formation or itching. At the beginning of an attack the blood pressure tends to fall and in some cases this fall is considerable. There is usually tachycardia and tachypnoea.

Lembeck (1953) was the first to find a high concentration of 5-HT in a portion of tumour removed from a case with these symptoms and this has been confirmed in subsequent cases. The amount of 5-HT in the blood is raised and there is an increased excretion of both 5-HT and 5-hydroxyindoleacetic acid (5-HIAA) in the urine. The estimation of this latter substance provides the best means of confirming the diagnosis. For this purpose all the urine passed in 24 hours is collected in a bottle containing 25 ml. glacial acetic acid and an aliquot is used for the estimation either by the method of Udenfriend, Titus and Weissbach (1955) or by the simplification of this method described by Macfarlane *et al.* (1956). The normal range by the latter method is 3 to 14 mg. 5-HIAA/24 hours; in cases of malignant carcinoid it is invariably raised and several hundred mg. may be excreted in 24 hours. A satisfactory simple test for excess 5-HIAA excretion has been described by Sjoerdsma, Weissbach and Udenfriend (1955) or a rough estimate may be made by paper chromatography (Jepson, 1958).

Intravenous infusion of 5-HT causes intestinal colic and diarrhoea, flushing and bronchoconstriction. These symptoms in patients with malignant carcinoid tumours are probably due therefore to the discharge of 5-HT from the tumour. This accords with the observation that patients with symptoms have tumours, most commonly liver secondaries, which would discharge into the systemic or pulmonary circulations, since 5-HT discharged into the portal circulation would largely be destroyed by amine oxidase in the liver. The cause of the cardiac lesions has so far not been explained. Microscopically there is a deposit of fibrin on the endocardium. The right side of the heart is affected much more frequently than the left; the pulmonary valve becomes stenosed and the tricuspid incompetent from contraction of the papillary muscle and chordae tendineae. The higher incidence of right heart lesions would be expected if they were caused by a substance secreted into the circulation and destroyed in the lungs as is 5-HT. Marked lesions on the left side have been observed in patients with septal defects and with pulmonary metastases. Chronic infusions of 5-HT and of 5-hydroxytryptophan into animals have failed to reproduce the condition.

In a small proportion of cases a pellagrinous rash has been reported. Nicotinamide is one of the products of normal tryptophan metabolism, being formed from it by the kynurenine pathway. Under normal circumstances hydroxyindole formation only accounts for about 1 % of dietary tryptophan metabolism; but this is increased when a carcinoid tumour is present and Sjoerdsma *et al* (1956) have reported a case in which 60% was diverted to this path. Symptoms of nicotinamide deficiency, and possibly also of impaired protein synthesis, might then be expected. Mental abnormalities are not a feature of the malignant carcinoid syndrome though there may be some emotional instability: no doubt the blood brain barrier protects the brain from circulating 5-HT.

Both Waldenström *et al.* (1956) and Sandler and Snow (1958) have found evidence that some cases of this syndrome are different in important respects from the majority. The former authors reported a case in which the flush was much longer in duration and brighter in colour than the usual flush seen in this condition, which is of dusky colour and often contains cyanotic patches. In the case they described it was similar to a histamine flush and the urine contained 4 to 8 mg. free histamine, 3 to 5 mg. 5-HT and 25 to 170 mg. 5-HIAA per day. The normal excretion of free histamine by the method used by these workers does not exceed 19 μg./day and that of 5-HT 100 μg./day. Sandler and Snow (1958) found a considerable amount of 5-hydroxytryptophan in the urine of a case with similar bright red flushes and a large excretion of both histamine and 5-HT in the urine. They suggested that these cases are examples of a distinct group having tumours which produce principally 5-HTP, and that this is decarboxylated in the kidney; the 5-HT formed would then largely escape oxidation by tissue amine oxidase and be excreted directly. In both cases described the tumour had the structural appearance of a carcinoid but contained no intracellular granules. The origin of the extra histamine in the urine is at present unexplained though two explanations have been put forward: 5-HT has been shown to be a weak histamine releaser (Feldberg and Smith, 1953) and might, in these cases, cause release of tissue histamine, but it has also been suggested that the tumour tissue may be active in decarboxylating histidine. Without further evidence neither of these explanations is convincing.

The treatment of cases of the malignant carcinoid syndrome is unsatisfactory. Surgical removal of as much of the neoplastic tissue as possible should be undertaken even if there are liver secondaries, which would normally be regarded as making a case of malignant disease inoperable, because when the amount of secreting tissue is reduced, symptoms are often less severe; but operation is not without risk as cases of fatal bronchospasm have occurred on administration of an anaesthetic. Symptomatic treatment with 5-HT antagonists (p. 140) has been tried with disappointing results. LSD, bromo-LSD and BAS have usually been found to have no effect on the symptoms, but recently some benefit has been reported from treatment with methysergide. Chlorpromazine sometimes appears to be of value but does not decrease 5-HIAA excretion. Phenylacetic acid, an inhibitor of 5-HTP decarboxylase, has been tried in 5 patients by Sandler *et al.* (1959) but without convincing results, though one patient showed some improvement during a short course. A number of other 5-HTP decarboxylase inhibitors are known (p. 128) and of these α-methyldopa would be worth a trial, though ill effects resulting from its hypotensive action and from the inhibition of decarboxylation of other aminoacids, might occur. Sjoerdsma *et al.* (1960) have given it in doses up to 6 G. per day to two patients and found that the excretion of 5-HIAA was markedly decreased and that of 5-HTP markedly increased while the drug was given, indicating an effective inhibition of 5-HT synthesis, but there are at present no reports on its effect on symptoms. A high protein diet and added nicotinamide will help to protect against the possibility of tryptophan deficiency. Reserpine causes some exacerbation of symptoms and a transient increase in 5-HIAA excretion. Iproniazid also causes an exacerbation of symptoms but reduces the excretion of 5-HIAA, presumably by depressing 5-HT oxidation. These results are those to be expected from the known actions of reserpine and iproniazid.

The course of the disease is often very prolonged and cases are known with a history of more than 20 years but once a cardiac lesion has developed, deterioration is usually rapid.

MENTAL DEFICIENCY

Phenylketonuria is an inherited condition due to a recessive gene and is associated with mental deficiency usually of a gross degree. There is a failure to oxidize phenylalanine to tyrosine which leads to a high blood phenylalanine concentration and to the formation and excretion in the urine of a number of products of phenylalanine metabolism normally not formed or only formed in small amounts. Of these the ones found in largest amounts are phenylacetic, phenylpyruvic and phenyllactic acids. In addition it has been shown (Pare, Sandler and Stacey, 1957, 1959) that the concentration of 5-HT in the blood and the daily excretion of 5-HIAA are both considerably below normal. There is thus a defect in hydroxyindole metabolism as well as in phenylalanine metabolism. Two explanations have been suggested: that the factor concerned in the oxidation of phenylalanine which is lacking is also required for the oxidation of tryptophan to 5-hydroxytryptophan, or that there is a depression of 5-HT synthesis by one or more of the products of abnormal phenylalanine metabolism. There is at present no convincing evidence in favour of either explanation although it has been shown that *in vitro* the three derivatives of phenylalanine mentioned above all depress decarboxylation of 5-HTP by kidney homogenates (Davison and Sandler, 1958). Nor is it known what relation this impairment of 5-HT synthesis has to the mental defect.

In some other forms of mental deficiency the amount of 5-HT in the blood is raised and there is probably an increase in 5-HIAA excretion (Pare, Sandler and Stacey, 1960). For example in a group of mentally defective patients with cerebral palsy the mean blood 5-HT concentration was more than double the normal value, whereas all mongols investigated had a normal blood 5-HT concentration. There is at present no explanation for the high values found in cerebral palsy and in a number of other kinds of mental deficiency.

BLOOD DISEASES

In various blood diseases the amount of 5-HT in the platelets is reduced (Hardisty and Stacey, 1957). This is due to a platelet defect, for when they are incubated with excess 5-HT the platelets fail to absorb it normally. The nature of the defect is not known: it is not associated with any deficiency in adenosine triphosphate which may be concerned in the binding of 5-HT in platelets (Born et al., 1958). Reduced platelet 5-HT does not appear to be responsible for the haemorrhagic manifestations in these diseases (Hardisty and Stacey, 1957).

In Hartnup disease there is a disturbance of tryptophan metabolism and of its absorption and excretion (Milne et al., 1960) but no disturbance of hydroxyindole metabolism has been reported.

ANTAGONISTS

Much work has been done on antagonism to 5-HT and it can only be briefly summarized here. Gyermek (1961) has reviewed the subject recently.

In 1953, Gaddum found that the action of 5-HT on the rat uterus was antagonized by lysergic acid diethylamide (LSD) (Fig. 14) but that contractions caused by acetylcholine and oxytocin were unaffected; the action was therefore specific. When doses are kept low the antagonist can be overcome by increasing the concentration of 5-HT and the antagonism is competitive. With larger doses LSD itself causes contractions. It also blocks the action of 5-HT on the rabbit's ear and on the circulation of the rat's kidney but only partially on the guinea pig ileum. This distinction has provided part of the evidence for the differentiation of D and M receptors by Gaddum and Picarelli (1957) discussed above (p. 133). In this classification LSD and phenoxybenzamine (dibenyline) behave as blockers of D-receptors which are thought to be situated on plain muscle cells. LSD is by no means the only derivative of lysergic acid which antagonizes the action of 5-HT on plain muscle. Its 2-bromo-derivative is equally active and has less tendency to stimulate the uterus and 1-methyl lysergic acid butanolamide (methysergide, UML491) is 4 times as active. This latter substance is very active *in vivo* and is reported to be of value in the symptomatic treatment of patients with the malignant carcinoid syndrome. Ergometrine, ergotoxine and dihydroergotamine are weak 5-HT antagonists.

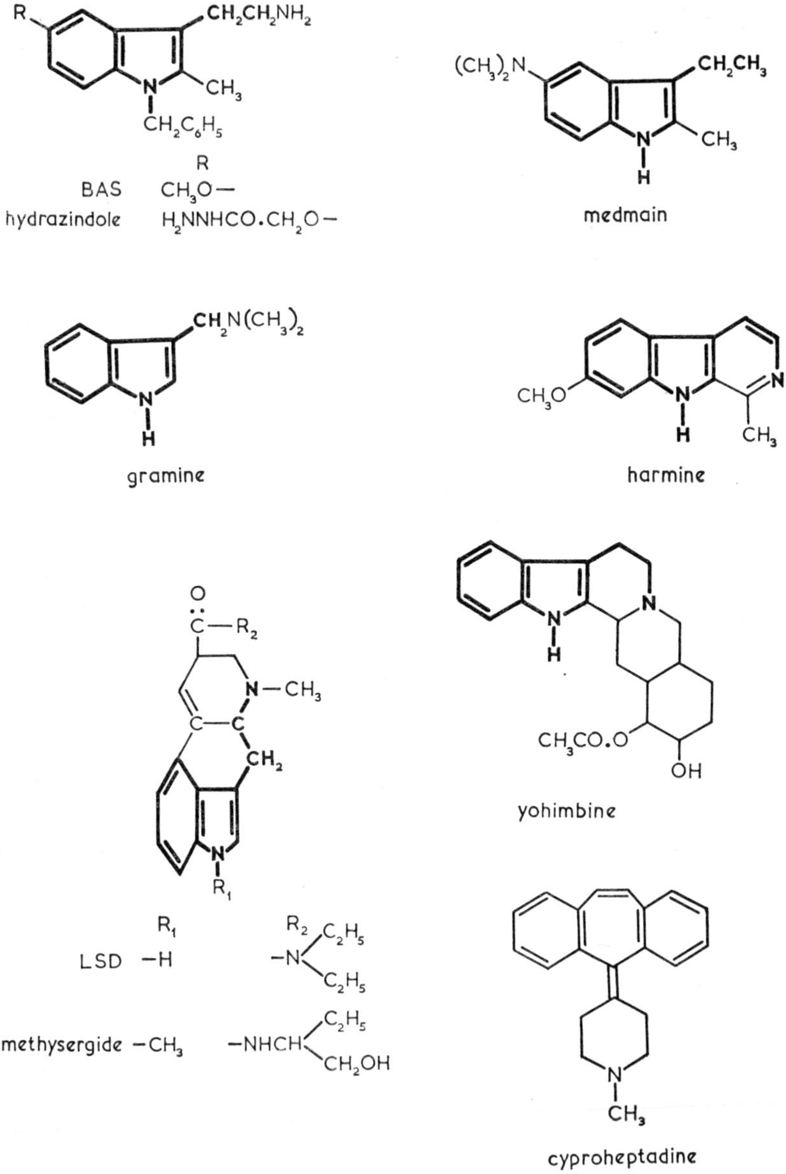

	R
BAS	CH₃O—
hydrazindole	H₂NNHCO.CH₂O—

medmain

gramine

harmine

yohimbine

	R₁	R₂
LSD	—H	—N(C₂H₅)(C₂H₅)
methysergide	—CH₃	—NHCH(C₂H₅)(CH₂OH)

cyproheptadine

FIG. 14. Some antagonists of 5-hydroxytryptamine

A number of indoles closely related to 5-HT have been tested on the rat uterus by Gaddum *et al.* (1955). Of these 5- and 6-benzyloxygramine were the most potent antagonists. Shaw and Wooley (1954, 1956) have prepared many more and tested them on a variety of preparations. On carotid artery rings and on the rat uterus 2-methyl-3-ethyl-5-dimethyl-aminoindole (medmain) was a very potent antagonist, while 1-benzyl-2-methyl-5-methoxytryptamine (BAS) was found to be especially active against the pressor action of 5-HT in dogs and to be a powerful and irreversible antagonist on the rat uterus. In a further series 1-benzyl-2-methyl-5-tryptaminoxyacethydrazide (hydrazindole) was found to have 20 times the activity of BAS in antagonizing the action of 5-HT on the rat uterus and in preventing diarrhoea caused by an injection of 5-HTP (Wooley, 1959). The structure of some of these compounds is given in Fig. 14 together with that of the naturally occurring alkaloids harmine and yohimbine which are less active than the other substances mentioned. Psilocybine, a naturally occurring indole discussed on p. 145, also antagonizes the actions of 5-HT on the rat uterus but is 80 to 100 times less potent than LSD.

Cypropheptadine [4 - (1:2 - 5:6 - dibenzo*cyclo*heptatrienylidene) - 1 - methyl-piperidine hydrochloride, Periactin] is a potent antagonist of 5-HT on the rat uterus, on the bronchial muscles of the guinea pig, of pressor effects in the dog and of increased capillary permeability in the rat. On the rat uterus it is said to be considerably more potent than LSD; its action is slow in developing and irreversible. It differs from other antagonists mentioned in being an active antihistamine (Stone *et al.*, 1961) and an anticonvulsant (Bodi *et al.*, 1960). Atropine, cocaine and morphine antagonize the action of 5-HT on guinea pig ileum and chlorpromazine, promethazine and diethazine on rat uterus.

After a large dose of 5-HT, plain muscle preparations show specific tachyphylaxis, that is subsequent doses have less effect though the tissue remains as sensitive to other spasmogens, such as acetylcholine, as it was before. Moreover tryptamine acts in the same way, large doses cause plain muscle to contract and cause tachyphylaxis to both 5-HT and tryptamine. This suggests that these two substances act on the same receptors.

The discovery of substances which block the action of 5-HT on plain muscle and vessels, directed attention to the possibility of blocking the action of 5-HT in the central nervous system. When injected intravenously only very large doses of 5-HT cause changes in behaviour; but as we have seen, there is evidence that it plays a part in cerebral function and 5-HT antagonists might conceivably be able to modify this action. Some of the compounds antagonizing the action of 5-HT on the rat uterus have central effects: LSD is an hallucinogen and medmain a convulsant. However, they have no stronger an effect on the rat uterus than their analogues 2-brom LSD and methyl medmain, which have no central actions. Benzyloxygramine and BAS are both effective antagonists of 5-HT probably acting on D receptors; benzyloxygramine has no central action and BAS is weakly sedative. These results might be explained by the failure of some compounds to reach the site of action of 5-HT owing to inability to penetrate the blood brain barrier or to destruction en route. The injection of 5-HT into the cerebral ventricles causes sedation and this can be antagonized by LSD, morphine and amphetamine (but not by 2-brom LSD, 5-hydroxygramine and methyl-medmain); elsewhere in the body LSD and morphine appear to block different receptors and amphetamine has no blocking action. It would therefore appear that either the 5-HT receptors in the brain are very different from those in peripheral organs or that these antagonists act on different receptors. Vogt *et al.* (1957) have shown, in support of this, that whereas the effect of 5-HT and LSD on spontaneous cerebral rhythms are antagonistic in some areas, they are synergistic in others. The position can at present be summarized by saying that there is no clear evidence that 5-HT antagonists which cause central effects do so by antagonizing endogenous 5-HT; but there is also no clear evidence that they do not.

SOME CHEMICALLY RELATED INDOLES

A large number of indoles related to 5-HT have been prepared and their pharmacological properties tested (Fig. 15). Most comparisons have been done on plain muscle preparations: rat uterus and rat stomach. For references and detailed reports of these the reader is referred to Vane (1959) and Barlow and Khan (1959). Only a few of the more important compounds will be discussed here.

Tryptamine has been found in normal human urine and is probably present in small amounts in brain and other tissues (see p. 26). It contracts plain muscle but is some hundreds of times less potent than 5-HT. Vane (1959) noticed that its action on the rat stomach, which contains amine oxidase, was potentiated more than 10 times by the amine oxidase inhibitor iproniazid but that of 5-HT was not. He suggested the following explanation. There is reason to believe that 5-HT does not readily pass through the cell membrane into the interior of cells and that the polar OH group is largely responsible for this. Tryptamine, with no OH group probably enters cells much more easily. If the plain muscle receptors are on the cell surface they will be equally accessible to both tryptamine and 5-HT but the local concentration of tryptamine will be kept down by more rapid diffusion into the cell and inactivation there. Iproniazid in these circumstances will have a bigger effect on the rate of inactivation of tryptamine than of 5-HT. Capacity to reach inactivating enzymes must therefore be added to the other factors which may influence structure-activity relationships.

The intravenous injections of tryptamine and of 5-HT into rats were found by Tedeschi *et al.* (1959) to produce similar overt peripheral effects such as blanching of the ears and paws followed by hyperaemia. Both caused chronic convulsions, but whereas those due to 5-HT appeared to be asphyxial as they followed a period of apnoea and were

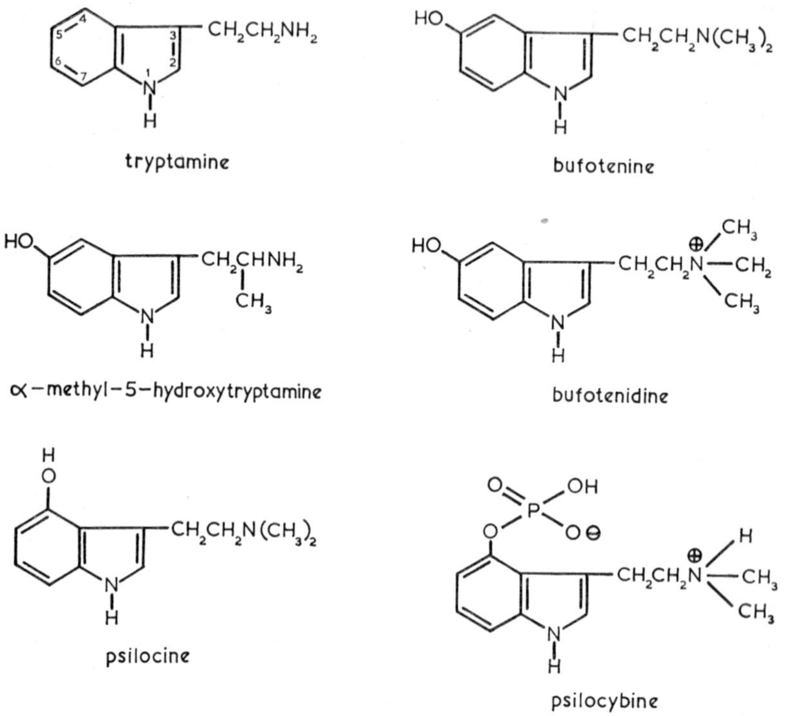

FIG. 15. Some indoles related to 5-hydroxytryptamine

accompanied by cyanosis, those due to tryptamine were not preceded by signs of respiratory embarrassment nor were they associated with cyanosis. Similar convulsions could be produced by the injection of 5-HTP into rats pretreated with iproniazid and this suggested that 5-HT, formed intracellularly from 5-HTP, and tryptamine were acting on the same receptors, which were not easily accessible to injected 5-HT. Iproniazid also potentiated the convulsant action of tryptamine. Here again differences in the actions of these two compounds are explicable as the result of differences in membrane penetration, in this case of the blood brain barrier. Intravenous injections of tryptamine (30 to 40 mg./kg.) in the cat, according to Nieuwenhuyzen (1936), causes catalepsy, a condition similar to that caused by the injection of 5-HT into the cerebral ventricles.

The secondary and tertiary amines formed from 5-HT by methyl substitution, both contract plain muscle but have somewhat less activity than 5-HT (Szara, 1961). The dimethyl derivative is known as bufotenine (Fig. 15) and is contained in the seeds of *Piptadenia peregrina* which is used as a snuff by South American Indians for its mental effects. Both bufotenine and the monomethyl compound are found in toad skin but neither have been found in mammals; both, like tryptamine, have similar effects to 5-HT on the blood pressure, respiration, bronchial smooth muscle and on the kidney, but are much weaker. The corresponding derivatives of tryptamine also contract plain muscle but are still weaker in their actions. Fabing and Hawkins (1956) found 16 mg. bufotenine/kg.i.v. to be hallucinogenic, though this is denied by Turner and Merlis (1959), who however agree with Szara (1957) that N'N'-dimethyltryptamine has no action by mouth but that 30 mg./kg.i.m. is powerfully hallucinogenic. They found the effect to be like that produced by LSD and mescaline but much shorter in duration, lasting less than 1 hour. Marrazzi and Hart (1955) using their two neurone transcallosal system found that bufotenine and 5-HT were among the most powerful inhibitors of central synaptic transmission, being considerably more active than adrenaline and noradrenaline.

The substitution of a methyl group on the α-carbon atom in the side chain of 5-HT only slightly reduces activity on the rat uterus. A similar change in the structure of tryptamine increases activity tenfold. This latter compound is not a substrate for amine oxidase and is in fact an amine oxidase inhibitor (Greig *et al.*, 1959). Its activity in the presence of an amine oxidase inhibitor is therefore unchanged and is of the same order as tryptamine under similar circumstances (Vane, 1959). In man it has mental effects like LSD (Szara, 1961) (see also p. 64).

The action of 6-hydroxytryptamine on the rat stomach is much weaker than that of 5-HT; that of 4-hydroxytryptamine is only slightly weaker and in many other pharmacological properties it resembles 5-HT (Erspamer *et al.*, 1960). The N'N'dimethyl derivative of 4-hydroxytryptamine is known as psilocine, the name being derived from psilocybine, an alkaloid obtained from the hallucinogenic mushroom, *Psilocybe mexicana* Heim (Fig. 15). Psilocybine was isolated by Hoffmann *et al.* (1958) and its pharmacological properties have been reported by Wiedmann, Taeschler and Konzett (1958). On isolated organs (auricles, small intestine, uterus, seminal vesicles) it has no action itself but blocks the action of 5-HT specifically: it has no blocking action against acetylcholine, histamine, adrenaline or nicotine. Intravenous injection leads to circulatory effects which, like those of 5-HT, are complex and vary from species to species: contraction of the cat's nictitating membrane, mydriasis, piloerection, tachycardia, tachypnoea, hyperthermia and hyperglycaemia. Doses of 10 to 50 mg./kg. are followed by diminished activity but the EEG has an alerted pattern. The mental effects in man are similar to those caused by eating the mushroom or by taking psilocine. These substances are structurally similar to LSD (Fig. 14) which is also a 4-substituted indole with a structure in which a dimethylethylamine chain can be discerned.

MELATONIN

Giarman and Friedman (1960) have estimated the 5-HT content of the pineal gland and found a high concentration in several mammalian species including man, and Lerner and his colleagues (1959) have isolated from the pineal of the ox an indole derivative to which they have given the name melatonin on account of its skin-lightening effect in the frog. This effect is brought about by the aggregation of the melanin granules about the nucleus of skin melanocytes and also by an indirect action inhibiting melanin formation. Melatonin is able to reverse the skin darkening action of the melanocyte stimulating hormone of the pituitary and it is 10^5 times as potent in this respect as adrenaline and acetylcholine, the most potent non-indolic substances known. Chemically it is N' acetyl-5-methoxytryptamine (Fig. 13) and is formed by the action of 5-hydroxyindole-o-methyltransferase on N'-acetyl-5-hydroxytryptamine. This enzyme has been found by Axelrod and Weissbach (1960) in the pineal of cow and monkey. N-acetylation in general diminishes the activity of amines and it is therefore remarkable that melatonin is some 50 times as active as 5-methoxytryptamine, while 5-hydroxytryptamine has a negligible effect on melanophores (Lerner and Case, 1960). In the rat, melatonin undergoes 6-hydroxylation forming 5-methoxy-6-hydroxytryptamine (Kopin *et al.*, 1960) and this is probably ultimately excreted as the sulphate or glucuronide. The oxidation product of melatonin, 5-methoxyindoleacetic acid, has also been found in the pineal but the importance of oxidation of the side chain in the elimination of melatonin is not known. The pineal also contains 5-methoxyindoleacetic acid formed, according to Kreder *et al.* (1960), not from melatonin but as an oxidation product of 5-methoxytryptamine.

Melatonin has no effect on the pigmentation of human skin and other actions have not yet been reported, but the finding of small amounts in peripheral nerves (Lerner *et al.*, 1959*b*) suggests that it may have some function in nerve metabolism.

IBOGAINE

Before concluding this section, brief mention may be made of this indole alkaloid. Plant extracts containing it are used in the Congo to overcome fatigue and in larger doses to cause excitement, confusion and possibly hallucinations. Its pharmacological actions have been described by Schneider and Sigg (1957). On injection into cats it causes excitement, rage and fear and in mice raises the electroshock threshold, thus acting as an anticonvulsant.

RELEASE

RESERPINE

Injection of reserpine (formula p. 49) into an animal is followed by a large increase in the excretion of 5-HIAA in the urine and a loss of 5-HT from sites where it is normally found: gastro-intestinal tract, brain, platelets and spleen.

In the intestine, depletion of 5-HT is accompanied by a reduction in the number of argentaffin cells. A comparison of the concentration of the amine with the number of argentaffin cells which can be identified histologically in various parts of gastro-intestinal tract of the guinea-pig normally and after reserpine is shown in Table 9. 5-HT is not the only

Table 9

Comparison of the numbers of argentaffin cells and the concentration of 5-HT in guinea pig gut

Cells were counted in diazo-stained sections of gut and the numbers per mm.^{3} mucous membrane calculated. Animals received either reserpine 0·8 mg./kg. s.c. daily for 6 days or an equal volume of the reserpine solvent.

	Normal		Reserpine treated	
	Cells/mm.^{3}	µg. 5-HT/g. tissue	Cells/mm.^{3}	µg. 5-HT/g. tissue
Stomach	600	1·9	30	0·3
Duodenum	8700	14·9	0	0·8
Jejunum	9300	7·9	85	1·0
Ileum	1400	5·1	0	0·75
Colon	390	4·0	20	0·43

(Jacobson and Stacey, unpublished)

amine to be released by reserpine. There is at the same time a reduction in the amount of catechol amines in brain, adrenals, heart, and sympathetic ganglia (p. 114). The changes in the concentration of 5-HT and noradrenaline in the rabbit brain stem are shown in Fig. 4 (p. 22) and discussed in Chapter 1 (p. 21). With large doses the fall is rapid during the first hour, continues for about 4 hours and the amount of amines then remains at a low level until about 36 hours after the injection, when a slow restitution begins. Fig. 16 shows the effect on platelet 5-HT and on the excretion of 5-HIAA in urine of a daily subcutaneous injection of 1 mg. reserpine into a human subject. With this much smaller dose maximum depletion is not reached until 48 hours after the injection but recovery is still very gradual. The prolonged effect of a reserpine injection contrasts strikingly with its rapid excretion; 2 to 4 hours after an injection, Hess, Shore and Brodie (1956) failed to find any in the brain though Plummer *et al.* (1957) using tritium labelled reserpine found appreciable amounts of activity up to 48 hours. It is unlikely that the prolonged action is due to the action of a slowly excreted metabolic product of reserpine for two reasons: no metabolic product has so far been identified which causes 5-HT release or the pharmacological effects

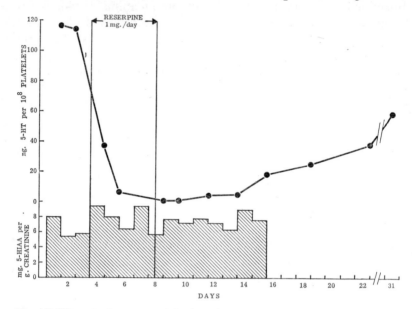

FIG. 16. Effect of subcutaneous injection of 1 mg. reserpine per day for three days on human platelet 5-hydroxytryptamine content and on 5-hydroxyindole-acetic acid excretion (expressed as mg. 5-HIAA per g. urine creatinine).

of reserpine, and the degree and duration of action is the same whether an animal is given 1 or 5 mg./kg., although in the latter case the amount of a metabolite formed would probably be much greater and its persistence in the body more prolonged. It appears that reserpine impairs the binding of these amines and this damage is only slowly repaired. The impaired absorption of 5-HT by platelets from a subject who had received reserpine (Table 10) is in accord with this. As to the nature of

Table 10

Effect of 1 mg. reserpine i.m. in man on the 5-HT content of the platelets and on their ability to absorb 5-HT

	in blood	ng. 5-HT per 10^8 platelets after incubation with 5-HT at 37° for 2 hours
Before reserpine	36	173
1 day after	14	39
3 days after	<1	36
9 days after	7	40

damage to the storage mechanism there is at present no evidence. The possibility that adenosine triphosphate is concerned in amine storage in the adrenal gland and in platelets has been referred to; and according to Hillarp (1960), release of catechol amines from the adrenal medulla after reserpine is accompanied by loss of adenosine phosphates; but reserpine causes no change in the adenosine triphosphate content of platelets (Born *et al.*, 1958) and only a partial loss from the intestine (Prusoff, 1961).

The pharmacological effects of reserpine administration are: sedation and loss of aggressiveness; miosis, ptosis and relaxation of the nictitating membrane; hypotension, bradycardia, hypothermia, salivation and diarrhoea. With prolonged administration in man symptoms of Parkinsonism appear: tremor, rigidity and a mask-like face. The development and duration of these effects corresponds to the changes in the concentration of the amines in the brain and not to the period of persistence of reserpine in the body, which is much shorter. This has led to the suggestion that the central effects of reserpine are mediated by its action on the binding of brain amines. (This subject is discussed in greater detail on page 22.) On the other hand there is evidence that some of the actions of reserpine are due to the loss of the transmitter, noradrenaline, from sympathetic nerves. Muscholl and Vogt (1958) found in experiments on rabbits and cats that after reserpine, stimulation of pre- or post-ganglionic fibres of the sympathetic system had little or no effect on the pupil or the nictitating membrane or on the size of the palpebral fissure, although these tissues were no less sensitive than normal to injected noradrenaline. Probably the hypotensive action of reserpine is largely due to this peripheral depletion of noradrenaline, though the central depression of vascular reflexes may play some part also (p. 315).

A large number of alkaloids related to reserpine have been isolated from *Rauwolfia serpentina* and from other species of Rauwolfia (Lewis, 1956). Brodie, Shore and Pletscher (1956) found only those having a sedative action released 5-HT. Pletscher has described benzoquinolizine derivatives which release 5-HT and have sedative properties. They are described and the structure of one of them, tetrabenzine, is given on page 50. These substances also release catecholamines but their action is more rapid in onset and of shorter duration than that of reserpine.

The *physiological release* of 5-HT is at present little understood. It is released into the intestinal tract as a result of raised intra-luminal pressure (p. 134) and from platelets during blood coagulation. This latter process appears to be closely related to the clotting mechanism as the release runs parallel with thrombin generation and with the disappearance of adenosine triphosphate from the platelets. Mechanical damage to platelets by entanglement in a clot is unnecessary as release

6

was found to be normal in the blood of a patient with afibrinogenaemia. In this blood no clot formed but the remaining stages of the clotting process were shown to be normal (Hardisty and Pinnigar, 1956).

Humphrey and Jacques (1954) were the first to observe that 5-HT was released with histamine from rabbits platelets during an antigen-antibody reaction. This has been confirmed and evidence is accumulating that 5-HT plays an important part in anaphylactic shock in the mouse. In this animal symptoms can be prevented by previous treatment with 5-HT antagonists.

DISTRIBUTION IN LOWER ANIMALS AND PLANTS

5-hydroxytryptamine is widely distributed throughout the animal kingdom. It is found in the gastrointestinal tract of all vertebrates. In invertebrates (Table 11) it is found in the salivary glands of those octopods (e.g. *Octopus vulgaris*) which have enterochromaffin cells and in the hypobranchial body of *Murex*. These tissues are related to the gastro-intestinal tract and the amounts in them is very considerable, in *Octopus vulgaris* for example it is 0·5 mg./gm. fresh tissue. High concentrations are also found in the skin of some, but not all, amphibia but here it is often associated with other hydroxyindoles, in particular the N'methylated compounds (Fig. 15) bufotenine, bufotenidine and dehydrobufotenine. The amounts in nervous tissue are smaller but it has been found in the ganglia and peripheral nerves of a great variety of invertebrates (Welsh and Moorehead, 1960). On the hearts of some crustacia it has an action similar to that of adrenaline in mammals and this has led (Florey and Florey, 1954) to the suggestion that in these animals it may be a transmitter. The increased strength of contraction of the excised heart of the molluscs *Venus mercenaria* and *Spisula solida* provide a very sensitive method of bioassay (p. 123). The anterior byssus retractor muscle of *Mytilus* is relaxed by it. Stimulation by cathodal pulses and by acetylcholine cause a contraction of this muscle, with delayed relaxation when the stimulus is discontinued. In the presence of 5-HT, relaxation is more rapid (for refs. see Twarog, 1960). The role, if any, of 5-HT in lower animals is far from clear but evidence is accumulating that makes a neurohumoral function seem likely.

The venom of the wasp, hornet and scorpion contain considerable amounts of 5-HT and this contributes to the pain of a sting, but in wasp venom it is not the only pain-producing substance; histamine and a substance resembling bradykinin are also present, and in hornet venom there is also much acetylcholine (p. 163). The sting of the bee, and the Portuguese man-of-war (*Physalia*) however, do not contain it and the stinging tentacles of the sea anemone contain little, though as much as 0·5 mg./gm. was found in the coelenteric tissues of the sea anemone *Calliactus parasitica* (Mathias et al., 1960).

5-HT is also present in the sting fluid of the common stinging nettle, *Urtica dioica*, where it is associated with acetylcholine and histamine, and in the trichomes of the pods of *Mucuna puriens*, which constitute cowhage. The only fruits which have been found to contain appreciable amounts are the banana, plantain, pineapple and tomato (Table 11).

Table 11

5-hydroxytryptamine in invertebrates and plants

		Ref.
Wasp venom (*V. vulgaris*)	0·32 mg./g. dry venom	1
Hornet venom (*V. crabo*)	10 to 20 mg./g. dry venom	10
Scorpion venom (*Leiurus quinquestriatus*)	2 to 4 mg./g. dry venom	2
Scorpion venom (*Buthotus minax*)	0·03 to 0·04 mg./g. dry venom	2
Cowhage trichomes (*Macuna puriens*)	0·15 mg./g.	3
Stinging nettle (*Urtica dioica*)	0·2 mg./ml. sting fluid	4
Sea anemone (*C. parasitica*) (coelenteric tissue)	0·5 mg./g. tissue	5
Venus mercenaria (visceral ganglia)	0·04 mg./g. tissue	6
Banana pulp	0·03 mg./g.	7
Banana peel	0·07 mg./g.	7
Pineapple juice	0·001 to 0·025 mg./ml.	8, 9
Tomato	0·012 mg./g.	7

1. Jaques and Schachter (1954)
2. Adam and Weiss (1959)
3. Bowden *et al.* (1954)
4. Brittain and Collier (1957)
5. Mathias *et al.* (1960)
6. Welsh and Moorhead (1960)
7. Waalkes *et al.* (1958)
8. Bruce (1960)
9. West (1960)
10. Bhoola *et al.* (1961)

These fruits contain enough for their consumption to affect excretion of 5-HIAA and they should be avoided when urine is collected for estimations. In mushrooms, bufotenine has been reported in *Amanita mappa* (Weiland and Motzel, 1953).

CONCLUSION

In the few years since 5-HT was first identified in living tissues the main facts of its biosynthesis and metabolism have been established and a very considerable body of information amassed about its distribution and pharmacological properties. From this it can be concluded that it is likely that it has a function in physiological processes in the mammalian gastro-intestinal tract and brain. In the gastro-intestinal tract there is a clear indication of the part 5-HT may play in maintaining peristalsis; as to its part in the brain we have not yet passed beyond the stage of unverified speculations.

REFERENCES

* Denotes review

ABRAHAMS, V. C. and PICKFORD, M. (1956). *Brit. J. Pharmacol.* **11**, 35, 44, 50
ADAM, K. R. and WEISS, C. (1959). *Nature (Lond.)*, **183**, 1398
AMIN, A. H., CRAWFORD, T. B. B. and GADDUM, J. H. (1954). *J. Physiol.* **126**, 596
ANNOTATION (1960). *Lancet*, **2**, 355
ARMSTRONG, D., DRY, R. M. L., KEELE, C. A. and MARKHAM, J. W. (1953). *J. Physiol.* **120**, 326
ÅSTRÖM, A. and SAMELIUS, U. (1957). *Brit. J. Pharmacol.* **12**, 410
AXELROD, J. and WEISSBACH, H. (1960). *Science*, **131**, 1312
BAKER, R. V. (1958). *J. Physiol.* **142**, 563
BAKER, R. V. (1959). *J. Physiol.* **145**, 473
BAKER, R. V., BLASCHKO, H. and BORN, G. V. R. (1959). *J. Physiol.* **149**, 55P
BARLOW, R. B. and KHAN, I. (1959). *Brit. J. Pharmacol.* **14**, 99, 265, 553
BENDITT, E. P., WONG, R. L., ARASE, M. and ROEPER, E. (1955). *Proc. Soc. exp. Biol. (N.Y.)* **90**, 303
BHARGAVA, K. P. and BORRISON, H. L. (1955). *J. Pharmacol.* **115**, 464
BHOOLA, K. D., CALLE, J. D. and SCHACHTER, M. (1961). *J. Physiol.* **159**, 167
BLACK, J. W., FISHER, E. W. and SMITH, A. N. (1958). *J. Physiol.* **141**, 22
BLASCHKO, H. and LEVINE, W. G. (1960). *Brit. J. Pharmacol.* **15**, 625
BODI, T., SIEGLER, P. E., GERSHENFELD, M., BROWN, E. B. and NODING, J. H. (1960). *Fed. Proc.* **19**, 195
BOGDANSKI, D. F., WEISSBACH, H. and UDENFRIEND, S. (1957). *J. Neurochem.* **1**, 272
BOGDANSKI, D. F., WEISSBACH, H. and UDENFRIEND, S. (1958). *J. Pharmacol.* **122**, 182
BORN, G. V. R. and GILLSON, R. E. (1959). *J. Physiol.* **146**, 472
BORN, G. V. R., INGRAM, G. I. C. and STACEY, R. S. (1958). *Brit. J. Pharmacol.* **13**, 62
BOWDEN, K., BROWN, B. G. and BATTY, J. E. (1954). *Nature (Lond.)*, **174**, 925
BRITTAIN, R. T. and COLLIER, H. O. J. (1957). *J. Physiol.* **135**, 58P
BRODIE, B. B., SHORE, P. A. and PLETSCHER, A. (1956). *Science*, **123**, 992
BRUCE, D. W. (1960). *Nature (Lond.)*, **188**, 147
BÜLBRING, E. and LIN, R. C. Y. (1958). *J. Physiol.* **140**, 381
BÜLBRING, E. and CREMA, A. (1958). *Brit. J. Pharmacol.* **13**, 444
BÜLBRING, E. and CREMA, A. (1959). *J. Physiol.* **146**, 29
*CLARK, W. G. (1959). *Pharmacol. Rev.* **11**, 330
COOPER, J. R. and MELCER, I. (1961). *J. Pharmacol. exp. Ther.* **132**, 265
DALGLIESH, C. E., TOH, C. C. and WORK, T. S. (1953). *J. Physiol.* **120**, 298
DAVIDSON, J., SJOERDSMA, A., LOOMIS, L. N. and UDENFRIEND, S. (1957). *J. Clin. Invest.* **36**, 1594
DAVISON, A. N. and SANDLER, M. (1958). *Nature (Lond.)*, **181**, 186
DAWES, G. S. and COMROE, J. H. (1954). *Physiol. Rev.* **34**, 167
DEL GRECO, F., MASSON, G. M. C. and CORCORAN, A. C. (1956). *Amer. J. Physiol.* **187**, 509
EBER, O. and LEMBECK, F. (1957). *Pflüg. Arch. ges. Physiol.* **265**, 563
ERSPAMER, V. (1953). *Arch. int. Pharmacodyn.* **93**, 293
*ERSPAMER, V. (1954). *Pharm. Rev.* **6**, 425
ERSPAMER, V. and ASERO, B. (1952). *Nature (Lond.)*, **169**, 800
ERSPAMER, V., GLASSER, A. and MANTEGAZZINI (1960). *Experientia (Basel)*, **16**, 505
ERSPAMER, V. and TESTINI, A. (1959). *J. Pharm. (Lond.)*, **11**, 618
EVANS, D. H. L. and SCHILD, H. O. (1953). *J. Physiol.* **122**, 63P
FABING, H. D. and HAWKINS, J. R. (1956). *Science*, **123**, 886
FASTIER, F. N., McDOWALL, M. A. and WAAL, H. (1959). *Brit. J. Pharmacol.* **14**, 527
FELDBERG, W. and SHERWOOD, S. L. (1954). *J. Physiol.* **123**, 148
FELDBERG, W. and SMITH, A. N. (1953). *Brit. J. Pharmacol.* **8**, 406
FELDBERG, W. and TOH, C. C. (1953). *J. Physiol.* **119**, 352

FEYERTER, F. (1953). Uber die peripheren endokrinen Drusen des Menschen. Vienna: Maudrich

FLOREY, E. and FLOREY, E. (1954). *Z. Naturforsch*, **9b**, 58

GADDUM, J. H. (1953). *Brit. J. Pharmacol.* **8**, 321

GADDUM, J. H. and GIARMAN, N. J. (1956). *Brit. J. Pharmacol.* **11**, 88

GADDUM, J. H., HAMEED, K. A., HATHAWAY, D. E. and STEPHENS, F. F. (1955). *Quart. J. exp. Physiol.* **40**, 49

GADDUM, J. H. (1953). *J. Physiol.* **119**, 363

GADDUM, J. H. and PICARELLI, Z. P. (1957). *Brit. J. Pharmacol.* **12**, 323

GADDUM, J. H. and PAASONEN, M. K. (1955). *Brit. J. Pharmacol.* **10**, 474

GARRETT, N. J. (1958). *Arch. int. Pharmacodyn.* **117**, 435

GIARMAN, N. J. and FREEDMAN, D. X. (1960). *Nature (Lond.)*, **186**, 480

GINZEL, K. H. and KOTTEGODA, S. R. (1953). *Quart. J. exp. Physiol.* **38**, 225

GINZEL, K. H. and KOTTEGODA, S. R. (1954). *J. Physiol.* **123**, 277

GINZEL, K. H. (1957). In '5-hydroxytryptamine'. Ed. Lewis. London: Pergamon

GOSSET, A. and MASSON, P. (1914). *Presse méd.* **22**, 237

GREIG, M. E., WALK, R. A. and GIBBONS, A. J. (1959). *J. Pharmacol.* **127**, 110

*GYERMEK, L. (1961). *Pharm. Rev.* **13**, 399

HAVERBACK, B. J. and BOGDANSKI, D. F. (1957). *Proc. Soc. exp. Biol. (N.Y.)* **95**, 392

HARDISTY, R. M. and STACEY, R. S. (1955). *J. Physiol.* **130**, 711

HARDISTY, R. M. and STACEY, R. S. (1957). *Brit. J. Haematol.* **3**, 292

HARDISTY, R. M. and PINNIGAR, J. L. (1956). *Brit. J. Haematol.* **2**, 139

HEDINGER, C. and LANGEMANN, H. (1955). *Schweiz. med. Wschr.* **85**, 541

HERTZLER, E. C. (1961). *Brit. J. Pharmacol.* **17**, 406

HERXHEIMER, H. (1955). *J. Physiol.* **128**, 435

HESS, S. M., SHORE, P. A. and BRODIE, B. B. (1956). *J. Pharmacol.* **118**, 84

HILLARP, N. A. (1960). *Nature (Lond.)*, **187**, 1032

HOFFMAN, A., HEIM, R., BRACK, A. and KOBEL, H. (1958). *Experientia (Basel)*, **14**, 107

HUGHES, F. B. and BRODIE, B. B. (1959). *J. Pharmacol.* **127**, 96

HUMPHREY, J. H. and JAQUES, R. (1954). *J. Physiol.* **124**, 305

HUMPHREY, J. H. and TOH, C. C. (1954). *J. Physiol.* **124**, 300

ISLER, P. and HEDINGER, C. I. (1953). *Schweiz. med. Wschr.* **83**, 4

JEPSON, J. P. (1958). In 'Chromatographic Techniques'. Ed. Ivor Smith. London: Heinemann

JAQUES, R. and SCHACHTER, M. (1954). *Brit. J. Pharmacol.* **9**, 49 and 53

KONZETT, H. (1956). *Brit. J. Pharmacol.* **11**, 289

KOPIN, I. J., PARE, C. M. B., AXELROD, J. and WEISSBACH, JR. (1960). *Biochim. biophys. acta*, **40**, 377

KOTTEGODA, S. R. and MOTT, J. C. (1955). *Brit. J. Pharmacol.* **10**, 66

KVEDER, S., MCISAAC, W. M. and PAGE, I. H. (1960). *Biochem. J.* **76**, 28*P*

KUNTZMAN, R., SHORE, P. A., BOGDANSKI, D. and BRODIE, B. B. (1961). *J. Neurochem.* **6**, 226

LANGENDORFF, H. and MELCHING, H. J. (1959). *Strahlentherapie*, **110**, 505

LEE, C. Y. (1960). *J. Physiol.* **152**, 405

LEMBECK, F. (1953). *Nature (Lond.)*, **172**, 910

LEMESSURIER, D. H., SCHWARTZ, C. J. and WHELAN, R. F. (1959). *Brit. J. Pharmacol.* **14**, 246

LERNER, A. B., CASE, J. D. and HEINZELMAN, R. V. (1959a). *J. Amer. chem. Soc.* **81**, 5264

LERNER, A. B., CASE, J. D., MORI, W. and WRIGHT, M. R. (1959b). *Nature (Lond.)*, **183**, 1821

LERNER, A. B. and CASE, J. D. (1960). *Fed. Proc.* **19**, 590

*LEWIS, G. P. (1958). Symposium on 5-hydroxytryptamine. London: Pergamon

LEWIS, J. J. (1956). *J. Pharm. (Lond.)*, **8**, 465

MACCANNON, D. M. and HORVATH, S. M. (1954). *Amer. J. Physiol.* **179**, 131

MACFARLANE, P. S., DALGLIESH, C. E., DUTTON, R. W., LENNOX, B., NYHUS, L. M. and SMITH, A. N. (1956). *Scot. Med. J.* **1**, 148

MARRAZZI, A. S. and HART, E. R. (1955). *J. nerv. ment. Dis.* **122**, 453

McCUBBIN, J. W., GREEN, J. H., SALMOIRAGHI, G. C. and PAGE, I. H. (1956). *J. Pharmacol.* **116,** 191

McISAAC, W. M. and PAGE, I. H. (1959). *J. biol. Chem.* **234,** 858

MATHIAS, A. P., ROSS, D. M. and SCHACHTER, M. (1960). *J. Physiol.* **151,** 296

MILNE, M. D., CRAWFORD, M. A., GIRÃO, C. B. and LOUGHRIDGE, L. W. (1960). *Quart. J. Med.* **29,** 407

MOTT, J. C. and PAINTAL, A. S. (1953). *Brit. J. Pharmacol.* **8,** 238

MUSCHOLL, E. and VOGT, M. (1958). *J. Physiol.* **141,** 132

NIEUWENHUYZEN, F. J. (1936). *Proc. Acad. Sci. Amst.* **39,** 1151

OUTSCHOORN, A. S. and JACOB, J. (1960). *Brit. J. Pharmacol.* **15,** 131

*PAGE, I. H. (1954). *Physiol. Rev.* **34,** 563

PAGE, I. H. and GLENDENING, M. B. (1955). *Obstet. and Gynec.* **5,** 781

PAGE, I. H. (1957). In '5-hydroxytryptamine'. Ed. Lewis. London: Pergamon

*PAGE, I. H. (1958). *Physiol. Rev.* **38,** 277

PAGE, I. H. and McCUBBIN, J. W. (1956). *Amer. J. Physiol.* **184,** 265

PANIGEL, M. and MAYER, M. (1959). *C. rend. Acad. Sc.* **248**(7), 1031

PARE, C. M. B., SANDLER, M. and STACEY, R. S. (1957). *Lancet,* **1,** 551

PARE, C. M. B., SANDLER, M. and STACEY, R. S. (1959). *Arch. Dis. Childh.* **34,** 177

PARE, C. M. B., SANDLER, M. and STACEY, R. S. (1960). *J. Neurol. Neurosurg. Psychiat.* **23,** 341

PARKS, V. J., SANDISON, A. G., SKINNER, S. L. and WHELAN, R. F. (1960). *J. Physiol.* **151,** 342

PARRATT, J. R. and WEST, G. B. (1957). *J. Physiol.* **137,** 169

PEART, W. S., ANDREWS, T. M. and ROBERTSON, J. I. S. (1961). *Lancet,* **1,** 577

PLUMMER, A. J., SHEPPARD, H. and SCHUBERT, A. R. (1957). In 'Psychotropic drugs'. Ed. Garratini and Ghetti. Amsterdam: Elsevier, p. 350

POULSON, E., BOWTROS, M. and ROBSON, J. M. (1960). *J. Endocr.* **20,** xi

PRUSOFF, W. H. (1960). *Brit. J. Pharmacol.* **15,** 520

PRUSOFF, W. H. (1961). *Brit. J. Pharmacol.* **17,** 87

RAPPORT, M. M. (1949). *J. biol. Chem.* **180,** 961

REID, G. and RAND, M. (1952). *Nature (Lond.),* **169,** 801

ROBSON, J. M., TROUNCE, J. R. and DIDCOCK, K. A. H. (1954). *J. Endocr.* **10,** 129

RODDIE, I. C., SHEPHERD, J. T. and WHELAN, R. F. (1955). *Brit. J. Pharmacol.* **10,** 445

SANDLER, M. and SNOW, P. J. D. (1958). *Lancet,* **1,** 137

SANDLER, M. DAVIES, A. and RIMINGTON, C. (1959). *Lancet,* **2,** 318

SCHINDLER, R., DAY, S. M. and FISCHER, G. A. (1959). *Cancer Res.* **19,** 47

SCHNECKLOTH, R., PAGE, I. H., DEL GRECO, F. and CORCORAN, A. C. (1957). *Circulation,* **16,** 523

SCHNEIDER, J. A. and SIGG, E. B. (1957). *Ann. N.Y. Acad. Sci.* **66,** 765

SHAW, E. N. and WOOLEY, D. W. (1954). *J. Pharmacol. exp. Ther.* **111,** 43

SHAW, E. N. and WOOLEY, D. W. (1956). *J. Pharmacol. exp. Ther.* **116,** 164

SJOERDSMA, A., WEISSBACH, H. and UDENFRIEND, S. (1955). *J. Amer. med. Ass.* **159,** 297

SJOERDSMA, A., WEISSBACH, H. and UDENFRIEND, S. (1956). *Amer. J. Med.* **20,** 520

SJOERDSMA, A., OATES, J. A., ZALTZMAN, M. S. and UDENFRIEND, S. (1960). *New Engl. J. Med.* **263,** 585

SMITH, S. E. (1960). *Brit. J. Pharmacol.* **15,** 319

SOURKES, T. L. (1954). *Arch. Biochem.* **51,** 444

SPECTOR, S., SHORE, P. A. and BRODIE, B. B. (1960). *J. Pharmacol. exp. Ther.* **128,** 15

SPIES, T. D. and STONE, R. E. (1952). *J. Amer. med. Ass.* **150,** 1509

SPINAZZOLA, A. J. and SHERROD, T. R. (1957). *J. Pharmacol. exp. Ther.* **119,** 114

STACEY, R. S. (1961). *Brit. J. Pharmacol.* **16,** 284

STEINER, F. A., SIEBENMANN, R. E., SANDRI, C. and HEDINGER C. (1957). *Experientia,* **13,** 500

STONE, C. S., WENGER, H. D., LUDDEN, C. T., STAVORSKI, J. and ROSS, C. A. (1961). *J. Pharmacol. exp. Ther.* **131,** 73

SULLIVAN, T. J. (1960). *Brit. J. Pharmacol.* **15,** 513

SULLIVAN, T. J. (1961). *Brit. J. Pharmacol.* **16,** 90

SZARA, S. (1957). In 'Psychotropic drugs'. Ed. Garratini and Ghetti. Amsterdam: Elsevier

SZARA, S. (1961). *Experientia (Base)*, **17**, 76

TEDESCHI, D. H., TEDESCHI, R. E. and FELLOWS, E. J. (1959). *J. Pharmacol. exp. Ther.* **126**, 223

THORSON, A., BIÖRCK, G., BJÖRKMAN, G. and WALDENSTRÖM, J. (1954). *Amer. Heart J.* **47**, 795

TRENDELENBURG, U. (1957). *J. Physiol.* **135**, 66; *Brit. J. Pharmacol.* **12**, 79

TURNER, W. J. and MERLIS, S. (1959). *Arch. Neurol. Psychiat. (Chicago)*, **81**, 121

TWAROG, B. M. and PAGE, I. H. (1953). *Amer. J. Physiol.* **175**, 157

TWAROG, B. M. (1960). *J. Physiol.* **152**, 236

UDENFRIEND, S. (1957). In '5-hydroxytryptamine'. Ed. Lewis. London: Pergamon

UDENFRIEND, S., TITUS, E. and WEISSBACH, H. (1955). *J. biol. Chem.* **216**, 499

UDENFRIEND, S. and WEISSBACH, H. (1958). *Proc. Soc. exp. Biol. (N.Y.)* **97**, 748

UDENFRIEND, S., WEISSBACH, J. and CLARK, C. T. (1955a). *J. biol. Chem.* **215**, 337

UDENFRIEND, S., WEISSBACH, J. and CLARK, C. T. (1955b). *Science*, **122**, 972

VANE, J. R. (1957). *Brit. J. Pharmacol.* **12**, 344

VANE, J. R. (1959). *Brit. J. Pharmacol.* **14**, 87

VOGT, M., GUNN, C. G. and SAWYER, C. H. (1957). *Neurology*, **7**, 559

WAALKES, T. P., SJOERDSMA, A., CREVELING, C. R., WEISSBACH, H. and UDENFRIEND, S. (1958). *Science*, **127**, 649

WALASZEK, E. J. and ABOOD, L. G. (1957). *Fed. Proc.* **16**, 133

WALDENSTRÖM, J., PERNOW, B. and SILWER, H. (1956). *Acta med. scand.* **156**, 73

WEISSBACH, H., LOVENBERG, W., REDFIELD, B. G. and UDENFRIEND, S. (1961). *J. Pharmacol. exp. Ther.* **131**, 26

WELSH, J. J. and MOORHEAD, M. (1960). *J. Neurochem.* **6**, 146

WEST, G. B. (1960). *J. Pharm. (Lond.)*, **12**, 768

WIEDMANN, H., TAESCHLER, M. and KONZETT, H. (1958). *Experientia (Basel)*, **14**, 378

WIELAND, T. and MOTZEL, W. (1953). *Liebigs Ann. Chem.* **581**, 10

WILSON, C. W. M. and BRODIE, B. B. (1961). *J. Pharmacol. exp. Ther.* **133**, 332

WOOLEY, D. W. (1959). *Biochem. Pharmacol.* **3**, 51

YUWEILER, A., GELLER, E. and EIDSUN, S. (1959). *Arch. Biochem.* **80**, 162

ZBINDEN, G., PLETSCHER, A. and STUDER, A. (1958). *Z. ges. exp. Med.* **129**, 615

CHAPTER 5

PHARMACOLOGICALLY ACTIVE PEPTIDES

(Kinins, Angiotensin, Substance P, Oxytocin and Vasopressin)

This chapter deals with a number of peptides of relatively simple structure which are either stored or formed in tissues. They are of considerable interest from a pharmacological point of view since their biological potencies are as great as those of acetylcholine or adrenaline. As yet, physiological roles can be ascribed with reasonable certainty only to oxytocin and vasopressin. The recent progress in the isolation and synthesis of these peptides, however, will undoubtedly accelerate the discovery of their significance in physiology and pathology. (Insulin and glucagon are discussed in chapter 6.)

KININS

The term kinin refers to a group of peptides, all of which are probably simple straight chain compounds, possibly with minor differences in structure. Kinin is released from a protein in plasma by a number of enzymes such as kallikrein and trypsin, and also occurs in a free or active form in certain venoms such as those of the wasp or hornet. Minute amounts lower the arterial blood pressure, contract most isolated smooth muscles and increase capillary permeability.

The study of kinins dates back to 1937 when it was shown by Werle, Götze and Keppler that kallikrein releases an active substance from an inactive precursor in plasma (Werle et al., 1937). This observation was made shortly after it was recognized that renin owed its hypertensive activity to the release of hypertensin from a globulin in plasma, and the early workers recognized the analogy between the action of kallikrein and renin (Werle et al., 1943).

KALLIKREIN AND KALLIDIN

The kallikreins are enzymes present in an active form in saliva and urine, and in an inactive form in pancreas, blood and intestine. The inactive form, kallikreinogen, is activated by changes in H^+ concentration, by proteolytic enzymes, or by acetone, presumably by the dissociation of an inactivating molecule from kallikrein (Frey et al., 1950). Recently, a similar enzyme has been found in an active form in high concentrations in the accessory sex glands of the guinea-pig (Bhoola et al., 1961). The different kallikreins display some chemical differences, particularly in their susceptibility to inactivation by various inhibitors, but they are all vasodilator agents, a property due to kallidin, the active peptide which they release from a protein in the α-2 globulin fraction of plasma (Werle, 1955, 1960). It is now known that the kallikreins possess a powerful esterolytic action on certain synthetic substrates (arginyl methyl esters) (Haberman, 1959; Contzen *et al.*, 1959; Werle and Kaufmann-Boetsch, 1960) but the exact nature of the bond which is split when kallidin is released from its natural substrate in plasma remains to be established.

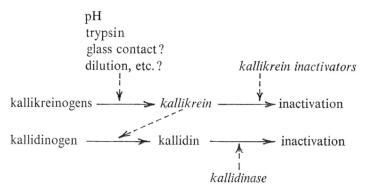

FIG. 17. Kallikrein-kallidin system in plasma.

The active substance released by kallikrein was shown to have all the pharmacological properties of kallikrein *in vivo*, and it was named substance DK (Darm kontrahierende Substanz), because unlike kallikrein, it also contracted many isolated smooth muscle preparations *in vitro*, in Tyrode's or Locke's solution (Werle *et al.*, 1937; Frey *et al.*, 1950; Werle, 1955). In 1948, Werle and Berek suggested that the name Substance DK be changed to kallidin, and that its precursor (or substrate for kallikrein) should be called kallidinogen (Werle and Berek, 1948).

The kallikrein system in blood is a complex one. Two similar, but distinct enzymes, exist as inactive precursors (kallikreinogens). In addition, there are two circulating kallikrein inactivators, and also a kallidinase, which inactivates kallidin (Frey *et al.*, 1950; Schachter, 1960). This system (Fig. 17), therefore, appears to be analogous in complexity to the enzymes involved in blood coagulation and clot lysis.

TRYPSIN AND BRADYKININ

In 1949, Rocha e Silva, Beraldo and Rosenfeld described the release of an active peptide from serum globulin by trypsin or snake venoms. They named the peptide bradykinin, because it caused a relatively slow contraction of the isolated guinea-pig ileum (Rocha e Silva *et al.*, 1949). (The contraction takes approximately 5 times as long to reach its maximum as it does when produced by acetylcholine or by histamine).

Although these workers distinguished this substance from acetylcholine, histamine, adenosine and other active substances (including kallikrein) known to be present in tissues, they were apparently unaware that kallikrein had already been shown to release a smooth muscle stimulant, substance DK (or kallidin) from a precursor in plasma. It is now apparent, however, that the peptides released by these different agents probably arise from the same substrate, and that the peptides themselves are closely related, if not identical (Mathias and Schachter, 1958; Schachter, 1960; Pierce and Webster, 1961).

TERMINOLOGY

It is unfortunate that smooth muscle stimulating peptides which were never distinguished from kallidin, were given new names (bradykinin, plasma kinin, pain-producing substance, urine kinin, etc.). The situation is complicated, however, by the fact (as described later) that these kallidin-like substances develop in plasma under a variety of conditions, and also exist in a free form in urine and other fluids. The formulation of a standard terminology will probably be made easier when the chemical structures of a number of these compounds are established and it becomes evident whether there is one or more molecular prototype.

In this review, the name kallidin or bradykinin is used when the peptide is released by the kallikreins or by trypsin (and snake venoms) respectively. The generic term, kinin, is used for kallidin-like peptides which develop in plasma or other fluids under various other conditions.

PROPERTIES OF KALLIDIN AND BRADYKININ

The different kallidins (released by the various kallikreins) and bradykinin (released by trypsin and snake venom) are undoubtedly all closely related or identical peptides (Mathias and Schachter, 1958; Schachter, 1960; Pierce and Webster, 1961). At present, only bradykinin released by trypsin from ox serum globulin and the kallidin released from human plasma by human urinary kallikrein have been isolated and their structures determined. These are described below. It is not improbable that the kinins will have minor variations in structure when prepared from serum or plasma of different mammals as is the case with vasopressin (du Vigneaud et al., 1953) and also with angiotensin (Elliott and Peart, 1956; Skeggs et al., 1956).

Pharmacology. Kallidin and bradykinin contract most isolated smooth muscle preparations such as the intestine of the guinea-pig, rabbit, cat and dog, but *relax* the duodenum of the rat. They are also all powerful vasodilators and also markedly increase capillary permeability (Rocha e Silva, 1960; Bhoola et al., 1960; Konzett and Stürmer, 1960; Elliott et al., 1960). The isolated rat uterus, though one of the most sensitive test preparations *in vitro*, is practically unaffected by brady-kinin *in vivo* (Berde and Saameli, 1961). Kallidin and bradykinin pro-duce bronchoconstriction in the guinea-pig on intravenous injection (Collier *et al.*, 1960; Bhoola, 1961) and contract the isolated tracheal chain of this animal, but fail to contract isolated bronchial muscle of dog or man (Bhoola *et al.*, unpublished). Bradykinin produces pain when applied to a blister base on human skin (Armstrong *et al.*, 1957). The potency of pure natural or synthetic bradykinin is of the same order as acetylcholine or oxytocin (Konzett *et al.*, 1960).

It is of interest that the bronchoconstrictor action of bradykinin in the guinea-pig is specifically suppressed by relatively small doses of acetylsalicylic acid, calcium acetylsalicylate, phenylbutazone, amido-pyrine and antipyrine (Collier *et al.*, 1960; Collier and Shorley, 1960). It has also been reported that phenylbutazone antagonizes the hypo-tensive action of bradykinin in the rabbit (Lecomte, 1959). However, none of these drugs specifically antagonized the actions of kallidin or bradykinin on capillary permeability or on isolated smooth muscles (Schachter, unpublished). Effective and specific antagonists, when avail-able, will help greatly in assessing the possible physiological or patho-logical role of these peptides.

Chemistry of bradykinin. Recently, Elliott, Lewis and Horton reported the isolation of pure bradykinin (trypsin on ox serum) by a combination of countercurrent fractionation, chromatography on carboxymethyl-cellulose, and paper electrophoresis. They concluded that it was an octapeptide containing the following amino acids in the molar propor-tions indicated—serine (1), glycine (1), phenylalanine (2), proline (2), and arginine (2) (Elliott *et al.*, 1960). Degradation analysis led them to conclude that this octapeptide had the structure H.Arg-Pro-Pro-Gly-Phe-Ser-Phe-Arg.OH. This compound was quickly synthesized and found, however, to be practically inactive (Boissonnas *et al.*, 1960; Schwyzer *et al.*, 1960). Boissonnas and his colleagues also synthesized a number of compounds related to this octapeptide and found that a nonapeptide with the same structure, but including an additional pro-line molecule in position 7, viz. H.Arg-Pro-Pro-Gly-Phe-Ser-Pro-Phe-Arg.OH, possessed potent bradykinin-like activity (Boissonnas *et al.*, 1960). Elliott and colleagues therefore re-examined their data and concluded that the natural bradykinin was in fact a nonapeptide with this structure (Elliott *et al.*, 1960). All the pharmacological properties previously described for impure preparations of bradykinin have been shown to reside in this nonapeptide (Konzett *et al.*, 1960).

Chemistry of kallidin. While this review was being written, Pierce and Webster (1961), in a preliminary report, described the isolation of kallidin released from human plasma by human urinary kallikrein. According to these workers, the incubation of urinary kallikrein and human plasma resulted in the release of 2 kallidins—one (kallidin I) identical with bradykinin (which is described above), and another (kallidin II) which had the same structure, but with an additional lysine molecule in the N-terminal position, i.e., a decapeptide (Pierce and Webster, 1961). Werle and his colleagues have also determined the structure of kallidin prepared by the action of salivary kallikrein on ox serum and found that it was the above decapeptide. They found that 8–10% only of the activity was due to the nonapeptide and concluded that the latter substance was not released by salivary kallikrein, but formed by enzymes in plasma during the preparation of the substrate by acidification (Werle, Trautschold and Leysath, 1961).

RELEASE OF KININ BY FOREIGN SURFACE, DILUTION, AND VARIOUS ENZYMES

In addition to the various kallikreins (in salivary gland, pancreas, blood, urine and intestine) and trypsin which release kallidin or brady-kinin from plasma, the release of a similar substance (kinin) by various physical or chemical processes has been recently demonstrated. These processes are briefly described below.

Human plasma rapidly generates a kinin on contact with glass (Armstrong *et al.*, 1957). Since this kinin produced pain when applied to a blister base on human skin it was called PPS (pain producing sub-stance). Anticoagulants such as heparin, citrate, or oxalate, do not prevent this 'activation' of plasma. PPS has so far not been distinguish-able from kallidin or bradykinin (Gaddum and Horton, 1959). Margolis found that plasma kinin does not develop when plasma of patients with Hageman trait (a condition characterized by a greatly prolonged clotting time in glass, but in which there is no abnormal tendency to bleeding) comes in contact with glass (Margolis, 1960). He attributes this kinin formation to activation of a substance which he called component A (or contact factor) and suggests that in the absence of Hageman factor, component A cannot be activated. The reader is referred to Margolis's article for details. Schachter has suggested that activated component A is closely related to, if not identical with serum kallikrein (Schachter, 1960).

Dilution. Serum or plasma of many mammals (especially ox and guinea-pig) rapidly develops kinin activity on dilution with Tyrode's solution (Schachter, 1956, 1960). Since this effect is prevented by soya bean trypsin inhibitor, or by heating plasma for 3 hours at 56–60°C., the release of kinin may be due to activation of serum kallikreinogen which then releases kallidin from its substrate in plasma.

Plasmin (or fibrinolysin) is a proteolytic enzyme which dissolves fibrin, and which exists in plasma as an inactive precursor, plasminogen; there are also several circulating inactivators of plasmin (antiplasmins) in plasma. Activators of plasminogen are present in urine and in extracts of many tissues. The activation of plasminogen results in increased fibrinolytic activity of plasma and occurs *in vivo* in physical (burns, haemorrhage) and emotional stress, and after injection of adrenaline. Activation *in vitro* may be brought about by dilution of plasma, by the addition of alcohol, ether or chloroform, or by various bacterial enzymes. Like kallikrein, plasmin with its precursor and inactivators, is part of a complex system analogous to that involved in blood coagulation. Plasmin is distinguishable from trypsin or kallikrein.

Various authors have claimed that plasmin is a potent releaser of kinin (Beraldo, 1950; Rocha e Silva, 1955; Lewis, 1958, 1959). It has been suggested, therefore, that conditions such as shock, adrenaline-induced vasodilatation, reactive hyperaemia, etc., which are accompanied by increased fibrinolytic activity in plasma, are due to kinin released by plasmin (Hilton, 1960). However, in experiments in which plasmin, trypsin, and serum kallikrein were compared, no correlation was found between the fibrinolytic activity of these substances and their ability to release kinin from plasma (Bhoola *et al.*, 1960). In fact, human plasmin, which was the most potent fibrinolytic agent, failed to release kinin from human plasma on incubation for periods up to 2 minutes; plasmin also failed to increase capillary permeability in guinea-pigs, a prominent property of kinin and kinin-releasing enzymes. It is likely, therefore, that kallikrein, and not plasmin, is the enzyme activated when there is a rapid release of kinin (Bhoola *et al.*, 1960).

Sweat. Human sweat has been shown to release a kinin from dog pseudoglobulin; also, when the subcutaneous space of the human forearm was perfused, kinin appeared in the perfusate when the body temperature was raised by heating the trunk and legs of the subject (Fox and Hilton, 1958). These authors concluded that the kinin was formed by an enzyme in sweat, and that it could fully account for the active dilatation of blood vessels which occurs during sweating. This conclusion, in our opinion, is not yet adequately warranted. Firstly, the above workers showed that human sweat released a kinin from dog pseudoglobulin. Human sweat, however, is a poor releaser when *human* plasma is used as a substrate and the guinea-pig ileum is the test preparation (Schachter, unpublished). Since some enzymes release a kinin from plasma of some animals but not from that of others (Schachter, 1960), it is necessary to show that human sweat is an effective releaser of kinin from human plasma; also, that this 'kinin' not only contracts isolated smooth muscles but does, in fact, dilate blood vessels.

Cerebrospinal fluid. In a series of recent papers it has been claimed that a kinin releasing enzyme, and kinin itself, appear in the cerebrospinal fluid of patients during migraine attacks and other neurological disturbances (Chapman et al, 1959, 1960). The CSF of normal dogs and monkeys, however, contains neither kinin nor kinin releasing enzymes (Schachter, unpublished). Chapman and colleagues maintain further, that kinin is released during the triple response induced by histamine in human skin, and also, after antidromic stimulation of dorsal nerve roots. Such striking observations must be confirmed, and precautions taken to ascertain that an increase in the concentration of kinin in perfusates or in body fluids is not secondary to vasodilatation, alteration in permeability, or to 'spontaneous' formation of kinin when body fluids come in contact with glass or are diluted (Schachter, 1960; Armstrong et al., 1957).

Permeability globulins (G-2). The permeability globulins (Miles and Wilhelm, 1960) are included here, because, in our opinion, they are identical with serum kallikrein and probably exert their permeability increasing action by the release of kallidin. The ether fractionation method used in the preparation of G-2 (permeability globulin) would activate serum kallikrein (Frey et al., 1950); also, the hypotensive activity, the permeability enhancing actions, and the sensitivity of G-2 and serum kallikrein (acetone activated) to inhibitors are identical. Keele and colleagues have in fact found that G-2 releases a kinin from plasma (Armstrong et al., 1957) although Lewis (1958) states that purified G-2 fails to do so. The latter negative finding may well be due to the possibility that plasma kininase is concentrated together with G-2, so that kinin release would not be apparent (due to rapid destruction) if G-2 is incubated with substrate for several minutes before testing the mixture for kinin.

Accessory sex glands. A powerful kinin releasing enzyme has recently been demonstrated in the coagulating and prostate glands of the guinea-pig (Bhoola et al., 1961). The kinin released by this enzyme closely resembles bradykinin, but shows some slight, though possibly significant differences in parallel pharmacological tests. Whereas extracts of guinea-pig coagulating and prostate glands release kinin from guinea-pig plasma and from that of rabbit, cat, dog and man, similar extracts from the prostate gland of these other mammals fail to release kinin. The kinin releasing system, therefore, cannot be a general mechanism regulating blood flow in the prostate gland. More likely, it has a function in the reproductive tract of the guinea-pig. Its ability to release a kinin from plasma is perhaps even irrelevant to its physiological role. The latter statement is supported by the fact that the kinin releasing enzyme in guinea-pig submaxillary gland releases kinin from the plasma of other mammals but not from its own (Schachter 1960).

Serum. A kinin releasing enzyme present in an *active* form in serum (man, ox) becomes evident when serum is incubated with the colostrum of women or cows (Guth, 1959; Werle, 1960). In this case the enzyme is in the serum and the substrate in colostrum. The substrate (kininogen) increases in cow colostrum for about 6 days after calving and decreases slowly from the 10th day for several weeks. The significance of these findings is not known.

KININS PRESENT IN FREE (OR ACTIVE) FORM

The kinins described above do not exist in tissues in an active form but are released (by the splitting of a chemical bond) from an inactive protein precursor in plasma or lymph. There are kinins, however, which exist in the free or active form in mammalian urine and in certain venoms. These are described briefly below.

Urinary kinin. The presence of a kinin-like substance in human urine was first described by Werle and Erdös (1954). Because they thought it differed slightly from kallidin they called it substance Z. Gaddum and Horton re-named it urinary kinin because they could not distinguish it from other kinins (Gaddum and Horton, 1959). Studies on the excretion of this kinin showed that it did not vary with changes in pH of urine (pH 5·5–7·3), or with urine secretion rate (0·26–18 ml./hr.). Also, the amount of urinary kinin excreted did not vary significantly during salivation (pilocarpine induced) or sweating (Horton, 1959). The origin or urinary kinin is not known.

Venom kinins. A kinin exists in wasp venom (*V. vulgaris*) in high concentrations together with histamine and 5-hydroxytryptamine (Jaques and Schachter, 1954; Schachter and Thain, 1954). It is pharmacologically indistinguishable from kallidin or bradykinin, but can be distinguished readily from them by paper or column chromatography, and by its inactivation by trypsin as well as by chymotrypsin (Mathias and Schachter, 1958; Holdstock *et al.*, 1957). Hornet venom (*V. crabro*) contains huge amounts of acetylcholine, together with 5-hydroxytryptamine, histamine, and a kinin which closely resembles kallidin and bradykinin, but which is distinguishable from them (and from wasp kinin) by being relatively less active on the isolated guinea-pig ileum (Bhoola *et al.*, 1961). The activity of partially purified preparations of wasp kinin suggests that this peptide is even more active than bradykinin (Holdstock *et al.*, 1957). There is no doubt that the venom kinins contribute to the inflammatory reactions resulting from stings inflicted by these insects. As yet, these kinins are the only ones which have been distinguished from kallidin and bradykinin.

POSSIBLE PHYSIOLOGICAL AND PATHOLOGICAL ROLES OF KININS

Because enzymes which release kinins are present in blood and various glandular organs, and because the substrate (or kinin precursor) is often present in blood and lymph, there have been many suggestions for their roles in physiology and pathology. The pharmacological properties of the kinins and of the enzymes which release them are such that they could participate in blood-flow regulation, inflammatory reactions, allergic phenomena, etc. These possibilities which have been critically discussed above will be subject to more crucial tests if specific antagonists of kinins become available. At present, drugs such as aspirin antagonize only the bronchoconstrictor action of bradykinin. It is of interest, therefore, that whereas antihistamine drugs greatly suppress anaphylactic bronchospasm in the guinea-pig, aspirin is without effect (Collier and Shorley, 1960).

The kinin releasing enzymes appear in high concentrations in various glandular secretions (e.g. saliva, pancreatic juice), and the possibility that they may have an exocrine function analagous to other enzymes of the gastrointestinal tract has received too little attention. The kallikreins have powerful esterolytic activity on synthetic substrates and they may have specific functions in the alimentary canal. The possibility must be considered also, that in some instances, the ability of an enzyme to release a kinin is irrelevant to its physiological action.

Other aspects of the kallikrein system in plasma which might be rewarding to study are those clinical conditions associated with oedema or urticaria, particularly those of a hereditary nature. It is well known that various disturbances (haemophilia, Christmas disease, etc.) are associated with the absence of a particular plasma protein. It would be of considerable interest if some diseases were associated with the absence of serum kallikrein, its circulating inactivators, or its precursor.

The revival of interest in the kallikreins and in similar kinin-releasing systems in the last 10 years has been rewarding towards understanding the chemistry, biochemistry, and pharmacology of these agents. It is likely that a better understanding of their roles in physiology and pathology will be achieved in the next decade.

ANGIOTENSIN

Angiotensin (hypertensin, angiotonin), like kallidin, is a polypeptide derived from an inactive precursor (angiotensinogen) belonging to the α-2 globulin fraction of plasma. It is considered to be the most powerful hypertensive substance known (Pickering, 1960). The enzyme, renin, which releases angiotensin from angiotensinogen was discovered in kidney extracts by Tigerstedt and Bergmann (1898), but it was not until 1940 that it was shown that its hypertensive action was indirect, that is, that it was due to angiotensin released by renin (Braun-Menendez *et al.*, 1940). Since then much has been learned of the biochemical properties of the renin-angiotensinogen system, the structures of angiotensins of different animals have been determined and synthesized (Skeggs *et al.*,

1956; Elliott and Peart, 1956; Rittel *et al.*, 1957), and their pharmacological properties have been studied in detail. The physiological and pathological significance of angiotensin remains, however, highly controversial.

RENIN AND ANGIOTENSIN

No interest was taken in renin from 1898 until 1934 when Goldblatt and his colleagues produced hypertension experimentally in animals by partial obstruction of the main renal arteries. The possible relevance of this observation to human hypertension was a new stimulus to research.

Renin has now been precisely located in the kidney. Cook and Pickering injected particles of magnetic iron oxide into the renal arteries of rabbits and then selectively removed the particles from a suspension of minced kidney cortex with an electro-magnet. The magnetic fraction consisted almost entirely of glomeruli; the non-magnetic, of tubules. By histological study and bio-assay they found that the highest concentrations of renin were in the outer glomeruli, less in the inner ones, and least in the tubules. They conclude that renin is located very close to the glomeruli, possibly in the juxtaglomerular cells described by Goormatigh (1944).

An effective substrate for renin, a tetradecapeptide containing 10 *different* amino acids, has been obtained by Skeggs and his colleagues by degrading angiotensinogen with trypsin. They have also verified the structure of this tetradecapeptide by synthesis and have shown that renin acts on its substrate between two leucine residues, a property not

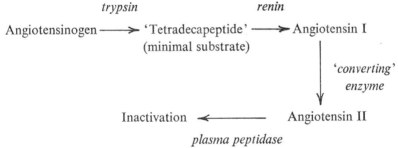

FIG. 18. Renin-angiotensin system.

known for any other enzyme. This action of renin yields angiotensin I, a decapeptide with the structure H.Asp-Arg-Val-Tyr-*Ileu*-His-Pro-Phe-His-Leu.OH. Another enzyme in plasma, the 'converting' enzyme, splits the Phe-His residues yielding the resulting pressor octapeptide, angiotensin II. Angiotensin II is split into inactive amino acid complexes by another peptidase in plasma (Skeggs, 1960). These stages in the release and inactivation of angiotensin are illustrated in Fig. 18.

The above angiotensins I and II were isolated from horse serum. Angiotensin has also been isolated from ox serum and is identical with horse angiotensin I, except that the fifth amino acid in the chain is valine instead of isoleucine (Elliott and Peart, 1956). The natural angiotensins are therefore referred to as ileu$_5$-angiotensin I and II (horse) and val$_5$-angiotensin I (ox). These different angiotensins and their amides have now all been synthesized together with many related compounds, including the corresponding angiotensin II of ox serum, which has not yet been isolated in the natural state (Schwarz *et al.*, 1957; Schwyzer, 1960).

PHARMACOLOGICAL PROPERTIES

In man, the intravenous injection of angiotensin in a dose of 0·1 µg./kg. produces, within 25 seconds, a significant rise in blood pressure which lasts for 2–5 minutes. It is about 10 times as active as adrenaline on a weight basis, there is no tachyphylaxis as there is with other hypertensive drugs, and the increased blood pressure may be maintained for hours by continuous intravenous infusion. It falls again within 2–4 minutes after the infusion is stopped. The hypertensive action is unaffected by ganglion-blocking, sympatheticolytic, or tranquillizing drugs (Meier *et al.*, 1957). The infusion of as little as 0·005 µg./min. into the femoral artery reduces the blood flow in both skin and muscle (Bock *et al.*, 1958). Angiotensin also has marked renal effects and its intravenous infusion markedly reduces urine flow and the excretion of Na^+ and K^+. The antidiuretic effect is apparently not due to the release of vasopressin since it has been shown to occur in a patient with diabetes insipidus (Peart, 1960).

In animals (rat, rabbit, cat, dog) the angiotensins produce a sharp rise in blood pressure and the pharmacological effects are like those described above in man. The nephrectomized rat is considered to be the most suitable animal for assay and val$_5$-angiotensin II is about 20 times as active as noradrenaline on this preparation. In the rabbit and cat there is a brief stimulating action on the intestine and uterus *in situ* after the intravenous administration of angiotensin (Gross and Turrian, 1960).

POSSIBLE ROLE OF RENIN-ANGIOTENSIN SYSTEM

There is a marked difference of opinion regarding the physiological or pathological significance of angiotensin.

According to some workers renin normally regulates glomerular filtration and is released in renal ischaemia or damage, thus maintaining or increasing the renal arterial pressure and hence filtration rate. If the ischaemia is slight, the increased renal pressure resulting from the release of renin would readjust the flow of blood to the glomerulus, and the amount of renin released would be maintained at a new level, possibly insufficient to raise the systemic blood pressure. Skeggs suggests further, that if kidney function is sufficiently impaired, then renin is released in amounts adequate to result in a persistent marked elevation of the systemic blood pressure, and that this is in fact what occurs in human malignant hypertension. In a group of 18 patients with benign hypertension, Skeggs found the average concentration of angiotensin in blood to be twice that of a normal group, and in 11 patients with malignant hypertension the average concentration was 20 times that in normals (Skeggs, 1960).

Peart and his colleagues, however, have failed to find evidence of the release of renin in severe human hypertension, or in that produced in animals by renal ischaemia, even when blood was collected by a catheter inserted into the renal vein. Peart also contends that there is indirect evidence against angiotensin being responsible for human hypertension in that (a) whereas intravenous infusions of angiotensin reduce skin blood flow as the systemic pressure rises, in human renal hypertension skin blood flow is either normal or greater than normal, (b) whereas infusions of angiotensin reduce urine flow and electrolyte excretion as the blood pressure rises, in human hypertension there is an increased output of water and sodium (Peart, 1960). Gross and Turrian are also of the opinion that there is no convincing evidence that renin acts on angiotensinogen *in vivo*, and suggest that the hypertensive action of angiotensin may be a pharmacological property irrelevant to its physiological role (Gross and Turrian, 1960).

SUBSTANCE P

Substance P was discovered by Euler and Gaddum (1931) while assaying acetylcholine in tissue extracts. They found that various extracts, particularly those of intestine and brain, contracted the atropinized rabbit's intestine. The polypeptide nature of substance P was suggested when it was shown to be inactivated by trypsin (Euler, 1936). This has been confirmed by the recent isolation of substance P in a pure form (Franz *et al.*, 1961).

Substance P, like kallidin and bradykinin, stimulates most smooth muscle preparations and also dilates blood vessels. It can be distinguished readily from the kinins, however, by parallel, pharmacological tests. A particularly useful preparation is the isolated rat duodenum which relaxes in response to kinins, but contracts to substance P; another, is the hen rectal caecum which contracts in the presence of minute amounts of substance P, but is practically insensitive to other polypeptides (Horton, 1959). The contraction of the isolated goldfish intestine in a microbath has recently been described as a sensitive and fairly specific test for substance P (Gaddum and Szerb, 1961).

DISTRIBUTION OF SUBSTANCE P

The presence of substance P in the gastrointestinal tract and brain has been confirmed, and there is no conclusive evidence that it occurs in other tissues, except for the retina, which contains high concentrations (Duner *et al.*, 1954). It is present in the wall of the entire digestive tract of many mammals (monkey—500 U/g>dog>horse>cattle>rat> guinea-pig>sheep>cat>pig—5 U/g). The highest concentrations are always found in the duodenum and jejunum, with progressively decreasing amounts from the jejunum to the ileum; the muscularis mucosae appears to contain more per gram of tissue than any other layer of the gut wall (Douglas *et al.*, 1951; Pernow, 1955; Amin *et al.*, 1954). There is also evidence of a correlation between the occurrence of ganglion cells in the intestine and substance P (Ehrenpreis and Pernow, 1953).

It is present in all parts of the central nervous system of mammals, but the concentrations in different regions vary over a range of more than 100 fold (see p. 2 and p. 33). Thus, the approximate amounts of substance P in units per gram in different parts of the human central nervous system is: substantia nigra (500–1000), ala cinerea (200–400), inferior colliculus (100–200), superior colliculus (40–80). However, the optic tract, corpus callosum, pyramids, olive and lateral geniculate body have less than 10 units per gram (Gaddum, 1960). Those areas of the central nervous system which contain relatively high concentrations of substance P contain little or no acetylcholine and choline acetylase, and this has given rise to the suggestion that it may be a non-cholinergic transmitter, in particular, that it is the chemical transmitter liberated by the first sensory neurone (Lembeck, 1953; Gaddum, 1960).

Substance P occurs in many vertebrates. It is present in the brain and intestine of fish, and its distribution in the brain of the dogfish is similar to that of mammals (Correale, 1959; Grabner *et al.*, 1959).

PHARMACOLOGICAL PROPERTIES

The main actions of substance P studied so far are its ability to contract intestinal and to relax vascular smooth muscle (Pernow, 1960). If administered systemically or intraventricularly it produces marked 'sedation', which along with its anti-convulsant action is considered to be an action on the central nervous system (Zetler, 1960).

According to some workers substance P acts on intestinal muscle in two ways. Firstly, by a 'direct' action on the muscle, and also, by stimulating the afferent nerve fibres which evoke the peristaltic reflex (Pernow, 1960). This view is based on the fact that substance P administered intraluminally elicits reflex intestinal peristalsis (prevented by hexamethonium), which fails to occur if the mucous membrane is removed (Beleslin and Varagic, 1958). Kosterlitz has shown, however, that the peristaltic reflex evoked by distension of the intestine, unlike that caused by substance P, is unaffected by hexamethonium (Kosterlitz, 1960). Endogenous substance P, therefore, cannot play an indispensable physiological role in the peristaltic reflex.

Substance P possesses powerful vasodilator activity, particularly in man and rabbit, although it is also active in the cat and dog (Pernow, 1960; Erspamer, 1961). Since the pure peptide contains 30,000–35,000 units/mg. (Franz et al., 1961), it may be calculated from the results of Erspamer that 0·006–0·02 μg./kg. injected intravenously will produce hypotension in the dog, and that 0·02–0·01 μg./kg./min. will cause marked vasodilatation in man (Erspamer, 1961).

The significance of effects of substance P such as sedation, potentiation of anaesthesia, anti-convulsant action, etc., which it exerts when administered in large amounts, and which are attributed to an action on the central nervous system (Zetler, 1960), is not clear. The preparations of substance P used for this purpose were extremely impure (9–17 units/kg.), and very large amounts were administered (up to 9000 units). The possibility cannot be disregarded that some of these effects are due to hypotension or to other active substances in the crude preparations.

CHEMISTRY OF SUBSTANCE P

Boissonnas and his colleagues have recently reported the isolation of substance P from horse intestine. Chromatographic purification was carried out on successive columns of the ion-exchange resins IR-45 and IRC-50, and on aluminium oxide and carboxymethylcellulose. Hydrolysis of the active material yielded large amounts of arginine and proline, but unlike bradykinin it also contained leucine, isoleucine and alanine. From preliminary degradation studies it was concluded that it was a straight-chain peptide, and unlike bradykinin, does not possess the C-terminal Phe-Arg.OH grouping (Franz et al., 1961).

FUNCTION OF SUBSTANCE P

It is at present impossible to ascribe a particular function to substance P. However, its potency and consistent presence in the intestine and nervous tissue of a wide variety of animals, suggests that it is of physiological significance.

OXYTOCIN AND VASOPRESSIN

In 1895 Oliver and Schäfer showed that injections of extracts of the pituitary gland markedly raised the blood pressure. By 1910 it was known that the substance which produced this effect was in the posterior part of the gland; also, that such extracts contracted uterine and other muscles, produced antidiuresis, and caused the ejection of milk from the lactating mammary gland (Berde, 1959). Approximately 20 years elapsed, however, before it became clear that these effects were due to specific substances other than histamine, and were, in fact, due to 2 substances—oxytocin and vasopressin (Kamm *et al.*, 1928). In 1953, when the isolation and synthesis of oxytocin and vasopressin was accomplished (du Vigneaud *et al.*, 1953; Tuppy, 1953), it was at last possible to ascertain which activities were due to oxytocin and which to vasopressin. Unlike the other peptides discussed in this chapter, there is some general agreement in ascribing certain physiological roles to them.

CHEMISTRY OF OXYTOCIN AND VASOPRESSIN

Oxytocin and vasopressin are octapeptide amides and both have a 20 membered ring with 5 amino acids, and a side chain with 3 amino acids (du Vigneaud *et al.*, 1953; Tuppy, 1953). Vasopressin differs from oxytocin only in 2 of its amino acids. Thus it has phenylalanine instead of *iso*leucine in the ring structure, and arginine instead of leucine in the side chain (Fig. 19). Vasopressin from hog pituitary, lysine vaso-pressin, contains lysine instead of arginine in the side chain; arginine vasopressin is the hormone in man, ox, camel, dog, sheep, rabbit and rat (van Dyke *et al.*, 1955).

CyS—Tyr—**Ileu**—Glu(NH$_2$)—Asp(NH$_2$)—CyS—Pro—**Leu**—Gly(NH$_2$)

Oxytocin

CyS—Tyr—**Phe**—Glu(NH$_2$)—Asp(NH$_2$)—CyS—Pro—**Lys**—Gly(NH$_2$)

Lys$_8$–Vasopressin

CyS—Tyr—**Phe**—Glu(NH$_2$)—Asp(NH$_2$)—CyS—Pro—**Arg**—Gly(NH$_2$)

Arg$_8$–Vasopressin

CyS—Tyr—**Ileu**—Glu(NH$_2$)—Asp(NH$_2$)—CyS—Pro—**Arg**—Gly(NH$_2$)

Arginine Vasotocin

1   2   3   4   5   6   7   8   9

FIG. 19. Structures of the known natural neurohypophysial hormones.

The availability of synthetic oxytocin and vasopressin has now made it possible to establish quantitatively the different pharmacological actions of each substance. As might be expected from their structural similarity there is in fact considerable overlap in their properties, and this is illustrated quantitatively in Fig. 20. Thus, a more basic group in position 8 increases the relative vasopressor activity of the molecule, whereas a less basic group, in that position enhances the relative oxytocic activity (Boissonnas, 1960). A compound with the ring structure of oxytocin and the side-chain of arginine vasopressin was synthesized by Katsoyannis and du Vigneaud (1958) with the view that its properties might provide insight into the structure/activity relationships of these peptides. This substance, called arginine vasotocin (Fig. 19), has both marked vasopressor and oxytocic activities— approximately 25% and 10% of the respective activities of arginine vasopressin and oxytocin (Katsoyannis and du Vigneaud, 1958). It has

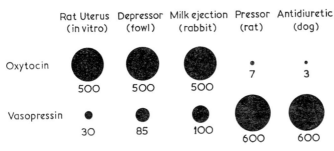

FIG. 20. Relative potencies of oxytocin and vasopressin in different tests. Black surface areas are proportional to potency in terms of the U.S.P. standard (after Berde, 1959).

recently been claimed that arginine vasotocin is actually present in the neurohypophysis of non-mammalian vertebrates (Heller, 1960). If this is the case, the peptide was synthesized before its existence in nature was known.

Oxytocin and vasopressin are inactivated by a variety of fluids and tissue homogenates. According to Hooper, oxytocinase and vasopressinase are different enzymes. Using human placental homogenates as a source of these enzymes he found that the enzyme destroying oxytocin was present in the soluble fraction, whilst the enzyme destroying vasopressin was predominantly in the mitochondrial and microsomal fractions (Hooper, 1960).

FORMATION AND RELEASE

Formation. It is now known, that the neurohypophysial hormones are secreted by neurones in the hypothalamus. The production of these hormones in the CNS is called neurosecretion. It appears that oxytocin and vasopressin are actually produced in the anterior hypothalamus and are merely stored in the neurohypophysis.

Experiments by Scharrer (1959) and by Bergmann (1958) have shown (in both invertebrates and vertebrates) that certain hypothalamic neurones produce granules of neurosecretion which are transported along the axons at a rate of about 3 mm./day. These granules are selectively stained by Gomori's chrome-alum-haematoxylin-phloxin reagent which shows that the supraoptic and paraventricular nuclei contain abundant neurosecretory material. The latter granules can be traced along the supraoptico-hypophysial axons to their endings within the neurohypophysis. These nerve endings are normally distended with stored neurosecretion which is massed around the capillaries of the neurohypophysis. Electron microscopy studies of the hypothalamo-neurohypophysial tract show that the axons contain dense granules of 600–3000 Å diameter (Green and Maxwell, 1959) which are probably the same neurosecretory granules which stain for light microscopy with Gomori's reagent. Appropriate physiological stimulation, e.g. prolonged thirst after water deprivation, depletes both the stainable granules and the content of assayable oxytocin and vasopressin (Sawyer and Roth, 1953; Scharrer and Scharrer, 1954). The ultracentrifugation of homogenates of neurohypophysial tissue shows that the oxytocic and vasopressor activities are associated with subcellular particles which are consistent in size and appearance with the dense granules seen in the axons with the electron microscope (Scharrer and Scharrer, 1954).

Oxytocin and vasopressin are thought to exist in a loose association with a 'carrier' protein which is probably the substance stained by Gomori's reagent. Since these peptides can be released by procedures such as dialysis against 0·1N acetic acid, electrodialysis, precipitation of the protein with trichloracetic acid, etc., it is very unlikely that they are held to a protein carrier by peptide bonds (Acher and Fromageot, 1957).

Release. Release of oxytocin and vasopressin occurs under many conditions. Amongst these are electrical stimulation of the supraoptico-hypophysial tract, dilatation of the uterus, suckling or mechanical stimulation of the teats, coitus, dehydration or increased osmolarity of plasma, after injection of acetylcholine, nicotine and other drugs, and haemorrhage (Berde, 1959). The evidence indicates that oxytocin and vasopressin are invariably released together, but not always in the same relative concentrations. The amount of oxytocin released is always greater than that of vasopressin, irrespective of the nature of the stimulus; this ratio, however, may vary from 4:1 after electrical stimulation of the hypothalamus to 100:1 during suckling (Harris, 1955).

The quantitative measurement of oxytocin and vasopressin release is a serious problem because of the lack of specificity of assay procedures. One method is to use the same animal as the source of oxytocin or vasopressin release and also for assay of the released hormones. Assay is performed by recording contractions of the animal's uterus or the rate of secretion of urine during release of the hormones. The effect produced on these organs may then be matched by injections of oxytocin and vasopressin. It is obvious that haemorrhage, for example, may result in the release of adrenaline, which will greatly influence the actions of simultaneously released pituitary hormones. Also, if blood is removed from an animal and then tested there are many other substances which may be present or which develop in shed blood which are oxytocic, or inhibit the action of oxytocin (e.g., kinins, 5-hydroxytryptamine, histamine and adrenaline are oxytocic; heparin and other substances reduce oxytocic activity).

The reader is referred to recent symposia for a critical assessment of the methods of assaying oxytocin and vasopressin in body fluids and tissues (Schachter, 1960; Heller and Caldeyro-Barcia, 1961).

PHARMACOLOGICAL PROPERTIES AND PHYSIOLOGICAL ROLE
Uterine contraction and milk ejection. It is now generally held that oxytocin plays a physiological role in parturition and in milk ejection during nursing.

There is a close similarity between the frequency, duration, and co-ordination of the uterine contractions following administration of minute amounts of oxytocin and those occurring in pregnancy (Caldeyro-Barcia and Poseiro, 1958), and there is also a marked increase in the sensitivity of the uterus to oxytocin at term (Fitzpatrick, 1957). Electrical stimulation of the supraoptico-hypothalamic tract in anaesthetized pregnant rabbits induces labour in a similar fashion to the intravenous administration of 50–200 mU of oxytocin (Cross, 1958). It is also of interest that the uterine reflex (evoked by dilatation of the uterus or cervix) which results in the release of oxytocin is readily elicited during labour or immediately post-partum, but not in non-pregannt animals (Cross, 1958).

There is much evidence that oxytocin also plays a physiological role in milk ejection. Only the milk in the large ducts of the lactating mammary gland can be extracted by the mechanical action of suckling or by milking. The greater part of the milk in the alveoli and finer ducts is, however, evacuated by the contractile action of the special myo-epithelial (or basket) cells which are of ectodermal origin. This forcing of milk into the large ducts is called 'let down' or milk ejection, and is accompanied by a rise of pressure in the mammary duct system. So sensitive is this reaction to oxytocin, that the intravenous injection of as little as 0·01 I.U. will produce a response in a lactating woman, and 0·00005 I.U. in a lactating rabbit (Berde and Cerletti, 1957). The latent period for the milk-ejection reaction in the rabbit is 7–15 seconds after intravenous injection of oxytocin, 13–25 seconds after electrical stimulation of the supraoptico-hypophysial tract, and 30–90 seconds after commencement of suckling (Harris and Pickles, 1953). These time relationships are in keeping with the reflex nature of oxytocin release and its subsequent humoral action on the myo-epithelial cells. Oxytocin may also have a true lactogenic effect since the involution of the mammary gland which occurs when a lactating mammal is deprived of its young can be delayed by injections of oxytocin (Benson and Folley, 1957).

Csapo (1961) has recently investigated the electrical and mechanical responses of uterine muscle exposed to oestrogens, progesterone, and to different ionic solutions. He suggests that Ca^{++} is the 'myoplasmic activator', and that oxytocin acts either as a Ca^{++} carrier resulting in the release of Ca^{++} from the myometrial muscle membrane, or that it modifies the distribution of membrane Ca^{++} by a special affinity for some component of the muscle membrane. He also observed that progesterone raised the membrane potential, and suggests that the progesterone treated uterus is resistant to oxytocin because progesterone causes Ca^{++} to be bound more firmly in the membrane. These results and the interpretation of them are, however, controversial (Kao, 1961).

Antidiuretic action. Vasopressin is now generally regarded as a hormone which is released during dehydration and other conditions, thus regulating water balance.

The injection of hypertonic saline into the carotid artery produces antidiuresis associated with the release of oxytocin and vasopressin (Jewell and Verney, 1957; Zuidema and Clarke, 1957). The latter hormone is, however, mainly or entirely responsible for the evoked antidiuresis. The exact nature and location of the osmoreceptive structure is unknown but they appear to be in the thalamus or hypo-thalamus. It is possible that the neurosecretory cells themselves are responsive to osmotic changes in their environment (Jewell and Verney, 1957). An abrupt decrease in circulating blood volume such as occurs in severe haemorrhage is a powerful stimulus for vasopressin release, and high concentrations are found in the blood of rapidly exsanguinated animals (Baratz and Ingraham, 1960; De Wied, 1960).

There is also evidence that the osmoreceptors respond to dilution of their chemical environment by inhibiting vasopressin release. For example, the infusion of hypotonic saline through the cerebral ventricles of a dog (that has not been water-loaded) initiates diuresis after a latency of about 30 minutes, a delay which probably depends upon the disappearance of circulating vasopressin and renal recovery from its action (Leusen and Lacroix, 1960). An increase in the circulating blood volume can also increase diuresis, presumably by likewise inhibiting vasopressin release (Welt, 1960).

It is generally accepted as suggested by Smith (1952) that the anti-diuretic response of the mammalian kidney is effected by an increase in the permeability of the distal tubule to water. Direct evidence for this view has been provided by the finding that fluid collected by micro-puncture is hypotonic in the distal tubule during water diuresis, but that it becomes progressively isotonic during the antidiuretic action of vasopressin (Gottschalk, 1960; Wirz, 1956). Ginetzinsky has recently presented evidence that vasopressin (or dehydration) causes a dissolution of the metachromatic intercellular substance between the epithelial cells of the distal tubules, which, he suggests, results in increased permeability. He suggests further that the intercellular substance is hyaluronic acid, and that vasopressin causes the secretion of hyaluronidase (which he detects in the urine during antidiuresis) from certain cells which then depolymerizes the intercellular hyaluronic acid (Ginetzinsky, 1958; Ginetzinsky et al., 1960). Ginetzinsky has described this phenomenon in the rat and dog. Recently, Dicker and Eggleton have performed experiments on man with results supporting Ginetzinsky's views (Dicker and Eggleton, 1961). They have shown that the intravenous administration of lysine—or arginine vasopressin at the peak of a water diuresis results in antidiuresis and in the excretion of hyaluronidase in the urine. Other workers, however, maintain that the 'hyaluronidase' concentration in urine simply reflects the degree of concentration of urine, and that it bears no other relationship to the administration of vasopressin (Berlyne, 1960; Sawyer, 1961).

Other actions. Oxytocin and vasopressin have a number of pharmacological activities of unknown significance (Fig. 20). It is doubtful whether the vasopressor activity of vasopressin is of physiological significance (it has simply been a useful test for the standardization of vasopressin preparations) and the same is true for the ability of oxytocin to increase the excretion of Na^+ and K^+. This effect is particularly marked in animals receiving simultaneous infusions of NaCl (Jacobson and Kellogg, 1956). The physiological significance of the hypotensive action of oxytocin is also unknown, as is the fact that both hormones are always released together, though in varying proportions. A challenging question on which some of these facts may have a bearing is the significance of oxytocin in the male.

REFERENCES

* Denotes review

*ACHER, R. and FROMAGEOT, C. (1957). In 'The Neurohypophysis', ed. H. Heller. London: Butterworth
AMIN, A. H., CRAWFORD, T. B. B. and GADDUM, J. H. (1954). *J. Physiol.* **126,** 596
ARMSTRONG, D., JEPSON, J. B., KEELE, C. A. and STEWART, J. W. (1957). *J. Physiol.* **135,** 350
BARATZ, R. A. and INGRAHAM, R. C. (1960). *Amer J. Physiol.* **198,** 565
BERGMANN, W. (1958). In 'Zweites Internationales Symposium über Neurosekretion', Berlin: Springer
BERALDO, W. T. (1950). *Amer. J. Physiol.* **171,** 371
*BERDE, E. (1959). 'Recent Progress in Oxytocin Research.' Springfield, Ill.: Thomas
BERDE, B. and CERLETTI, A. (1957). *Gynaecologia,* **144,** 275
BERDE, B. and SAAMELI, K. (1961). *Nature (Lond.),* **191,** 83
BELESLIN, D. and VARAGIC, V. (1958). *Brit. J. Pharmacol.* **13,** 321
BENSON, G. K. and FOLLEY, S. J. (1957). *J. Endocr.* **16,** 189

BERLYNE, G. M. (1960). *Nature (Lond.)*, **185,** 389
BHOOLA, K. D. (1961). Ph.D. Thesis, London University
BHOOLA, K. D., CALLE, J. D. and SCHACHTER, M. (1960). *J. Physiol.* **152,** 75
BHOOLA, K. D., CALLE, J. D. and SCHACHTER, M. (1961). *J. Physiol.* **159,** 167
BHOOLA, K. D., COLLIER, H. O. J., SCHACHTER, M. and SHORLEY, P. G. (In press)
BHOOLA, K. D., MAY MAY YI, R., MORLEY, J. and SCHACHTER, M. (1961). *J. Physiol.* **159,** 34P
BHOOLA, K. D. and SCHACHTER, M. (1961). *J. Physiol.* **157,** 20P
BOCK, K. D., KRECKE, H. J. and KUHN, H. M. (1958). *Klin. Wschr.* **36,** 254
BOISSONNAS, R. A. (1960). In 'Polypeptides which affect smooth muscles and blood vessels', ed. Schachter, M. London: Pergamon
BOISSONNAS, R. A., GUTTMANN, ST., JAQUENOD, P. A., KONZETT, H. and STÜRMER, E. (1960). *Experientia (Basel)*, **16,** 326
BRAUN-MENENDEZ, E., FASCIOLO, J. C., LELOIR, L. F. and MUNOZ, J. M. (1940). *J. Physiol. (Lond.)*, **98,** 223
CALDEYRO-BARCIA, R. and POSEIRO, J. J. (1959). *N. Y. Acad. Sci.* **75,** 813
CHAPMAN, L. F., GOODELL, H. and WOLFF, H. G. (1959). *Fed. Proc.*, **18,** 95
CHAPMAN, L. F., GOODELL, H. and WOLFF, H. G. (1959). *Arch. Neurol.* **1,** 557
CHAPMAN, L. F., RAMOS, A. O., GOODELL, H., SILVERMAN, G. and WOLFF, H. G. (1960). *Arch. Neurol.* **3,** 223
COLLIER, H. O. J., HOLGATE, J. A., SCHACHTER, M. and SHORLEY, P. G. (1960). *Brit. J. Pharmacol.* **15,** 290
COLLIER, H. O. J. and SHORLEY, P. G. (1960). *Brit. J. Pharmacol.* **15,** 601
CONTZEN, C., HOLTZ, P. and RAUDONAT, H. W. (1959). *Naturwissenschaften*, **46,** 402
COOK, W. F. and PICKERING, G. W. (1960). In 'Polypeptides which affect smooth muscles and blood vessels', ed. Schachter, M. London: Pergamon
CORREALE, P. (1959). *Arch. int. Pharmacodyn.* **119,** 435
CROSS, B. A. (1958). *J. Endocr.* **16,** 237 and 261
*CSAPO, A. (1961). 'Oxytocin', eds. Heller, H. and Caldeyro-Barcia, R. London: Pergamon
DE WIED, D. (1960). *Acta physiol. pharmacol. neerl.* **9,** 69
DICKER, S. E. and EGGLETON, M. G. (1961). *J. Physiol.* **157,** 351
DOUGLAS, W. W., FELDBERG, W., PATON, W. D. M. and SCHACHTER, M. (1951). *J. Physiol.* **115,** 63
DUNER, H., EULER, U. S. VON and PERNOW, B. (1954). *Acta physiol. scand.* **31,** 113
DU VIGNEAUD, V., LAWLER, H. C. and POPENOE, E. A. (1953). *J. Amer. chem. Soc.* **75,** 4880
DU VIGNEAUD, V., RESSLER, C., SWAN, J. M., ROBERTS, C. W., KATSOYANNIS, P. G. and GORDON, S. (1953). *J. Amer. chem. Soc.* **75,** 4879
EHRENPREIS, T. and PERNOW, B. (1953). *Acta physiol. scand.* **27,** 380
ELLIOTT, D. F., HORTON, E. W. and LEWIS, G. P. (1960). *J. Physiol.* **153,** 473
ELLIOTT, D. F., HORTON, E. W. and LEWIS, G. P. (1960). *Biochem. Biophys. res. Comm.* **3**(1), 87
ELLIOTT, D. F., LEWIS, G. P. and HORTON, E. W. (1960). In 'Polypeptides which affect smooth muscles and blood vessels', ed. Schachter, M. London: Pergamon
ELLIOTT, D. F., LEWIS, G. P. and HORTON, E. W. (1960). *Biochem. J.* **74,** 15P
ELLIOTT, D. F., LEWIS, G. P. and HORTON, E. W. (1960). *Biochem. J.* **76,** 16P
ELLIOTT, D. F. and PEART, W. S. (1956). *Nature (Lond.)*, **177,** 527
ERSPAMER, V. (1961). *Ann. Rev. Pharmacol.* **1,** 175
EULER, U. S. VON (1936). *Arch. exp. Path. Pharmak.* **181,** 181
EULER, U. S. VON and GADDUM, J. H. (1931). *J. Physiol.* **72,** 74
FITZPATRICK, R. J. (1957). In 'The Neurohypophysis', ed. Heller, H. London: Butterworth
FOX, R. H. and HILTON, S. M. (1958). *J. Physiol.* **142,** 219
FRANZ, J., BOISSONNAS, R. A. and STÜRMER, E. (1961). *Helv. chim. Acta*, **44,** 881
FREY, E. K., KRAUT, H. and WERLE, E. (1950). 'Kallikrein (Padutin)'. Stuttgart: Enke

GADDUM, J. H. (1960). In 'Polypeptides which affect smooth muscles and blood vessels', ed. Schachter, M. London: Pergamon

GADDUM, J. H. and HORTON, E. W. (1959). *Brit. J. Pharmacol.* **14,** 117

GADDUM, J. H. and SZERB, J. C. (1961). *Brit. J. Pharmacol.* **17,** 451

GINETZINSKY, A. G. (1958). *Nature (Lond.)*, **182,** 1218

GINETZINSKY, A. G., KRESTINSKAYA, T. V., NATOCHIN, J. V., SAX, M. G. and TITOVA, L. K. (1960). *Physiol. bohemoslov.* **9,** 166

GOORMATIGH, N. (1944). 'La Fonction des Artérielles Renales.' Louvain: Fonteyn

GOTTSCHALK, C. W. (1960). *Circulation,* **21,** 861

GRABNER, R., LEMBECK, F. and NEUHOLD, K. (1959). *Arch. exp. Path. Pharmak.* **236,** 331

GREEN, J. D. and MAXWELL, D. S. (1959). In 'Comparative Endocrinology', ed. Gorbman, A. New York: John Wiley

GROSS, F. and TURRIAN, H. (1960). In 'Polypeptides which affect smooth muscles and blood vessels', ed. Schachter, M. London: Pergamon

GUTH, P. S. (1959). *Brit. J. Pharmacol.* **14,** 549

HABERMAN, E. (1959). *Arch. exp. Path. Pharmak.* **236,** 492

HARRIS, G. W. (1955). In 'Neural Control of the Pituitary Gland'. London: Arnold

HARRIS, G. W. and PICKLES, V. R. (1953). *Nature (Lond.)*, **172,** 1049

HELLER, H. (1960). *Acta endocr. (Kbh.)* **34,** suppl. 50, p. 51

HILTON, S. M. (1960). In 'Polypeptides which affect smooth muscles and blood vessels', ed. Schachter, M. London: Pergamon

HOLDSTOCK, D. J., MATHIAS, A. P. and SCHACHTER, M. (1957). *Brit. J. Pharmacol.* **12,** 149

HOOPER, K. C. (1960). In 'Polypeptides which affect smooth muscles and blood vessels', ed. Schachter, M. London: Pergamon

HORTON, E. W. (1959). *Brit. J. Pharmacol.* **14,** 125

JACOBSON, H. N. and KELLOGG, R. H. (1956). *Amer. J. Physiol.* **184,** 376

JAQUES, R. and SCHACHTER, M. (1954). *Brit. J. Pharmacol.* **9,** 53

JEWELL, P. A. and VERNEY, E. B. (1957). *Proc. roy. Soc. B.* **240,** 197

KAMM, O., ALDRICH, T. B., GROTE, I. W., ROWE, L. W. and BUGBEE, E. P. (1928). *J. Amer. chem. Soc.* **50,** 573

KAO, C. Y. (1961). 'Oxytocin', eds. Heller, H. and Caldeyro-Barcia, R. London: Pergamon

KATSOYANNIS, P. G. and DU VIGNEAUD, V. (1958). *J. biol. Chem.* **233,** 1352

KONZETT, H. and STÜRMER, E. (1960). *Brit. J. Pharmacol.* **15,** 544

KONZETT, H., STÜRMER, E., LEWIS, G. P., SHORLEY, P. G. and COLLIER, H. D. J. (1960). *Nature (Lond.)*, **188,** 998

KOSTERLITZ, H. W. (1960). In 'Polypeptides which affect smooth muscles and blood vessels', ed. Schachter, M. London: Pergamon

LECOMTE, J. (1959). *Acta allerg. (Kbh.)*, **14,** 408

LEMBECK, F. (1953). *Arch. exp. Path. Pharmak.* **219,** 197

LEUSEN, I. and LACROIX, E. (1960). *Arch. int. Physiol.* **68,** 372

LEWIS, G. P. (1958). *J. Physiol.* **140,** 285

LEWIS, G. P. (1959). *J. Physiol.* **147,** 458

MARGOLIS, J. (1960). *J. Physiol.* **151,** 238

MATHIAS, A. P. and SCHACHTER, M. (1958). *Brit. J. Pharmacol.* **13,** 326

MEIER, R., GROSS, F., TRIPOD, J. and TURRIAN, H. (1957). *Experientia (Basel),* **13,** 361

MILES, A. A. and WILHELM, D. L. (1960). In 'Polypeptides which affect smooth muscles and blood vessels', ed. Schachter, M. London: Pergamon

OLIVER, G. and SCHÄFER, E. A. (1895). *J. Physiol.* **18,** 277

PEART, W. S. (1960). In 'Polypeptides which affect smooth muscles and blood vessels', ed. Schachter, M. London: Pergamon

PERNOW, B. (1955). In 'Polypeptides which stimulate plain muscle', ed. Gaddum, J. H. Edinburgh: Livingstone

PERNOW, B. (1960). In 'Polypeptides which affect smooth muscles and blood vessels', ed. Schachter, M. London: Pergamon

PICKERING, G. W. (1960). In 'Polypeptides which affect smooth muscles and blood vessels', ed. Schachter, M. London: Pergamon

PIERCE, J. V. and WEBSTER, M. E. (1961). *Biochem. Biophys. res. Comm.* **5**, 353

RITTEL, W., ISELIN, B., KAPPELER, H., RINIKER, B. and SCHWYZER, R. (1957). *Helv. chim. Acta*, **40**, 614

ROCHA E SILVA, M. (1955). In 'Polypeptides which stimulate plain muscle', ed. Gaddum, J. H. Edinburgh: Livingstone

ROCHA E SILVA, M. (1960). In 'Polypeptides which affect smooth muscles and blood vessels', ed. Schachter, M. London: Pergamon

ROCHA E SILVA, M., BERALDO, W. T. and ROSENFELD, G. (1949). *Amer. J. Physiol.* **156**, 261

SAWYER, W. H. (1961). *Ann. Rev. Pharmacol.* **1**, 225

SAWYER, W. H. and ROTH, W. D. (1953). *Fed. Proc.* **12**, 125

SCHACHTER, M. (Unpublished)

SCHACHTER, M. (1956). *Brit. J. Pharmacol.* **11**, 111

*SCHACHTER, M. (1960). In 'Polypeptides which affect smooth muscles and blood vessels', ed. Schachter, M. London: Pergamon

SCHACHTER, M. and THAIN, E. M. (1954). *Brit. J. Pharmacol.* **9**, 352

SCHARRER, B. (1959). In 'Comparative Endocrinology', ed. Gorbman, A. New York: John Wiley

SCHARRER, E. and SCHARRER, B. (1954). *Recent Progr. Hormone Res.* **10**, 183

SCHWARZ, H., BUMPUS, F. M. and PAGE, I. H. (1957). *J. Amer. chem. Soc.* **79**, 5697

SCHWYZER, R. (1960). In 'Polypeptides which affect smooth muscles and blood vessels', ed. Schachter, M. London: Pergamon

SCHWYZER, R., RITTEL, W., SIEBER, P., KAPPELER, H. and ZUBER, H. (1960). *Helv. chim. Acta*, **43**, 1130

SKEGGS, L. T. (1960). In 'Polypeptides which affect smooth muscles and blood vessels', ed. Schachter, M. London: Pergamon

SKEGGS, L. T., KAHN, J. R. and SHUMWAY, N. P. (1956). *J. exp. Med.* **103**, 295

SKEGGS, L. T., LENTZ, K. E., KAHN, J. R., SHUMWAY, N. P. and WOODS, K. R. (1956). *J. exp. Med.* **104**, 193

SMITH, H. W. (1952). *Fed. Proc.* **11**, 701

TIGERSTEDT, R. and BERGMANN, P. G. (1898). *Skand. Arch. Physiol.* **8**, 223

TUPPY, H. (1953). *Biochim. biophys. Acta*, **11**, 449

VAN DYKE, H. B., ADAMSONS, K. and ENGEL, S. L. (1957). 'The Neurohypophysis.' London: Butterworth

WELT, L. G. (1960). *Circulation*, **21**, 1002

WERLE, E. (1955). In 'Polypeptides which stimulate plain muscle', ed. Gaddum, J. H. Edinburgh: Livingstone

WERLE, E. (1960). In 'Polypeptides which affect smooth muscles and blood vessels', ed. Schachter, M. London: Pergamon

WERLE, E. and BEREK, U. (1948). *Angew. Chem.* **60A**, 53

WERLE, E. and ERDÖS, E. G. (1954). *Arch. exp. Path. Pharmak.* **223**, 234

WERLE, E., GÖTZE, W. and KEPPLER, A. (1937). *Biochem. Z.* **289**, 217

WERLE, E. and HAMBÜCHEN, R. (1943). *Arch. exp. Path. Pharmak.* **201**, 311

WERLE, E. and KAUFMANN-BOETSCH, B. (1960).

WERLE, E., TRAUTSCHOLD, I. and LEYSATH, G. (1961). *Hoppe-Seyl. Z.* **326**, 174

WIRZ, H. (1956). *Helv. physiol. Acta*, **14**, 353

ZETLER, G. (1960). In 'Polypeptides which affect smooth muscles and blood vessels', ed. Schachter, M. London: Pergamon

ZUIDEMA, G. D. and CLARKE, N. P. (1957). *Amer. J. Physiol.* **188**, 616

CHAPTER 6

HYPOGLYCAEMIC AGENTS AND DIABETES MELLITUS

Before considering the various hypoglycaemic agents used in diabetes mellitus it will be as well to start with a few remarks aimed towards a definition of the disease. The ancients and physicians of the middle ages recognized it as a wasting condition associated with passing copious amounts of sweet urine. It is perhaps important to point out that even today our definitions are not as precise as we should like, largely because we remain ignorant of the real aetiology of the disease. We can, of course, exclude from the diagnosis conditions where the urine contains glucose at normal levels of blood sugar, due to impaired tubular reabsorbtion; and we can record that certain relatively rare metabolic and endocrine disorders may be complicated by the appearance of diabetes mellitus, for example Cushing's disease, acromegaly, haemosiderosis and so on. But the great bulk of the cases of the idiopathic condition accepted as diabetes mellitus seems to fall into two categories. First, there are the cases who have the classical wasting disease so long recognized, with thirst, polyuria, glycosuria and a tendency to ketosis. Some 20% of diabetics attending clinics are made up of such patients, who may be regarded as insulin dependent and prone to ketosis. Second, under the present conditions of society, not only in Europe and the Western Hemisphere, but also in Africa and Asia, it is clear that many persons have glycosuria without intense thirst or wasting—indeed many of them, but not *all*, are obese and often without complaints about their health and glycosuria is found unexpectedly at some routine examination: blood sugar examinations follow and then glucose tolerance tests. Most clinicians diagnose diabetes mellitus if the patient, after an overnight fast, shows a 'true' blood sugar above 100 mg./100 ml. and when this is supported by a blood sugar in excess of 180 mg./100 ml. during a standard glucose tolerance test (50g. by mouth, in Great Britain), or if the concentration $2\frac{1}{2}$ hours after taking the glucose is higher than the fasting level. Such cases—whose disease usually begins in middle or late life, and whose survival does not depend upon insulin therapy and who are not prone to ketosis—make up 70–80% of our diabetic clinics.

However, while known diabetics show an incidence of about $\frac{1}{2}$%, when community surveys have been carried out, several per cent of the population have been found to be glycosuric. Among these latter, diabetes can be detected, (i.e. recognized for the first time) on the above blood sugar criteria in $\frac{1}{2}$% of the original population. On closer questioning, a third or more of these new patients have symptoms and signs associated with diabetes or its vascular, neurological or renal complications, and the rest are symptomless, though suffering from hyperglycaemia and glycosuria. Having glucose tolerance tests defined as diabetic, current clinical practice dictates that such patients are kept under surveillance and their disease controlled if possible, because they are thought to be prone to develop the disabling complications of diabetes if left with high blood sugars.

There the matter seemed to stand until the results of population surveys repeatedly drew attention to the fact that in our society today a surprisingly high proportion of persons show glycosuria and diabetic glucose tolerance curves on some occasion or another. Thus it has recently been reported by Malins and the Birmingham group of General Practitioners interested in a diabetic detection drive (Malins, 1961) that 10% of their randomly selected group—127 persons *previously agly-cosuric*—showed diabetic glucose tolerance curves. This sort of information is not unique and there are many other clues which suggest either that the diabetic diathesis is much more common than the 0·5–1% accepted, perhaps because of the rising standards of living, or that our criteria for diagnosis are too loose.

This means that there must be a reappraisal of diabetes in the near future and that the present review must be seen for what it is: remarks reflecting our views at the time of writing, set in a changing scene. Proceeding in this vein, it seems to us that the most likely resolution of the present difficulty about the diagnosis may come from the wider use of the intravenous glucose tolerance test rather than the oral method. Studies of peripheral glucose metabolism in normal subjects suggest that over half the 50 g. glucose load taken by mouth finds its way into the muscles—a higher proportion in thin subjects and less in fat. But with intravenous loading a much smaller proportion (20%) of the administered 25 g. of glucose finds its way into the peripheral tissues, much of the rest presumably going into the liver. Lundbaek (1961) has shown that intravenous tests may become abnormal within a few hours of administration of glucocorticoids, suggesting that the liver glycogen deposited by such steroids may be affecting the glucose assimilation by that organ. That these changes are apparent before there is any change in the general level of glucose, implies that the intravenous test may be a very sensitive indicator of abnormal glucose metabolism. Furthermore, Lundbaek has produced information that the intravenous glucose tolerance test, flatter in diabetics than normals, is unaffected by reducing body weight: that is, the diabetic tendency is still detected with this test under conditions where oral tests have reverted towards normal. In other words, the intravenous test may detect diabetes earlier than and detect it, despite dietary treatment, better than the oral glucose tolerance test. If this is substantiated, we must expect a definition of diabetes mellitus in these terms to be more precise and gain wider acceptance. Further studies of diabetes in man will inevitably be concerned more with the metabolism of different tissues than with simple blood levels of sugar.

But, while the prevalence of the disease still tantalizes us and the diagnosis is still difficult in border-line cases, as an introduction to what follows, certain principles can be stated about the treatment needed day in and day out for the many diabetics whose expectation of life has been extended by the discovery of insulin and of antibacterial chemotherapy and antibiotics. Dietary intake remains the central theme of therapy— if the patient is on insulin, intake must be geared to the dose; if the patient is on oral antidiabetic compounds, the intake must be regulated to prevent increasing obesity. For those diabetics who show hyperglycaemia with ketosis, insulin is necessary—for those who cannot be controlled by diet alone, oral antidiabetic drugs, such as the sulphonylureas and the biguanides, are available as an alternative.

We have not here attempted to give the clinical indications for one therapy or the other. These have been well reviewed elsewhere and our opinions are already recorded. The plan has been to consider the different therapeutic agents first as chemicals—now possible even for insulin. In the case of the hormone, we trace its physiology—production, storage, release, transport and distribution, before trying to consider its relationship to the pathological state of diabetes and its metabolic effects. Partly because it is another pancreatic polypeptide, and partly because it may come to have some therapeutic value in the treatment of insulin overdosage, we digress to consider glucagon. We then turn to consider the oral synthetic hypoglycaemic drugs in current use, their development, chemistry, pharmacology and mode of action.

INSULIN

The name 'insuline' was given to the hormone of the islets of Langerhans (de Meyer, 1909) 12 years before the proof of its existence was obtained by Banting and Best (1922) and 16 years before it was isolated and obtained in crystalline form (Abel *et al.*, 1927).

Insulin is produced and stored in the β-cells of the islets of Langerhans from which it is discharged into the pancreatico-duodenal vein, carried in the blood into and through the liver and then distributed throughout the body. The 'life cycle' of insulin from its formation to its destruction, possibly in action, offers a fascinating glimpse of some of the self-regulatory mechanisms of the body. So far, only limited aspects of the various stages of this life cycle have been unravelled.

7

CHEMISTRY

The discovery by Sanger (1960) and his co-workers in Cambridge of the precise order in which the 51 amino-acids are arranged to make up the molecule of insulin was incidentally also the first description of the structural formula of any protein. The weight of the insulin molecule is about 6000. It consists of two chains containing 21 and 30 amino-acids respectively, linked by the disulphide bridges of two cystine residues.

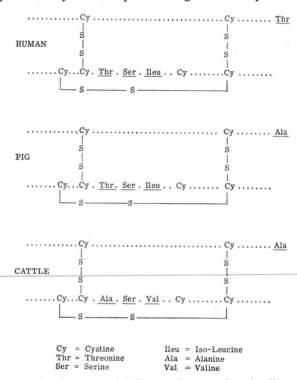

Cy = Cystine	Ileu = Iso-Leucine
Thr = Threonine	Ala = Alanine
Ser = Serine	Val = Valine

FIG. 21. The structural differences between three insulins. Only the disulphide bridges and the different amino acid arrangements are shown; the remainder of the molecule is similar in the insulins derived from different species (for full details of the molecule, see Sanger, 1960).

There is a further disulphide bridge in the shorter (A) chain. It is within this latter disulphide ring that the major variations occur in the amino-acid composition of insulins from different species; differences also occur in the terminal amino-acid of the longer (B) chain. These particular areas are clearly not essential for biological activity, but are concerned with immune reactions. Indeed, many different peptides with insulin-like activity have been derived from insulin by a variety of degradation procedures (Nichol, 1960). This indicates that the complete molecule is not essential for biological activity. It has been known for a long time that biological activity is lost if the disulphide bridges are broken, either by oxidation or by reduction. This might occur naturally by interaction with glutathione or cysteine. It occurs also as the result of radiation damage when insulin is labelled with [131]I. A more precise knowledge of the molecular requirements for insulin-like activity offers the prospect of producing synthetic insulin-like compounds.

INSULIN PRODUCTION

The factors concerned in the synthesis of insulin are at present under investigation in several laboratories. The pathways by which amino-acids are built up into the protein structure of the insulin molecule are being traced with the help of ^{14}C or tritium-labelled amino-acids (Ashmore, 1961; Humbel *et al.*, 1961). This work is still in its very early stages but should offer a much greater insight into the ability of the pancreas to respond adequately to stimuli calling for changes in insulin production or release. These techniques will, incidentally, also provide a source of labelled material for further studies on insulin, unhampered by the many disadvantages which arise at present from the use of ^{131}I labelled insulin.

The metabolism of the β-cells themselves is also relevant to the problem of insulin synthesis. Many enzymes have been detected in the β-cells and their relative activities assessed by histochemical methods (Lacy, 1961). Again, it is not yet possible to attach precise meaning to the relatively high oxidative capacity of these cells or to the very intriguing discovery of the presence in the β-cells of glucose-6-phosphatase which had previously been thought to be limited only to liver, kidney and intestinal mucosa (Lazarus, 1959). It may be that certain co-factors produced as the result of the carbohydrate metabolism of the β-cells themselves become available for protein synthesis and so influence the synthesis of insulin. It may also be that some of the intermediary products of metabolism, such as citrate, could act as chelating agents for zinc, releasing free insulin from its zinc-protein complex in which it exists in the pancreas (Maske, 1957); or, possibly alterations in the steering of glucose-6-phosphate metabolism, partly controlled by the glucose concentration of the blood reaching the β-cells, partly by other pace-making enyzme reactions at this site, may exert a profound influence on insulin production. Although much of this is at present speculative, techniques are becoming available which will make it possible to test some of these possibilities. Histochemistry and electron microscopy have shown changes in β-cell granulation and in the Golgi apparatus in response to changes in blood sugar concentration and to stimulation by the sulphonylureas, changes which are thought to be related to 'insulinogenic' activity (Lacy and Hartroft, 1959; Batts, 1959; Volk and Lazarus, 1959).

INSULIN STORAGE

About 200 units of insulin or more can be extracted from the human pancreas, the amount varying with age and the clinical condition of the patient (Wrenshall *et al.*, 1952). Reduced amounts are obtained from the pancreas of patients who become diabetic during active growth, but normal amounts are found in the pancreas of patients in whom the diabetes began later in life. Recently, using a microbiochemical technique, Lacy (1961) separated the islets from the acinar tissue of the rabbit pancreas. He found the insulin content of a single β-cell to be 1·7 micro-units (plasma insulin activity, using the same assay technique is 50 to 350-micro-units per ml.).

Some means must exist to prevent a sudden discharge from the pancreas of this large and potentially dangerous amount of insulin. It has been known for many years that the combination of insulin with zinc and a small basic protein such as protamine, results in the formation of a slow-release insulin. Both zinc and proteins of this type occur in relatively high concentrations in the pancreas. It is almost certain that the granules seen histologically in the β-cells represent a conglomeration of such insulin-zinc-protein complexes. The immediate mechanisms within the β-cells which may cause a release of insulin from this complex have already been outlined.

The stimulus for insulin secretion in the body is a rising blood sugar concentration (Foà, 1956). The smoothness and rapidity of the response suggest that insulin is released in a controlled and graded manner from preformed stores rather than newly synthesized whenever a demand for it arises.

The rate at which insulin appears in the circulation in rats has been deduced from the rate at which anti-insulin sera of known titre had to be infused to maintain a high steady blood sugar. At present the estimate lies between 1·2 and 2·6 units per hour per kg. of body wt. (Armin *et al.*, 1960).

INSULIN TRANSPORT

To reach its target tissues, insulin must enter the blood stream. In the blood it interacts with several of the plasma protein fractions, most of it being associated, as shown on electrophoresis, with the β-globulins. β-globulin may be the vehicle which picks up insulin and puts it down at its site of action. It has also been suggested that the small, basic proteins of the blood may act as such a carrier (Antoniades, 1958). In this form, insulin may be protected against destructive mechanisms and used as a circulating store. (The relation of insulin to other proteins in the blood will be discussed in another section.)

DISTRIBUTION IN THE BODY

From the pancreas, insulin enters the pancreatico-duodenal vein. The concentration of insulin in the vein rises when insulin secretion is stimulated by hyperglycaemia (Anderson *et al.*, 1959) or by the administration of the sulphonylureas (Goetz and Egdahl, 1958).

The vein carries insulin directly into the liver, where a varying proportion (up to 40%) is trapped, inactivated or destroyed (Mortimore and Tietze, 1959). The removal of insulin by the liver is reflected in the observation that the insulin concentration in femoral vein blood is always less than in pancreatic vein blood. This arrangement, of insulin having to pass through the liver, has the further advantage that it acts as a potential buffer mechanism against the sudden release of an overwhelming amount of insulin and may also offer the endogenously secreted insulin the opportunity to act directly on the main glucose producing organ of the body.

Young (1961) has made the very intriguing observation that the insulin-like activity in the blood is related to its state of oxygenation. He found greater activity in arterial blood than in blood obtained simultaneously from the pancreatic vein. The activity in drawn venous blood is increased when this is subsequently oxygenated *in vitro*. The significance of this observation is at present obscure, but the mechanism may play some part in protecting insulin from destruction in its journey through the liver.

Using trace amounts of ^{131}I insulin, it has been found that the labelled hormone is concentrated in the renal tubular cells and to a lesser extent in the liver, but little is excreted in the urine.

To exert its action, insulin has to leave the blood and become 'fixed' at its site of action. The term 'fixation' was applied by Stadie *et al.* (1952) to the process by which insulin remained attached to the rat diaphragm after dipping this tissue for a few seconds into a solution containing insulin. Within the last 2 years, methods have been developed to study, in human subjects, the factors concerned with the movement of insulin out of the blood and on to the tissues (Briggs *et al.*, 1960). Essentially, the method consists of the injection of 0·1 unit of ^{131}I-labelled insulin into the brachial artery and its recovery from an antecubital vein draining predominantly muscle. The fraction of the injected dose which fails to return is assumed to have been 'fixed' by the forearm tissues. In normal subjects, about 14% of the injected insulin is fixed during one passage through the forearm. A smaller proportion of the injected dose disappears from the blood in diabetic patients and in some non-diabetic acromegalics. These changes may be due to a faster blood flow through the forearm giving it less time to escape from the blood; or to insulin 'binding' substances in the plasma; or to changes at the site of action of insulin, preventing its 'fixation'. Such patients also show a diminished glucose uptake in response to the injected insulin.

Very recently, evidence that insulin is 'fixed' to muscle has been obtained by injecting radioactive insulin into the brachial artery of a monkey and assaying the radioactivity in various muscle fractions obtained at biopsy a few minutes after the injection. Using the technique described by McCollister and Randle (1961) it was found that radioactivity was concentrated on the isolated muscle membranes but none was found in the muscle protein fraction (Butterfield *et al.*, 1961a).

INSULIN DESTRUCTION

Insulin is destroyed in the body by at least two mechanisms. One of these is its degradation by a sequence of proteolytic enzymes acting as an 'insulinase' (Mirsky and Broh-Kahn, 1949). The highest insulinase activity is found in liver and kidneys; some is also found in muscle. Liver insulinase activity is increased by a high carbohydrate diet and reduced by fasting, hypophysectomy and thyroidectomy (Mirsky *et al.*, 1955). It is doubtful whether insulinase plays any part at all in the development of diabetes or that therapeutic doses of the sulphonylureas inhibit this enzyme system.

A more specific destructive inactivation of insulin is due to the disruption of its disulphide bridges. Naturally occurring compounds, such as glutathione or cysteine, are capable of doing this (du Vigneaud *et al.*, 1931). It is interesting to speculate whether insulin is 'used up' in some such fashion by interaction with the sulphydryl groups of the cysteine radicle of cell membrane proteins.

The rate of insulin degradation can be deduced from the change in radioactivity of the plasma after an injection of ^{131}I-labelled insulin. In man, 50% of the circulating insulin disappears every 40 minutes (Berson *et al.*, 1956). In untreated diabetic patients, the rate of degradation is the same, but in patients previously treated with insulin, the fall in plasma insulin is delayed. This is due to the binding of insulin to antibody in the plasma which protects it from destruction, even though it reduces its physiological activity. (See page 190.)

INSULIN ASSAY

The ideal and only specific assay would be a chemical one, based on the whole structure or some unique chemical property of the insulin molecule itself. It is not yet feasible to do this with the small amounts of insulin present in blood, but investigations along these lines are now well advanced.

Until such an 'absolute' method is available, bioassays have to be employed. Because they measure many other factors acting as activators or inhibitors of insulin in the blood, it is best to talk of 'insulin-like' activity of the plasma or serum (but the temptation to pronounce this as the words 'ILA', 'PILA' or 'SILA' should be strongly resisted!)

To date, the most specific assay of plasma insulin in man is a radio-immunological assay, employing ^{131}I-labelled beef-insulin and an anti-insulin serum produced by sensitizing guinea pigs to protamine-zinc beef-insulin (Berson and Yalow, 1960). It is based on the fact that human plasma insulin can displace some of the radioactive beef-insulin from the complex formed between it and the beef-insulin anti-serum. This may be shown schematically as:

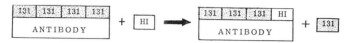

SCHEMATIC REPRESENTATION OF INSULIN RADIO-IMMUNO ASSAY

[131] = radioactive insulin

[HI] = human insulin (not radioactive)

FIG. 22. One molecule of human insulin displaces one molecule of [131]-iodine labelled beef insulin from its combination with beef-insulin-antibody. The concentration of radioactive iodine liberated gives a measure of insulin originally present in the serum.

After incubating the plasma with a tracer dose of ^{131}I beef-insulin and beef-insulin anti-serum, an aliquot of the mixture is chromatographed and the separated protein fractions scanned for radioactivity. ^{131}I-insulin bound to the antibody, moves with the proteins away from the site of

Table 12

INSULIN ACTIVITY OF NORMAL HUMAN PLASMA
(from Randle and Taylor, 1960)

METHOD OF ASSAY	PLASMA INSULIN ACTIVITY (micro-units/ml.)	COMMENT	REFERENCE
In vivo			
ADHA rat: blood glucose	100	Fasting	
	350	After glucose (2.5 hr.)	Bornstein (1950)
ADA mouse: blood glucose	800 - 1,150	Acid-ethanol extract. Fasting	Baird and Bornstein (1959)
	1,700 - 3,700	Acid-ethanol extract. After food	
In vitro			
Rat diaphragm -			
(a) Glucose uptake	10 - 140	Undiluted plasma. Fasting	Vallance-Owen & Hurlock (1954)
	100 - 800	One hour after oral glucose	Wright (1957); Seltzer & Smith (1959)
	100 - 4,600	Diluted plasma. Fasting	Willebrands & Groen (1956); Willebrands, van der Geld & Groen (1958)
	1,000 - 2,000	Acid-ethanol extract. Fasting	Baird and Bornstein (1957)
	1,000 - 20,000	Diluted plasma; 2.5 hr. after glucose	Randle (1954a, 1957)
(b) (^{14}C) Glycine incorporation into protein	2,000 - 10,000	Diluted plasma; 2.5 hr. after glucose	Manchester, Randle & Young, (1959)
Rat epididymal fat pad -			
(a) Glucose uptake	250 - 1,000	Undiluted or diluted plasma	Beigelman & Antoniades (1958)
(b) $^{14}CO_2$ production from (^{14}C) glucose	50 - 350	Undiluted plasma. Fasting	Martin, Renold & Dagenais (1958)
Immunochemical	64 - 98	Fasting	Yalow and Berson (1959)
	236 - 302	After glucose (1 hr.)	

ADHA - adrenalectomized, hypophysectomized, and made diabetic with alloxan.

ADA - adrenalectomized and treated with alloxan.

application, but the ^{131}I-insulin displaced from the complex and therefore 'free', remains at the origin. This free ^{131}I-insulin is proportional to the amount of insulin in the test sample.

The same workers have now extended the method to the assay of endogenous plasma insulin in diabetic patients treated with beef insulin, using human ^{131}I-insulin and guinea-pig anti-beef insulin serum (Berson and Yalow, 1961).

At the present time, however, the most widely used techniques for plasma insulin assay employ either the rat diaphragm (Vallance-Owen and Hurlock, 1954; Randle, 1954), or the epididymal fat pad (Martin *et al.*, 1958).

The rat diaphragm technique is based on the stimulation of glucose uptake by insulin and is thought to give a measure of 'insulin-like' activity. It measures not only insulin, but also factors which stimulate or inhibit insulin and any other agents in the plasma that may enhance or reduce the glucose uptake by the diaphragm. A simplified version of this method was recently described by Rafaelson (1961): he measures the increase in the glycogen content of the rat diaphragm $2\frac{1}{2}$ hours after an intraperitoneal injection of the insulin-containing plasma. It is comparable in sensivity to the methods employing isolated tissues.

In the method described by Martin *et al.* (1958) the fatty sheet attached to the rat epididymis is incubated with glucose of which only the first carbon atom is labelled with ^{14}C. In adipose tissue, insulin stimulates the direct oxidation of glucose to CO_2 via the hexose monophosphate shunt.

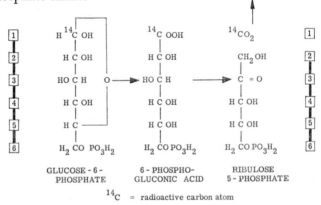

^{14}C = radioactive carbon atom

Fig. 23. The basis for insulin assay by the epididymal fat pad. The amount of radioactive $^{14}CO_2$ produced by direct oxidation of the first carbon atom of glucose through the 'hexose monophosphate shunt' is directly proportional to the concentration of insulin.

This is conveniently determined by measuring the specific activity of the $^{14}CO_2$ produced from glucose-1-^{14}C during the incubation. The increase in specific activity of the CO_2 is proportional to the concentration of insulin.

The action of insulin on adipose tissue is thought to be less affected than that on the rat diaphragm by the other factors present in the plasma and therefore to represent more nearly total insulin levels.

To avoid such interfering factors, various methods of extraction and purification of plasma insulin have been devised. These include the acid-ethanol extraction which has been used commercially for many years to prepare insulin from the pancreas, and more recently the use of ion-exchange resins (Antoniades *et al.*, 1960). With suitable resins, insulin is retained on the resin while most of the proteins are washed off. The insulin is then washed off the resin with 0·3 M. citric acid so that finally, after several such treatments, the ratio of insulin to total protein is increased by a factor of $1·5 \times 10^6$ (Antoniades, 1958).

Although it will probably not be long before these bioassays are replaced by specific chemical estimations, their very imperfection has proved of great value. The present interest in anti-insulin factors is largely the result of the discrepancies found between these different methods of insulin assay.

INSULIN ANTAGONISTS IN PLASMA

Although plasma antagonists interfere with the absolute measurement of insulin, it has been possible to turn this to good account in defining the different types of antagonists present in plasma and in assessing their possible role in the development of diabetes.

In uncontrolled diabetic patients, there appear to be three hormone-dependent antagonists.

Vallance-Owen has studied an antagonist associated with the albumin fraction of plasma (Vallance-Owen *et al.*, 1958). This factor may depend on the presence of the pituitary gland and on adrenal cortical steroids. A high level of the antagonist occurs not only in uncontrolled diabetic patients, but also in the plasma of prediabetic subjects. The factor inhibits the action of insulin on muscle, but not on adipose tissue.

In this connection it is of particular interest that the fat pad technique often indicates high levels of plasma insulin, even in young, untreated, ketotic diabetics, in whom the rat diaphragm assay shows apparently reduced insulin levels. These observations by Steinke *et al.* (1961) have led to the suggestion that in some subjects there may be a genetically determined over-production of insulin antagonists and that overt diabetes develops when the β-cells of the pancreas are no longer able to produce enough insulin to neutralize the circulating antagonist (Vallance-Owen and Lilley, 1961).

Hormone dependent antagonists have also been found in the α_1 and α_2 globulin fractions (Field and Stetten, 1956; Taylor, 1961). They appear to be related to diabetic ketosis. The α_1 antagonist disappears when ketosis is brought under control, but the α_2 antagonist has occasionally been found in the serum of normal subjects. The α_1 fraction inhibits insulin-stimulated glucose uptake of the rat diaphragm; the α_2 fraction is capable of reducing glucose uptake of the rat diaphragm below control levels whether or not insulin is present in the incubating medium.

It is interesting to reflect on the possible meaning behind this bewildering variety of so-called antagonists. Insulin is clearly a very active and valuable hormone. It is known that, in common with other peptides, only part of the complete molecule is necessary for biological activity. The remainder of the molecule is capable of interacting with other proteins which may act as the carriers for the essential part of the molecule. Perhaps different carrier proteins react at different rates, both in their formation and dissolution of the complex and this may be of value in preventing too sudden a metabolic change following a release of insulin from the pancreas.

It may be that insulin can act on a tissue only if it has first been attached to it by a tissue-specific carrier—a concept analogous to the tissue specificity of iso-enzymes (Annotation, 1960). In this connection it is of great interest that immunological differences have been demonstrated in one and the same animal between its circulating plasma insulin and the insulin extracted from its own pancreas (Slater *et al.*, 1961). These differences may reflect the association of insulin with different carrier proteins.

A further possibility is that insulin-antagonist complexes exist to protect insulin from degradation or to hold insulin in the plasma to keep it available as an emergency store, ready for immediate action.

Protein synthesis is under close genetic control. Small changes in protein structure, genetically determined, may be sufficient to alter the kinetics of insulin-antagonist 'binding' and play an important part in the development of diabetes.

INSULIN ANTIBODIES

Insulin antibodies may be regarded as distinct from the insulin-antagonists described above, because they appear only when insulin has been administered to a patient. As a protein, insulin can be expected to have antigenic properties. Nevertheless, it came as a surprise to most clinicians to learn that antibodies can be demonstrated in the serum of most patients on insulin therapy, because clinical manifestations attributable to this type of antibody reaction appear to be rare. These serum antibodies are present in the globulin fraction of the serum protein. They bind insulin tightly, preventing its transfer from the bloodstream to its site of action, and may account for the severe insulin resistance of some patients whose plasma could bind hundreds of units of beef insulin (Berson and Yalow, 1960). This type of insulin resistance responds to treatment with cortisone, the steroid presumably interfering with the association of insulin with the antibody. The management of such patients presents many difficulties. During the resistant phase they may require over 1,000 units of insulin per day to control the hyperglycaemia and ketosis; but, severe and persistent hypoglycaemia may occur when the resistance suddenly ceases and large amounts of insulin, previously bound to the antibody, are set free in the plasma. There is little species-specificity in these circulating antibodies, so that attempts at treatment with insulin from different animal sources meet with little success.

'Conventional' allergic reactions to insulin due to 'reagin' type antibodies may also occur. They take the form of local or, rarely, generalized, skin reactions, after insulin injections. This type of antibody can be demonstrated by patch-testing on the skin. It is not certain, however, that these reactions are due to insulin at all, because highly purified, crystalline insulin preparations from the same animal species do not provoke such reactions in the same patients. It is therefore almost certain that some other protein in the commercial insulin preparation causes these reactions.

Experimentally, insulin antibody formation has been induced in guinea pigs by sensitizing them to beef insulin (Moloney and Coval, 1955). The serum from such guinea pigs is used in the immuno-assay of plasma insulin and for the experimental production of acute insulin deficiency in rats and other animals (Armin *et al.*, 1960).

MECHANISM OF ACTION OF INSULIN

Insulin lowers the blood sugar concentration and promotes the synthesis of glycogen, fat and protein in different tissues.

How are these actions connected with one another and are they all brought about by one single basic action of insulin?

This problem of the precise action of insulin has been discussed and debated for many years but as yet no single mechanism has been put forward which will satisfy all the observed effects of insulin (Fisher, 1960; Randle and Young, 1960; Park *et al.*, 1959; Goldstein and Levine, 1960).

Current views favour a primary action on cell permeability rather than an effect on intra-cellular enzymes concerned directly with glucose utilization. They are based largely on the work of Levine and his colleagues (Goldstein and Levine, 1960) who showed that insulin speeds the movement of many sugars into the cell and that this movement is not dependent upon the subsequent metabolic fate of the sugar. This is in contrast to the theory proposed by Cori (1945), who suggested that insulin acts primarily on the enzyme hexokinase within the cell, accelerating the phosphorylation of glucose to glucose-6-phosphate. This suggestion, however, is no longer tenable because it has been shown that insulin leads to the accumulation not of hexose phosphates but of free glucose within the cell (Park *et al.*, 1959). This could not happen if hexokinase had been stimulated, but is in keeping with the view that insulin facilitates the movement of glucose across the cell membrane into the cell.

From studies on the glucose uptake of forearm tissues in man, we believe that there is a tissue glucose threshold (Butterfield, 1961), i.e. that the glucose concentration of the blood and extracellular fluid must be above a certain minimum level (the threshold) if glucose is to shift from the extra-cellular fluid into the tissues. In normal fasting subjects this threshold is 70–90 mg./100 ml., almost the same as the fasting blood sugar; the uptake of glucose by the tissues is therefore negligible in the fasting state. In diabetic subjects, the threshold is much higher, being again almost the same as the systemic blood sugar, and glucose uptake is again negligible. In insulin-sensitive subjects the intra-arterial injection of insulin lowers the threshold very quickly and thus increases the glucose uptake.

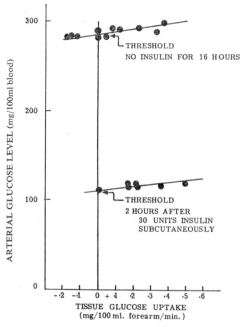

FIG. 24. Tissue glucose uptake in a diabetic patient. Insulin lowers the tissue glucose threshold so that glucose is taken up from the blood at much lower concentrations.

These concepts are in harmony with the general hypothesis that insulin acts by increasing cell permeability to glucose.

METABOLIC CHANGES IN DIABETES MELLITUS

A more detailed consideration of our present views on the relative importance of the effect of insulin on the metabolism of various tissues is based on our studies on normal and diabetic subjects and on the experimental production, in rats, of acute insulin deficiency with anti-insulin serum.

The metabolic changes are largely the consequence of lack of effective insulin action on certain tissues. At one time, contending theories of peripheral under-utilization and hepatic overproduction of glucose were put forward to account for the hyperglycaemia. It is now apparent that both these factors play a part and that there is a temporal and quantitative relationship between them.

In the absence of insulin, the threshold for the movement of glucose into cells is raised and the glucose uptake of such tissues is reduced (Butterfield, 1961). Meanwhile, however, the liver continues to produce glucose as before (from glycogen and from non-carbohydrate sources) so that glucose begins to accumulate in the blood and extra-cellular fluid. The raised glucose concentration can, to some extent, exceed the raised cell threshold and glucose can once again enter the cell. At this stage, there is a moderate hyperglycaemia with minimal glycosuria and the physiological state may be described as 'peripheral under-utilization with normal hepatic glucose production'. If insulin deficiency is severe and the tissue threshold is higher than the renal threshold, glucose begins to spill over into the urine and is wasted; it follows, therefore, that the liver must increase its production of glucose if it is to maintain the high blood sugar needed to overcome the raised tissue glucose threshold. At this stage there is thus a high blood sugar with heavy glycosuria and the stage of 'under-utilization and over-production' of glucose has been reached (Mahler, 1961).

The effect of insulin on the glucose output by the liver is still not entirely clear. It is certainly reduced several hours after treatment with insulin has been started, but the immediate effect is less certain. While some claim that insulin greatly reduces the output (Jacobs *et al.*, 1958; Madison and Unger, 1958), others have not found it so (Mahler *et al.*, 1959). These differences may be resolved by other observations (Dunn *et al.*, 1960) which suggest that insulin, while not actually reducing the hepatic glucose output, restrains the increase in glucose release from the liver which normally occurs when the blood sugar falls.

At this point it is pertinent to consider which are the tissues principally affected by insulin lack and responsible for the rise in blood sugar as the result of their under-utilization of glucose. Muscle and adipose tissues are quantitatively the most important tissues in the body known to respond immediately to insulin.

Muscle has for long been regarded as the main site of glucose utilization and it certainly responds briskly to injected insulin with an increase in glucose uptake. Furthermore, unpublished studies in our department indicate that diabetic muscles fail to accept glucose from the bloodstream after a glucose load; this probably largely accounts for the abnormality of the glucose tolerance curve. But how does insulin-lack affect the level of the blood sugar in *fasting* subjects? In 1956 Andres, Cader and Zierler showed that normal resting muscle takes up very little glucose, an observation which we have repeated and confirmed many times. It is difficult then, to attribute a rising blood sugar under these conditions to the under-utilization of glucose by muscle.

Adipose tissue, however, is known to be exquisitively sensitive to insulin lack. Without insulin, glucose utilization is inadequate and this in turn initiates profound disturbances of lipid metabolism. Under-utilization of glucose by adipose tissue could, in part at least, account for the hyperglycaemia. In addition, many of the complications of diabetes are obviously related to changes in lipid metabolism.

The other major glucose consuming organ in the body is the brain, but the general concensus of opinion is, that its glucose uptake is not affected directly by either the presence or the absence of insulin.

It would thus appear that the hyperglycaemia of diabetes must be attributed in the first place to under-utilization of glucose by various tissues but particularly by adipose tissue. At a later stage the hyperglycaemia is maintained or even further increased by overproduction by the liver of glucose from non-carbohydrate precursors. The new glucose molecules are ultimately derived from an increased catabolism of protein. This yields amino-acids and, by transamination in the liver, pyruvate is produced. Two molecules of pyruvate so formed are then resynthesized in the liver to one molecule of glucose.

$$2(C_3H_4O_3) + 4H \longrightarrow C_6H_{12}O_6$$
$$\text{Pyruvate} \longrightarrow \text{Glucose}$$

The hydrogen required for this synthesis is derived from the oxidation of hydrogen-rich fatty acids. Within the cell, hydrogen is made available in the form of the reduced coenzymes triphosphopyridine nucleotide (TPNH) and diphosphopyridine nucleotide (DPNH). TPNH takes part in the initial step of the synthesis of pyruvate to glucose. This is the conversion of pyruvate to phospho-enol-pyruvate by a process of CO_2 fixation.

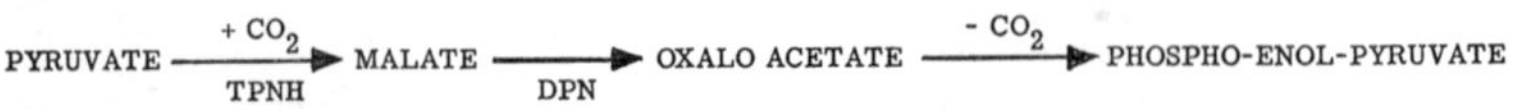

$$\text{PYRUVATE} \xrightarrow[\text{TPNH}]{+ CO_2} \text{MALATE} \xrightarrow[\text{DPN}]{} \text{OXALO ACETATE} \xrightarrow{- CO_2} \text{PHOSPHO-ENOL-PYRUVATE}$$

FIG. 25. CO_2 fixation: the initial step of gluconeogenesis in the liver.

By a reversal of the glycolytic pathways, phospho-enol-pyruvate is then converted to phospho-glycerate. At this stage another hydrogen is introduced, this time by DPNH, to reduce glycerate to the triose phosphates glyceraldehyde and dihydroxy-acetone phosphate. Two molecules of these triosephosphates combine to yield glucose-6-phosphate, from which the liver finally produces a new molecule of glucose.

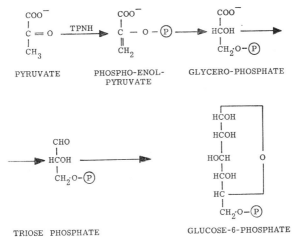

FIG. 26. A simplified version of the Embden Meyerhof pathway followed in gluconeogenesis.

As mentioned above, in the absence of insulin there is an increased catabolism of protein. Korner and Manchester (1960) showed that insulin affects the incorporation of amino-acids into muscle proteins, apparently independently of its action on glucose. Normally, in the presence of insulin, the amino-acids formed from the intracellular breakdown of protein are resynthesized into tissue-protein. In the absence of insulin, the process of amino-acid incorporation into protein is reduced and the amino-acids accumulating in the cell escape into the plasma and are carried to the liver where they become available for transamination to pyruvate. The nitrogen of the protein is wasted and appears in the urine as urea.

Fatty acids come to the liver from the adipose tissues. In the fat cells, triglyceride fat is constantly breaking down to fatty acids and the acids are then resynthesized to triglycerides by esterification with glycero-phosphate. Insulin lack, by reducing the entry of glucose into fat cells, reduces the production of glycero-phosphate. The breakdown of triglycerides continues and the fatty acids which cannot now be re-synthesized to triglyceride, accumulate in the fat depots, are discharged into the blood and carried to muscle and liver. The free fatty acids which are not used by muscle for energy metabolism are carried to the liver, there to be partly resynthesized to triglyceride and long-chain fatty acids and partly to be oxidized via acetoacetyl-CoA. Some of the acetoacetyl CoA forms ketone bodies, viz., acetoacetate and β-hydroxy-butyrate. These diffuse into the blood and are also used by muscle for the production of energy. As long as muscle can metabolize these ketone bodies, there will be no ketosis. But when insulin deficiency is severe and fatty acids flood to the liver from the depots, acetoacetate begins to accumulate in the blood and the resulting ketonaemia and ketonuria aggravate the already existing metabolic disturbances of hyperglycaemia and glycosuria.

In the liver, the ability to synthesize long-chain fatty acids is lost as soon as ketone bodies begin to accumulate. The pathway of fatty acid synthesis differs from that of its catabolism.

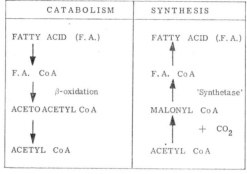

CoA = Coenzyme A

FIG. 27. Synthesis of fatty acids. (This is not simply a reversal of their catabolism but involves different enzymes and co-factors.)

It had been thought that the limiting factor in fatty acid synthesis is TPNH (Siperstein, 1959). But recently, considerable doubt has been thrown on this suggestion by the fact that TPNH is generated to the same extent by the livers of normal and diabetic rats (Abraham *et al.*, 1959). Some very recent work on acute insulin deficiency in rats induced by anti-insulin serum suggests an alternative explanation (Ashmore and Mahler, 1961). Acetoacetate is formed in the liver early in acute insulin deficiency and its appearance is associated with impairment of long chain fatty acid synthesis. It is conceivable that acetoacetyl CoA may act as a structural competitor with malonyl CoA for the enzyme 'fatty acid synthetase' and so block the synthesis of these fatty acids. This would be a satisfying explanation for the inhibition of a synthetic process by its own product of oxidation.

In summary, adipose tissue appears to be the important insulin-sensitive tissue. In a normal man, about 20% of the body weight is fat, but even a thin man rarely has less than 10% fat. In insulin deficiency, the threshold of this tissue to the entry of glucose is raised. To overcome this and to restore normal function, the glucose concentration in the

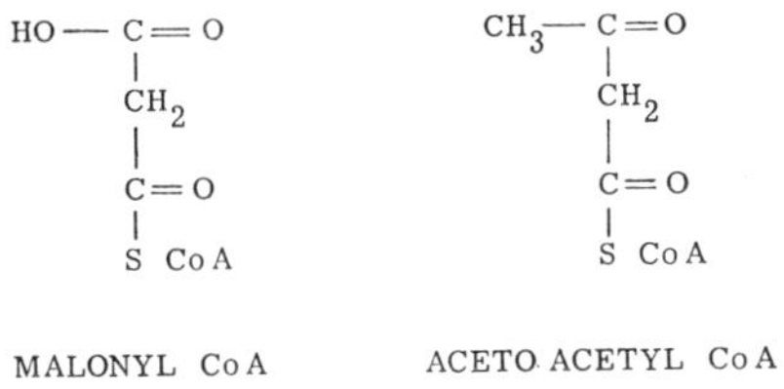

FIG. 28. Structural similarity of the co-enzymes involved in fatty acid metabolism.

blood and extra-cellular fluid must increase (Winegrad and Renold, 1958). Much of the extra glucose released from the liver is derived by gluconeogenesis from amino-acids. When the fat depots are starved of glucose, fatty acids escape into the blood and are carried to the liver, where they are oxidized to yield the hydrogen required for gluconeo-genesis. Insulin lowers the threshold to glucose, fat synthesis in the fat depots is restored and in due course, the hepatic glucose output returns to normal; the other metabolic disturbances, such as ketosis and protein wastage, also return to normal. Throughout these disturbances, muscle appears to act as a metabolic banker: it abstracts from the circulation the excess of any available substrate which it may then use to provide energy, but contributes its own amino-acids when required to maintain a stable metabolic economy.

VIEWS ON DIABETES MELLITUS

Until recently, diabetes was assumed to be simply due to an absolute deficiency of insulin secretion by the pancreas. But as we have already indicated, the recognition of insulin antagonists has stimulated many new concepts of diabetes.

Thus the diminished insulin content of the pancreas may merely reflect the exhausted state of the β-cells after vain attempts to neutralize excessive amounts of circulating antagonists. Obesity, which is generally thought to contribute to the development of diabetes, may in fact be the consequence of an excess of antibody-bound insulin, free to act only upon adipose tissue. It may be that some of the complications of diabetes, particularly those affecting the endothelium of the blood vessels, may similarly arise as the result of an excess rather than a lack of circulating insulin.

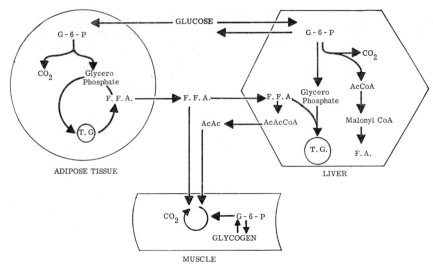

NORMAL

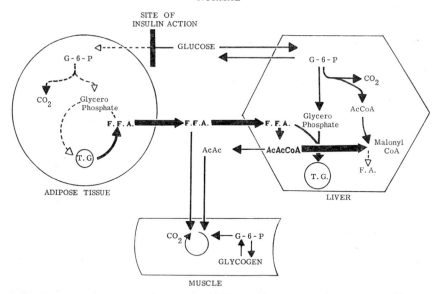

DIABETIC

FIG. 29. A suggested relationship between fat and carbohydrate metabolism in vivo. Fat, present in adipose tissue as triglycerides (T.G.), breaks down to short-chain free fatty acids (F.F.A.) which are re-esterified to triglyceride in the presence of adequate amounts of glycero-phosphate. In the absence of insulin, inadequate amounts of glucose enter the fat cell with subsequent lack of glycero-phosphate for re-esterification. The free fatty acids escape into the blood and are carried to the liver, there to be partly esterified to triglyceride and partly to be oxidized and converted through aceto-acetyl CoA (AcAcCoA) to aceto-acetate (AcAc) which can be mopped up by muscle. When the amount of free fatty acids released overwhelms the liver, AcAcCoA accumulates and inhibits the normal process of long-chain fatty acid synthesis (F.A.) taking place via malonyl CoA. For further details, see text. (Adapted from Renold and Cahill, 1960.)

Such re-appraisals of the fundamental causes of diabetes have the merit of offering a fresh approach to the treatment of diabetes, particularly with respect to the prevention of diabetic complications. The incidence of these complications is still disappointingly high in spite of apparently satisfactory control of the hyperglycaemia.

Because of this unsatisfactory state, a great deal of attention is now given to the early diagnosis of asymptomatic 'latent' diabetes and to the detection of 'pre-diabetes'. The latent diabetic, although free from symptoms, shows the characteristic diabetic response to laboratory tests such as the glucose tolerance test. Subjects with a strong family history of diabetes are suspected of being in the prediabetic state. They often have an abnormal glucose tolerance test according to the stringent criteria laid down by Conn (1958).

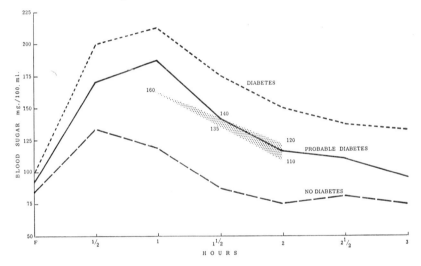

FIG. 30. Significance of glucose tolerance curves.
The glucose tolerance is abnormal if the blood sugar concentration is above 160, 140 and 120 mg./100 ml. at 1, 1½ and 2 hours respectively, after a standard glucose load.
It is normal, if the values lie below 160, 135 and 110 mg./100 ml. at these same times.
The shaded area indicates the response of a group of people who will probably develop diabetes at some future date. (From Conn, 1958.)

To expose the abnormality, the ordinary glucose tolerance test may have to be augmented by the addition of 50 mg. of cortisone given 8½ and 2 hours before the glucose load. With this method, many prediabetics have been detected. Also, mothers whose babies weigh more than 10 lbs. at birth are very likely to develop diabetes sometime later, and a very high proportion of these mothers have an abnormal cortisone-glucose tolerance test.

Can the future development of diabetes be prevented if treatment with insulin or other hypoglycaemic agents is started in this prediabetic state?

The approach to this problem depends a great deal on the concepts of the precipitating causes of diabetes. Plans to study this problem were discussed at great length at the 4th Congress of the International Diabetic Federation in 1961.

GLUCAGON

The name 'glucagon' was given in 1923 to a factor found in a pancreatic extract which caused a rise in blood sugar (Kimball and Murlin, 1923); it was thought to be the same substance as that which caused a transient rise in blood sugar when crude insulin preparations were injected intravenously (Macleod, 1922; Collip, 1923).

ORIGIN

There is a great deal of evidence to support the view that glucagon is secreted in the pancreas by the alpha-cells of the islets of Langerhans (Foà and Galansino, 1960); it has also been found in the mucosa of the stomach and the duodenum of the dog and rabbit (Sutherland and de Duve, 1948) and in other tissues, including lymphatic tissue and skin (Rao and De, 1955).

CHEMISTRY

In 1953 glucagon was isolated from the pancreas and crystallized by Staub and his co-workers at the Lilly Laboratories. These workers showed it to be a polypeptide with a minimum molecular weight of 3482 (Bromer *et al.*, 1957).

$$
\begin{array}{ccc}
\text{NH}_2 & \text{NH}_2 & \text{NH}_2 \\
| & | & |
\end{array}
$$

LEU. ASP. SER. ARG. ARG. ALA. GLU. ASP. PHE. VAL. GLU. TYR. LEU. MET. ASP. THR.
|
TYR. LYS. SER. TYR. ASP. SER. THR. PHE. THR. GLY. GLU. SER. HIS.
|
NH_2

FIG. 31. The sequence of amino-acids in glucagon.

The molecule consists of 29 amino-acids in a single chain. It differs in its amino acid composition from insulin in containing no cystine, proline or isoleucine, but it contains methionine and tryptophan which are absent from insulin. Glucagon is more resistant to alkali than insulin and is not susceptible to cystine reduction. It is not destroyed by whole blood, but is rapidly removed from the circulation by the liver and other tissues.

Several degradation products have been prepared, but so far none have been found to possess a glucagon-like action. It is, therefore, probable that the complete molecule is required for biological activity.

ACTION OF GLUCAGON

The hyperglycaemic action of glucagon is the result of mobilization of liver glycogen (Bürger and Kramer, 1929), with subsequent outpouring of free glucose from the liver (Myers *et al.*, 1952). The height and duration of the blood sugar response are dependent on the availability of glycogen stores in the liver (Rossi *et al.*, 1957) and on the dose of glucagon injected (Butterfield *et al.*, 1960). The smallest dose, injected intravenously, to give a definite, reproducible effect on blood sugar, is 0·5 μg. per kg. body weight. Recently, a considerable release of glucose from the liver in man has been achieved by as little as a total of 0·5 to 1·0 μg. injected directly into the liver through a catheter wedged in a hepatic vein (Rees *et al.*, 1961). The mobilization of glycogen is brought about by the activation of the enzyme phosphorylase; the details of this process have been described by Sutherland and his co-workers (Rall *et al.*, 1956) and by Berthet (1959).

Phosphorylase catalyzes the degradation of glycogen to glucose-1-phosphate; in the process, the enzyme becomes inactivated. Reactivation of the enzyme is brought about by a 'cyclic adenosine monophosphate'. This co-factor is formed in the presence of ATP and magnesium as the result of the action of glucagon on a particulate fraction of the cell (see Fig. 12, p. 108). The same nucleotide has recently been shown to activate another enzyme—phosphofructokinase—which is one of the enzymes concerned in the glycolytic pathway (Mansour and Menard, 1960). Glucagon activates only liver and heart phosphorylase and phosphofructokinase. It has no effect on these enzymes in skeletal muscle. Intra-arterial injection of glucagon in physiological doses does not affect the glucose uptake of human forearm tissues (Butterfield *et al*, 1960; Ginsburg *et al.*, 1960). In these studies on the human forearm, plethysmographic measurements showed no change in muscle blood-flow. But a big increase in liver blood flow measured by the bromsulphalein excretion technique was observed in dogs after systemic or intra-portal injection of glucagon (Shoemaker *et al.*, 1959).

The action of glucagon on phosphorylase stimulation is similar to that of adrenaline in its biochemical detail. Adrenaline, however, also activates the phosphorylase of skeletal muscle. Moreover, ergotamine blocks the action of adrenaline on glycogenolysis, but does not affect glucagon.

ASSAY

The most sensitive and specific test available at present depends on a radio-immunological assay similar to that of insulin (Unger *et al.*, 1961). It is claimed that as little as 50 μμg. of glucagon can be estimated by this technique. This represents about 6×10^9 molecules of glucagon and is 400 times as sensitive as the immunological insulin assay.

GLUCAGON IN PLASMA

Using such a specific immune assay, it was found that the level of glucagon in femoral vein plasma averaged 44 μg./100 ml. and the glucagon level in the pancreatico-duodenal vein averaged 65 μg./100 ml. (Unger *et al.*, 1961). There was almost always a gradient across the liver. The glucagon level in the pancreatico-duodenal vein rose in response to insulin-induced hypoglycaemia and returned rapidly to normal after an intravenous injection of glucose (Vuylsteke and de Duve, 1957).

PHYSIOLOGICAL ROLE OF GLUCAGON

Glucagon is secreted by the pancreas and carried in the blood to the liver, where it exerts its physiological function. It fulfils, therefore, the criteria by which it may be regarded as a hormone.

The significance of glucagon in the general metabolism of the body is not entirely clear. The most reasonable hypothesis concerns its counterplay with insulin in glucose homeostasis: hypoglycaemia caused by insulin is followed by an increase in hepatic glucose output, stimulated by glucagon. But there is nothing to suggest that glucagon plays a part in the aetiology of human diabetes or that it affects its clinical course. Glucagon has been found to have two other actions in the body:

(i) The motility both of the stomach and of the colon is drastically reduced within a few minutes of the injection of glucagon and gastric secretion is diminished (Sporn and Necheles, 1956). This effect persists while glucagon is infused, but ceases within a few minutes of termination of the infusion.

(ii) Glucagon also enhances the renal clearance of a number of electrolytes, but again, this effect is transient. It is thought to be due to an action on the renal tubules and not related to the hyperglycaemia (Elrick *et al.*, 1958).

CLINICAL APPLICATIONS

The response to physiological doses of glucagon has been used to study the carbohydrate metabolism of diabetic patients (Butterfield *et al.*, 1960). Patients, whose diabetes is under good control, whether by insulin or sulphonylureas, show a normal rise in blood sugar after glucagon. From this it is inferred that their glycogen stores are adequate; an observation of considerable value, since the ability of the liver to synthesize glycogen is lost early in insulin deficiency (Renold *et al.*, 1953).

Glucagon has also been used for the treatment of hypoglycaemia due to an excess of insulin (Elrick *et al.*, 1958). 5 mg. of glucagon, injected intramuscularly, produces a rise in blood sugar adequate to terminate the hypoglycaemic manifestations, but without causing the excessively high blood sugar levels which generally occur after the conventional treatment with 25, 50 or sometimes even 100 grams of glucose.

Prolonged infusions of glucagon have been given to a group of patients with rheumatoid arthritis. The relief obtained was very slight and transient, but the side effects, particularly vomiting, were prolonged and distressing (Ezrin *et al.*, 1958). Glucagon has also proved of some value in certain types of glycogen storage diseases if given several times a day and particularly if given immediately after meals. When given in this way, it may help to prevent the trapping of the absorbed glucose as glycogen in the liver and may also help to prevent spontaneous hypoglycaemic attacks.

In general, however, it may be said that there is at present no clear indication for the routine clinical use of glucagon.

SYNTHETIC HYPOGLYCAEMIC AGENTS

The search for effective hypoglycaemic agents has an interesting and varied history. Claims that they were of value in the treatment of diabetes were made for innumerable compounds before insulin became available. Many were quite valueless; some caused severe damage to the liver or kidney, though several did appear to reduce glycosuria. But the majority of these latter compounds were merely diuretic agents, thus reducing the urinary glucose concentration without in any way diminishing the daily wastage of glucose in the urine (von Noorden, 1901).

After the discovery of insulin in 1922, its large scale production made it readily available to diabetic patients all over the world. Consequently, interest in other forms of treatment fell off, particularly as it was generally considered that diabetes is no more than the clinical manifestation of insulin deficiency and that all its clinical aspects could be dealt with completely by adequate treatment with insulin.

It was also unfortunate that just about that time a guanide derivative (Synthalin), which appeared to be a promising oral hypoglycaemic agent, caused a number of deaths from severe liver damage. This fact, when compared to the safety and effectiveness of insulin, stopped further serious research along these lines.

Thirty years later, clinical experience of the treatment of diabetes had reached the point where the introduction of a hypoglycaemic agent, effective by oral administration, was eagerly accepted and could be subjected to careful clinical trials. The sulphonylureas were introduced in 1954 and the biguanides followed shortly thereafter.

Since the introduction of these compounds, a vast amount of pharmacological, biochemical and clinical research has been done and many entirely different compounds examined for hypoglycaemic activity. However, the compounds now in use still belong to only one or other of these two groups. Their properties and uses have been reviewed by

Duncan and Baird (1960) and by Creutzfeldt and Söling (1961). The effectiveness of salicylates in the treatment of diabetes was discovered in 1877 (Müller, 1877) and rediscovered in 1957 (Reid *et al.*, 1957). They are proving to be of some practical value in combination with other oral hypoglycaemic drugs (Stowers *et al.*, 1959).

THE SULPHONYLUREAS

The accidental discovery of the hypoglycaemic properties of sulphanilyl thiadiazoles by Janbon in 1942, their systematic study by Loubatières in France during the war and the equally accidental discovery of the hypoglycaemic properties of sulphonylureas in 1954 is now well known and requires no re-telling (Duncan and Baird, 1960).

CHEMISTRY

The relation between chemical structure and hypoglycaemic activity of these compounds has been reviewed recently (Mahler, 1960). The sulphonylureas are substituted urea derivatives.

Hundreds of sulphonylureas with various side chains and rings have been synthesized and tested for hypoglycaemic activity and the main ones are shown in Table 13.

Table 13.

SULPHONYL UREA DERIVATIVES

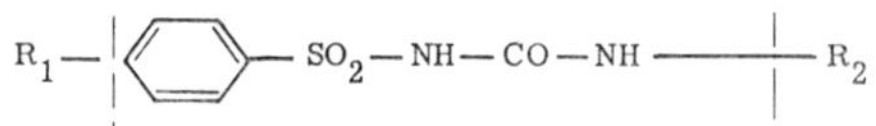

$R_1 -$ [benzene ring] $- SO_2 - NH - CO - NH -$ R_2

R_1		R_2
H_2N	CARBUTAMIDE	C_4H_9
CH_3	TOLBUTAMIDE	C_4H_9
Cl	CHLORPROPAMIDE	C_3H_7
$CH_3\text{-}C(=O)$	ACETOHEXAMIDE	C_6H_6

From the various substitutions and subsequent pharmacological trials, certain general rules concerning the relationship of hypoglycaemic activity to chemical structure have been established. Substitution in the benzene ring with a halogen such as chlorine, yields potent and long acting compounds, e.g. chlorpropamide, but hypoglycaemic activity is lost if many other simple radicals, such as $-OH$, $-CH_2OH$, $-NO_2$ are used. Maximum activity is found in compounds in which the hydrogen of the other $-NH_2$ group of the urea radical is replaced by an alkyl group containing 3 to 6 carbon atoms (e.g. butyl). This confers lipophilic properties on the whole molecule and is essential if it is to have any hypoglycaemic action at all.

TOLBUTAMIDE, CHLORPROPAMIDE AND ACETOHEXAMIDE

At the present time, the safest and most effective of the sulphonylureas are tolbutamide and chlorpropamide. They are the only two in common use. Because they do not possess an aminogroup attached to the benzene ring, they are without the antibacterial properties of the sulphonamides; but, probably for the same reason, they do not have the toxic actions of the sulphonamides on the bone marrow. Carbutamide, the first sulphonylurea to be used, has such an aminogroup and, although effective, proved to be toxic. Its use has been condemned.

After oral administration, peak blood levels are achieved within 4 hours. The rate of disappearance of these drugs from the blood varies considerably, tolbutamide having a half-life of 5 hours, while that of chlorpropamide is about 35 hours. The effective blood levels of these compounds range from 1 to 20 mg./100 ml. Between these limits, there is a direct relationship between the concentration of the drug in the blood and its hypoglycaemic effects. At greater concentrations, however, no further hypoglycaemic response is obtained. This is probably related to the fact that more than half of the drug in the blood may be bound to protein and is pharmacologically inactive. The drugs are distributed in the body in a volume corresponding to the extra-cellular fluid.

Tolbutamide is metabolized in the body to an inactive compound by carboxylation in the para position; 10–30% of the drug exists in the plasma in this inactive form. Chlorpropamide, however, because of its chlorine group in that position, cannot be inactivated in the same way. Elimination from the body is entirely by renal excretion, both of the active and inactive forms.

Very recently, a new sulphonylurea, acetohexamide, has come into clinical use and may take its place alongside chlorpropamide and tolbutamide (Anderson *et al.*, 1961). This compound is an analogue of metahexamide which was a very effective hypoglycaemic agent, but had to be withdrawn by the manufacturers when several cases of severe liver damage had been reported following its use at high dose levels. Acetohexamide has now had a clinical trial for over a year without any such undesirable effects. It disappears from the blood more slowly than tolbutamide and 50% of a single dose is excreted in the urine in 24 hours. The metabolite, which is excreted in the urine also has some hypoglycaemic actions in the dog and rat. Evidence so far indicates that the mechanism of action of acetohexamide is similar to that of tolbutamide and it appears to have the same indications for clinical use so that success may be expected in diabetes developing in middle life. The daily dosage of acetohexamide ranges from 250–1,500 mg. The average dose is of the order of 750 mg./day, given in divided doses.

MODE OF ACTION

The mode of action of the sulphonylureas is by no means settled. There is now very good evidence that they stimulate the secretion of insulin. Raised plasma insulin levels have been found in the pancreatico-duodenal vein and in peripheral veins (Vallance-Owen *et al.*, 1959) after sulphonylurea administration. In very mild diabetics, the carbohydrate tolerance was restored to normal by the long continued use of tolbut-amide (Fajans, 1961) and a reduction in the tissue glucose threshold, similar to that caused by insulin, was found in diabetic patients after 9 days of treatment with tolbutamide (Butterfield *et al.*, 1958). In juvenile diabetics and in totally depancreatized animals, the sulphonylureas do

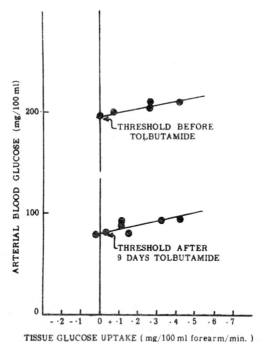

FIG. 32. The effect of tolbutamide on tissue glucose threshold of a diabetic patient.

not lower the blood sugar; nor have they any effect when such patients or experimental animals are given an injection of insulin.

It is clear, therefore, that the ability of these drugs to lower the blood sugar depends on the presence of a normal pancreas.

The initial fall in blood glucose is not accompanied by an increase in glucose utilization (Stadie, 1958), but is the result of a reduced glucose output by the liver (Ashmore *et al.*, 1958; Tarding and Schambye, 1960; Jacobs *et al.*, 1958). The reduction in hepatic glucose output may be due to the insulin released from the pancreas or it may be the result of the effect of the drug directly on the liver. The only stumbling block in accepting the first possibility is the uncertainty of the immediate effect of insulin on the release of glucose from the liver; but it has been suggested that insulin does have such an action if it reaches the liver through the portal vein in small amounts at a time (Madison and Unger, 1958).

Direct effects of the sulphonylureas on many aspects of liver metabolism have been demonstrated *in vitro* but are thought to be of little consequence in relation to their hypoglycaemic activity (Creutzfeldt and Söling, 1961).

CLINICAL USE

Thousands of patients have now been treated with various sulphonylureas and the indications for their use have become well established.

Best results have been obtained in patients whose diabetes began in middle age, who are overweight (which indicates that they have good supplies of endogenous insulin), who do not develop ketosis and who have had their disease for not more than 5 years. They represent about 10% of all patients attending diabetic clinics in Great Britain and the United States. These compounds are not effective in diabetics with severe insulin deficiency and may be disappointing in long standing diabetes, where the beta-cells are presumably exhausted. In general, they are of no value in juvenile diabetics, but occasional successes have been reported in young patients in whom the diabetes was of very recent (2–3 weeks) onset.

As would be expected from their pharmacological behaviour in the body, tolbutamide must be given three times a day, but chlorpropamide needs only to be taken once a day. Chlorpropamide in doses greater than 0·5 gm. may give rise to gastro-intestinal side effects and if a greater dose is required, it should be divided. A reasonable maintenance dose of chlorpropamide is 250–350 mg./day. Tolbutamide is not quite as active on a weight for weight basis, and 0·5 gm. two or three times a day is generally required. The maximal response usually occurs on the first day of treatment, but occasionally no response may be seen for several days.

One of the current clinical problems in the use of sulphonylureas is the occurrence of so-called 'secondary failure'. By definition, this refers to patients who, after a period of at least one month of satisfactory treatment, lose their responsiveness to the drug. Some recent figures from the Joslin Clinic (Marble and Camerini-Davalos, 1961) show that secondary failure occurred in 20% of 300 patients. Excluding various exogenous factors, such as faulty selection of patients for treatment, or dietary indiscretions, only 5% could be attributed to true failure to respond to the drug after initial satisfactory control.

It is very interesting and of considerable importance that patients who have resumed insulin after a period of tolbutamide therapy showed no increase in insulin requirement and no deterioration of glucose tolerance.

TOXIC AND SIDE EFFECTS

Toxic effects of tolbutamide and chlorpropamide are remarkably rare. A few minor reactions such as rashes and gastro-intestinal upsets may occur in 1–2% of patients and may occasionally necessitate stopping the drug. Serious marrow depression is very rare, but transient leucopenia and hypoplastic anaemia have been reported; a few cases of thrombocytopenic purpura have occurred in patients on chlorpropamide. An intriguing side effect of tolbutamide and chlorpropamide is the conspicuous flushing which occurs in some patients after taking alcohol.

LONG TERM TREATMENT WITH SULPHONYLUREAS

The sulphonylureas, particularly tolbutamide and chlorpropamide, have been widely used for the last 5–6 years. In Great Britain, their use is confined mainly to middle-aged or elderly patients whose diabetes cannot be controlled adequately by diet alone. In other countries, particularly Germany, the sulphonylureas are given more freely and less emphasis is placed upon dietary restriction.

Such differences in the approach to the management of diabetes will make it difficult to assess the long term results of drug treatment. The touchstone of successful treatment is the prevention of the complications of diabetes such as obliterative vascular disease, retinopathy, nephropathy and neuropathies. If the action of these drugs is indeed a stimulation of insulin secretion by the pancreas, without exhausting the β-cells, then the prognosis of patients taking these drugs should be no worse than if they were taking insulin; it may even be better, if endogenous insulin has a more physiological action than injected insulin of animal origin.

BIGUANIDES

Shortly after the unfortunate experiences with the diguanidines—Synthalin A and Synthalin B—a series of synthetic biguanides were found to have hypoglycaemic properties when tested in animals; but it is not surprising that at that time no clinical trials were undertaken. However, almost 30 years later the search for new oral antidiabetic compounds was in full swing. Now the appraisal, by clinical trial, of a new biguanide, phenformin, was acceptable, particularly as two other guanides, viz. chlorhexidine ('Hibitane') and proguanil hydrochloride

('Paludrine') both without hypoglycaemic action, had already shown that they could be used with safety over long periods.

CHEMISTRY

The biguanides are derived from two moles of guanidine with the elimination of one mole of ammonia. They have two guanide groups in apposition and differ, thus, from the diguanidines which may be

Table 13. Formulae of some guanide derivatives.

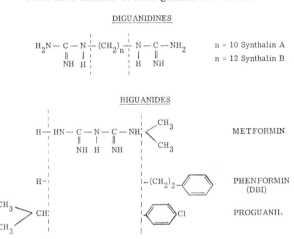

considered as being made up of two terminal guanidine molecules separated from each other by an intervening chain of methylene groups. If more than one amino group of the biguanide molecule is substituted hypoglycaemic activity is lost; but one or both hydrogen atoms of the same amino group may be substituted (Mahler, 1960).

FATE IN THE BODY

Relatively little is known about the metabolism of the biguanides in the body. Cohen and Costerousse (1961) studied the autoradiographs of mice after administration of ^{14}C labelled dimethyl biguanide (metformin). They observed that it had a particular affinity for the intestinal mucosa, not only after oral, but even after subcutaneous or intravenous administration. The metabolic half-life of phenformin labelled with radioactive sulphur is about 6 hours. Most of the injected compound is excreted unchanged in the urine.

HYPOGLYCAEMIC ACTION

After oral administration, the blood glucose concentration begins to fall within 2 hours and the effect persists for 6–14 hours. Unlike the sulphonylureas, the magnitude and duration of the fall increases with increasing dosage. In practice, the dose range is limited by the appearance of gastro-intestinal disturbances, particularly vomiting. The maximum single dose tolerated is about 400 mg.

Only diabetic patients respond to phenformin with hypoglycaemia. This applies to the middle aged, overweight diabetic as well as to the juvenile diabetic. Normal subjects show no change in blood sugar even after maximal doses of phenformin (Fajans *et al.*, 1960).

The action of the biguanides at cell level is at present under active investigation, but no clear picture has emerged yet. The original hypothesis, that phenformin interferes with the cytochrome system (Williams *et al.*, 1957) has now been shown to have been based on the use of a large excess of the drug; smaller, though still adequate, doses of phenformin do not have this action, and this interference is not caused by metformin at any dose level.

Using the technique for metabolic studies on the human forearm previously described (Butterfield and Holling, 1959) it was found that effective oral treatment with phenformin reduced the tissue glucose threshold; but no effect on glucose uptake by these tissues occurred after the direct injection of the drug into the brachial artery. From these and other studies it was concluded that, *in vivo*, phenformin has no significant direct action of its own on the peripheral tissues but exerts its blood-sugar lowering effects by augmenting the action of insulin (Butterfield *et al.*, 1961b).

CLINICAL APPLICATION

The place of the biguanides in the treatment of diabetes is not yet fully defined. Diabetic patients of all types may respond to them.

In general, the biguanides are not given to patients who respond adequately to diet alone or to the sulphonylureas. There is clearly a general feeling that they are not as safe as the sulphonylureas. Serious toxic effects, are, however, very rare. But the biguanides often cause gastro-intestinal upsets, particularly nausea and vomiting, which have not infrequently been severe enough to force the withdrawal of the drug.

The biguanides are probably finding their place as adjuvants to insulin or the sulphonylureas (Bewsher and Stowers, 1961). The recently introduced timed-disintegration capsules (Radding and Zimmerman, 1961) are said to cause less dyspepsia and to produce smoother control of the insulin-requiring diabetic (Fabrykant and Ashe, 1961). The biguanides are particularly useful in patients who require uncomfortably large doses of insulin. They can reduce the insulin requirement by up to 25%, but they cannot replace insulin entirely.

The biguanides have been of value in the management of secondary failure to sulphonylurea therapy. In such patients there would appear to be a true potentiation between the sulphonylureas and the biguanides

(Bewsher and Stowers, 1961). Some patients on phenformin easily become ketotic and have raised plasma lactic and pyruvic acid concentrations (Walker and Linton, 1959). This does not seem to occur so frequently with metformin.

REFERENCES

* Denotes review

ABEL, J. J., GEILING, E. M. K., ROUILLER, C. A., BELL, F. K. and WINTERSTEINER, O. (1927). *J. Pharmacol. exp. Ther.* **31**, 65
ABRAHAM, S., MATTHES, K. J. and CHAIKOFF, I. L. (1959). *Biochim. biophys. Acta*, **36**, 356
ANDERSON, E., WHERRY, F. and BATES, R. W. (1959). *Fed. Proc.* **18**, 4
ANDERSON, R. C., ROOT, M. A. and WELLES, J. S. (1961). Report of Lilly Research Laboratories
ANDRES, R., CADER, G. and ZIERLER, K. L. (1956). *J. clin. Invest.* **35**, 671
ANNOTATION (1960). *Lancet*, **2**, 1311
ANTONIADES, H. N. (1958). *Science*, **127**, 593
ANTONIADES, H. N., BEIGELMAN, P. M. and RENOLD, A. E. (1960). In 'Hormones in Human Plasma'. Ed. Antoniades, H. N. Boston: Little, Brown
ARMIN, J., GRANT, R. T. and WRIGHT, P. H. (1960). *J. Physiol. (Lond.)*, **153**, 146
ASHMORE, J. (1961). Personal communication
ASHMORE, J., CAHILL, G. F., JR., EARLE, A. S. and ZOTTU, S. M. (1958). *Diabetes*, **7**, 1
ASHMORE, J. and MAHLER, R. F. (1961). To be published
BANTING, F. G. and BEST, C. H. (1922). *J. Lab. clin. Med.* **7**, 251
BATTS, A. (1959). *Ann. N.Y. Acad. Sci.* **82**, 302
BERSON, S. A., YALOW, R. S., BANNAN, A., ROTHSCHILD, M. A. and NEWERLY, K. (1956). *J. clin. Invest.* **35**, 170
BERSON, S. A. and YALOW, R. S. (1960). In 'Hormones in Human Plasma'. Ed. Antoniades, H. N. Boston: Little, Brown
BERSON, S. A. and YALOW, R. S. (1961). In Proc. IVth Congr. Intern. Diabet. Fed., Geneva
*BERTHET, J. (1959). *Amer. J. Med.* **26**, 703
BEWSHER, P. and STOWERS, J. M. (1961). In Proc. IVth Congr. Intern. Diabet. Fed., Geneva
BRIGGS, J. H., BUTTERFIELD, W. J. H., GARRATT, C. J., PEARSON, J. D. and WHICHELOW, M. J. (1960). In 'Radioaktive Isotope in Klinik und Forschung. IV.' Ed. Fellinger, K. and Höfer, R. Munich: Urban and Schwarzenberg
BROMER, W. W., SINN, L. G., STAUB, A. and BEHRENS, D. K. (1957). *Diabetes*, **6**, 234
BÜRGER, M. and KRAMER, H. (1929). *Z. ges. exp. Med.* **69**, 57
BUTTERFIELD, W. J. H. (1961). *Brit. med. J.* **1**, 1705
BUTTERFIELD, W. J. H., CAMERON, J. S., GARRATT, J., McCOLLISTER, D. L. (1961a). Unpublished observations
BUTTERFIELD, W. J. H., FRY, I. K., WHICHELOW, M. J. (1960). *Guy's Hosp. Rep.* **109**, 95
BUTTERFIELD, W. J. H., FRY, I. K. and HOLLING, H. E. (1958). *Diabetes*, **7**, 449
BUTTERFIELD, W. J. H., FRY, I. K. and WHICHELOW, M. J. (1961). *Lancet*, **2**, 563
BUTTERFIELD, W. J. H. and HOLLING, H. E. (1959). *Clin. Sci.* **18**, 147
COHEN, Y. and COSTEROUSSE, O. (1961). In Proc. IVth Congr. Intern. Diabet. Fed., Geneva
COLLIP, J. B. (1923). *Amer. J. Physiol.* **63**, 391
CONN, J. W. (1958). *Diabetes*, **7**, 347
CORI, C. F. (1945). *Harvey Lect.* **41**, 253

CREUTZFELDT, W. and SÖLING, H. D. (1961). 'Oral Treatment of Diabetes'.
   Berlin: Springer-Verlag
*DUNCAN, L. J. P. and BAIRD, J. D. (1960). *Pharmacol. Rev.* **12**, 91
DUNN, A., STEELE, R., ALTSZULER, N., DE BODO, R. C., ARMSTRONG, D. T. and
   BISHOP, J. S. (1960). In Proc. 1st Intern. Congr. Endocrinol., Copenhagen
ELRICK, H., HUFFMAN, E. R., HLAD, C. J., WHIPPLE, N. and STAUB, A. (1958).
   J. clin. Endocr. **18**, 813
EZRIN, C., SALTER, J. M., OGRYZLO, M. A. and BEST, C. H. (1958). *J. Canad.
   med. Ass.* **78**, 96
FABRYKANT, M. and ASHE, B. I. (1961). *Metabolism*, **10**, 684
FAJANS, S. S. (1961). In Proc. IVth Congr. Intern. Diabet. Fed., Geneva
FAJANS, S. S., MOORHOUSE, J. A., DOORNEBOS, H., LOUIS, L. H. and CONN, J. W.
   (1960). *Diabetes*, **9**, 194
FIELD, J. B. and STETTEN, D., JR. (1956). *Amer. J. Med.* **21**, 339
FISHER, R. B. (1960). *Brit. med. Bull.* **16**, 224
FOÀ, P. P. (1956). Ciba Found. Coll. Endocr. **9**, 55. London: Churchill
FOÀ, P. P. and GALANSINO, G. (1960). In 'Clinical Endocrinology. I.' Ed. Astwood,
   E. B. New York: Grune and Stratton
GINSBURG, J., GALBRAITH, H. J. B. and PATON, A. (1960). In 'Mechanism of
   Action of Insulin.' Eds. Young, F. G., Broom, W. A. and Wolff, W. F.
   Oxford: Blackwell Scientific Publications
GOETZ, F. C. and EGDAHL, R. G. (1958). *Fed. Proc.* **17**, 55
*GOLDSTEIN, M. S. and LEVINE, R. (1960). In 'Clinical Endocrinology. I.' Ed.
   Astwood, E. B. New York: Grune and Stratton
HUMBEL, R. E., RENOLD, A. E., HERRERA, M. G. and TAYLOR, K. W. (1961).
   Endocrinology, **69**, 874
JACOBS, G., REICHARD, G. A., GOODMAN, E. H., JR., FRIEDMANN, B. and WEIN-
   HOUSE, S. (1958). *Diabetes*, **7**, 358
KIMBALL, C. P. and MURLIN, J. R. (1923). *J. biol. Chem.* **58**, 337
KORNER, A. and MANCHESTER, K. L. (1960). *Brit. med. Bull.* **16**, 233
LACY, P. E. (1961). In Proc. IVth Congr. Intern. Diabet. Fed., Geneva.
LACY, P. E. and HARTROFT, W. S. (1959). *Ann. N.Y. Acad. Sci.* **82**, 287
LAZARUS, S. S. (1959). *Proc. Soc. exp. Biol. (N.Y.).* **102**, 303
LUNDBAEK, K. (1961). Proc. Brit. Diabet. Assoc., Birmingham
MADISON, L. L. and UNGER, R. H. (1958). *J. clin. Invest.* **37**, 631
MAHLER, R. F. (1960). *Brit. med. Bull.* **16**, 250
MAHLER, R. F. (1961). In Proc. IVth Congr. Intern. Diabet. Fed., Geneva
MAHLER, R. F., SHOEMAKER, W. C. and ASHMORE, J. (1959). *Ann. N.Y. Acad.
   Sci.* **82**, 452
MALINS, J. M. (1961). Proc. Brit. Diabet. Assoc., Birmingham
MANSOUR, T. E. and MENARD, J. S. (1960). *Fed. Proc.* **19**, 50
MARBLE, A. and CAMERINI-DAVALOS, R. A. (1961). In Proc. IVth Congr. Intern.
   Diabet. Fed., Geneva
MARTIN, D. B., RENOLD, A. E. and DAGENAIS, Y. M. (1958). *Lancet*, **2**, 76
MASKE, H. (1957). *Diabetes*, **6**, 335
MCCOLLISTER, D. L. and RANDLE, P. J. (1961). *Biochem. J.* **78**, 27P
MACLEOD, J. J. R. (1922). *J. metab. Res.* **2**, 149
MEYER, DE J. (1909). *Arch. Fisiol.* **7**, 96
MIRSKY, I. A. and BROH-KAHN, R. H. (1949). *Arch. Biochem.* **20**, 1
MIRSKY, I. A., PERISUTTI, G. and JINKS, R. (1955). *Endocrinology*, **56**, 484
MOLONEY, P. J. and COVAL, M. (1955). *Biochem. J.* **59**, 179
MORTIMORE, G. E. and TIETZE, F. (1959). *Ann. N.Y. Acad. Sci.* **82**, 329
MÜLLER, G. (1877). *Berl. klin. Wschr.* **14**, 29
MYERS, J. D., KIBLER, R. F. and TAYLOR, W. J. (1952). *Fed. Proc.* **11**, 111
NICHOL, D. S. H. W. (1960). In 'Mechanism of Action of Insulin'. Ed. Young, F. G.,
   Broom, W. A. and Wolff, W. F. Oxford: Blackwell Scientific Publications
NOORDEN, C. H. VON (1901). 'Die Zuckerkrankheit und ihre Behandlung,' 3rd ed.
   Berlin: Hirschwald

PARK, C. R., REINWEIN, D. HENDERSON, M. J., CADENAS, E. and MORGAN, H. E. (1959). *Amer. J. Med.* **26**, 674
RADDING, R. S. and ZIMMERMAN, S. J. (1961). *Metabolism,* **10**, 238
RAFAELSON, O. J. (1961). In Proc. IVth Congr. Intern. Diabet. Fed., Geneva
RALL, T. W., SUTHERLAND, E. W. and WOSILAIT, W. D. (1956). *J. biol. Chem.* **218**, 483
RANDLE, P. J. (1954). *Brit. med J.* **1**, 1237
RANDLE, P. J. and TAYLOR, K. W. (1960). *Brit. med. Bull.* **16**, 209
*RANDLE, P. J. and YOUNG, F. G. (1960). *Brit. med. Bull.* **16**, 237
RAO, M. R. R. and DE, N. N. (1955). *Acta Endocr. (Kbh.).* **18**, 299
REES, J. R., CAMERON, J. S. and JOHNSON, A. M. (1961). *Lancet,* **2**, 804
REID, J., MACDOUGALL, A. I. and ANDREWS, M. M. (1957). *Brit. med. J.* **2**, 1071
*RENOLD, A. E. and CAHILL, G. F. (1960). In 'The Metabolic Basis of Inherited Disease'. Ed. Stanbury, J. B., Wyngaarden, J. B. and Fredrickson, D. S. New York: McGraw Hill
RENOLD, A. E., TENG, C. T., NESBETT, F. B. and HASTINGS, A. B. (1953). *J. biol. Chem.* **204**, 533
ROSSI, E., VASSELLA, F., SCHWAMM, H., HUG, G. and GITZELMANN, R. (1957). *Int. Z. Vitaminforsch.* **28**, 118
SANGER, F. (1960). *Brit. med. Bull.* **16**, 183
SHOEMAKER, W. C., VAN ITALLIE, T. B. and WALKER, W. F. (1959). *Amer. J. Physiol.* **196**, 315
SIPERSTEIN, M. D. (1959). *Amer. J. Med.* **26**, 685
SLATER, J. D. H., SAMAAN, N., FRASER, R. and STILLMAN, D. (1961). *Brit. med. J.* **1**, 1712
SPORN, J. and NECHELES, H. (1956). *Amer. J. Physiol.* **187**, 634
STADIE, W. C. (1958). *Diabetes,* **7**, 61
STADIE, W. C., HAUGAARD, N. and VAUGHAN, M. (1952). *J. biol. Chem.* **199**, 729
STEINKE, J., TAYLOR, K. W., GUNDERSEN, K. and RENOLD, A. E. (1961). *Lancet,* **1**, 30
STOWERS, J. M., CONSTABLE, L. W. and HUNTER, R. B. (1959). *Ann. N.Y. Acad. Sci.* **74**, 689
SUTHERLAND, E. W. and DE DUVE, C. (1948). *J. biol. Chem.* **175**, 663
TARDING, F. and SCHAMBYE, P. (1960). In 'The Mechanism of Action of Insulin'. Eds. Young, F. G., Broom, W. A. and Wolff, F. W. Oxford: Blackwell Scientific Publications
TAYLOR, K. W. (1961). In Proc. IVth Congr. Intern. Diabet. Fed., Geneva
UNGER, R. H., EISENTRAUT, A. M., McCALL, M. S. and MADISON, L. L. (1961). In Proc. IVth Congr. Intern. Diabet. Fed., Geneva
VALLANCE-OWEN, J., DENNES, E. and CAMPBELL, P. N. (1958). *Lancet,* **2**, 336
VALLANCE-OWEN, J., JOPLIN, G. F. and FRASER, R. (1959). *Lancet,* **2**, 584
VALLANCE-OWEN, J. and HURLOCK, B. (1954). *Lancet,* **1**, 68
VALLANCE-OWEN, J. and LILLEY, M. D. (1961). *Lancet,* **1**, 806
VIGNEAUD, DU V., FITCH, A., PEKAREK, E. and LOCKWOOD, W. W. (1931). *J. biol. Chem.* **94**, 233
VOLK, B. W. and LAZARUS, S. S. (1959). *Ann. N.Y. Acad. Sci.* **82**, 319
VUYLSTEKE, C. A. and DE DUVE, C. (1957). *Arch. int. Pharmacodyn.* **111**, 437
WALKER, R. S. and LINTON, A. L. (1959). *Brit. med. J.* **2**, 1005
WILLIAMS, R. H., TYBERGHEIN, J. M., HYDE, P. M. and NEILSEN, R. L. (1957). *Metabolism,* **6**, 311
WINEGRAD, A. I. and RENOLD, A. E. (1958). *J. biol. Chem.* **273**, 1233
WRENSHALL, G. A., BOGOCH, A. and RITCHIE, R. C. (1952). *Diabetes,* **1**, 87
YOUNG, F. G. (1961). In 'Cell Mechanisms in Hormone Production and Action'. Memoirs of the Society for Endocrinology No. 11. Cambridge University Press

8

CHAPTER 7

DIURETICS AND ELECTROLYTE BALANCE

The action of diuretic drugs is intimately connected with the physiology and pathology of body water and of electrolytes, and therefore it is necessary to give a brief summary of relevant aspects of this branch of metabolism.

BODY WATER

The proportion of body water to the total body weight varies considerably according to the age and build of the subject, the extremes being a maximum of 70% in the normal infant and a minimum of 45% in the obese adult. Normal voluntary muscle, which accounts for about 30% of the total body weight, contains 70% water, whereas fat and bone contain only a small amount. Body water can be divided into the intracellular and the extracellular fluids, the former being the more variable according to body build. Extracellular fluid averages 20% of the total body weight, and can be subdivided into 5% within the vascular compartment and 15% within the interstitial compartment in direct contact with body cells. These two fractions are only separated by the capillary wall which allows free diffusion of water and electrolytes but impedes the passage of plasma proteins. The composition of these two fractions differs especially in protein content, but there is a slight difference in electrolyte concentration governed by the Donnan equilibrium. Since plasma proteins behave as weak acids at physiological pH, interstitial fluid contains a slightly lower cation content and a slightly higher anion content than plasma water. The average electrolyte composition of plasma and of interstitial and intracellular fluid is given in Fig. 33.

The plasma proteins produce a constant colloid osmotic pressure or oncotic pressure between plasma and interstitial fluid, amounting to an average value of 30 mm. Hg. This would cause movement of water into the vascular compartment, but is balanced by the hydrostatic pressure of blood within the capillaries tending to force fluid into the interstitial compartment. The balance is presumably in favour of the interstitial fluid at the proximal end of the capillary, and in favour of the vascular compartment at the distal end, owing to the slight fall of hydrostatic pressure along the length of the capillary. Plasma albumin is quantitatively the most important fraction of plasma protein, and because of its comparatively small molecular weight has a disproportionate importance in the maintenance of the plasma oncotic pressure. Expansion of the interstitial compartment, with eventual formation of overt clinical oedema, is therefore favoured by a fall in plasma albumin and a rise in capillary hydrostatic pressure.

There are, in addition, several discontinuous fractions of extracellular fluid which cannot strictly be classified as either plasma or interstitial fluid. These include cerebrospinal and intraocular fluids, the small quantities of fluid in the synovial, pericardial, pleural and peritoneal cavities, the fluid in lymphatics, and finally that within the gastro-intestinal tract.

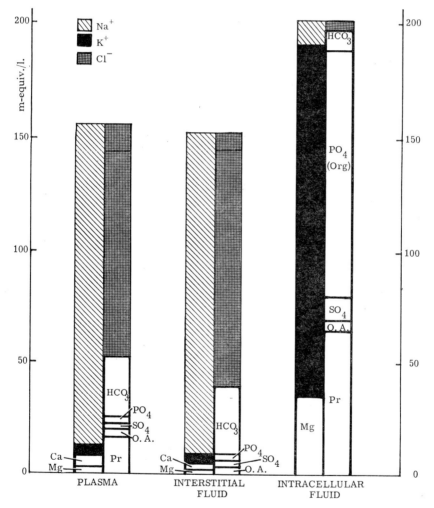

FIG. 33. Average ionic concentrations of plasma, interstitial fluid, and muscle intracellular fluid. The osmolality of plasma, interstitial fluid, and intracellular fluid are all equal, averaging 290 mOsm./l. Since a large proportion of intracellular anions are either poorly ionized or colloidal, the total concentration of intracellulae electrolytes is greater than that of extracellular fluid. The scale is in m-equiv./l. O.A.=organic acid. PO_4 (Org.)=intracellular phosphatic esters, and Pr=ionized protein.

The sum of these fractions is normally less than 5% of the total body weight, but may become much greater in disease. The pleural and peritoneal cavities are especially liable to contain considerable quantities of fluid either as a result of inflammation or as serous effusions in conditions associated with severe oedema.

Intracellular fluid accounts for 25%–45% of body weight, the proportion varying according to the relative mass of voluntary muscle which has a high water content, and of adipose tissue which contains very little water. This fluid is the sum of the water contained in all body cells, and varies considerably in composition in different organs or tissues. Voluntary muscle, which accounts for about 30% of body weight, is quantitatively by far the most important fraction of the intracellular compartment. From the point of diuretic action, the composition of kidney cells is of great importance but is less easily analysed than that of muscle, as it is difficult to avoid errors from inclusion of fluid within the lumen of the renal tubules. The average composition of the intracellular fluid of voluntary muscle is given in Fig. 33. It is seen that the average total ionic strength of anions plus cations is 304 m-equiv./l. for interstitial fluid and 402 m-equiv./l. for muscle cell intracellular water. This difference of composition, combined with the fact that when tissues are placed *in vitro* in an extracellular medium under conditions which inhibit metabolism they invariably swell from increase of fluid content, led to the hypothesis of hypertonicity of intracellular fluid (Robinson and McCance, 1952). It was suggested that water tends to pass continuously into cells, but is actively extruded by metabolic processes. Maffly and Leaf (1959) have conclusively shown that almost all tissue, including muscle, heart, liver and brain, is isosmotic with interstitial fluid, and thus there is no tendency for fluid to accumulate within the intracellular compartment at the expense of interstitial fluid and plasma. The only tissue found to be hypertonic was kidney, and this was entirely due to the hypertonicity of the renal medullary area, to be described later. Many intracellular anions, including organic phosphate esters and intracellular proteins, and some intracellular cations, especially magnesium, are polyvalent, and it is impossible to equate ionic strength and osmotic activity. The osmolality of intracellular fluid, excluding that of the renal medulla, is identical with that of the interstitial fluid, amounting, in healthy subjects, to values between 285 and 310 mOsm./l.

THE ELECTROLYTES OF BODY FLUIDS

As shown in Fig. 33, the electrolyte composition of intra- and extracellular fluids is completely dissimilar. Intracellular fluid contains about 36 times the concentration of potassium and 23 times the concentration of magnesium compared with interstitial fluid, whereas the latter has

14 times the concentration of sodium contained in intracellular water. These substantial ionic gradients are not due to impermeability of the cell membrane to cations, as injection of radioisotopes has shown there is free exchange of cations between the two compartments. The difference in concentration is maintained by active extrusion of sodium from cells, possibly combined with active inward transport of potassium. The concentration gradient of the two cations is dependent on metabolic energy, and the gradients are reduced by factors injurious to cellular metabolism, e.g. cold and metabolic poisons. The same changes occur during cellular injury from serious chronic disease, e.g. severe congestive heart failure, cirrhosis of the liver and prolonged tuberculosis, when the potassium content of cells is reduced and the sodium content increased. In addition, there is a tendency to generalized hypo-osmolality of body fluids, sometimes to values less than 250 mOsm./l. This is shown clinically by a fall in plasma sodium content to values of 120 m-equiv./l. or even less. The changes in plasma are almost certainly secondary to reduction of the osmolality of intracellular fluid, the primary defect being within the cell and causing abnormalities of ionic content of intracellular water. This change in composition of body fluids has profound effects on the efficiency of diuretic drugs.

Similarly, the anionic content of intra- and extracellular fluids is completely dissimilar. The main anions of interstitial fluid are chloride and bicarbonate, with much smaller amounts of inorganic phosphate, sulphate, organic acids and protein. Intracellular fluid contains large quantities of protein and phosphatic esters behaving as anions, with only very small amounts of chloride. As described in the section on acid-base balance, the intracellular fluid is more acidic than plasma and, therefore, the bicarbonate content is considerably less than in extracellular fluid. These anions vary in diffusibility across the cell membrane, chloride being freely diffusible, whereas the cell membrane is impermeable to proteins and phosphatic esters. Inorganic phosphate, sulphate and bicarbonate ion occupy an intermediate position, diffusibility being considerably less than that of chloride. The gross difference in chloride composition between the intra- and extracellular compartments is explained by exclusion of chloride from the cell interior by the high concentration of non-diffusible organic anions within the intracellular fluid. The relative diffusibility of anions across the cells of the renal tubules is of major importance in relation to diuretic action.

THE REACTION OF BODY FLUIDS

Changes in acid-base balance also considerably influence the action of diuretics. The pH of arterial blood is maintained within narrow limits in the healthy subject at values from 7·35 to 7·45. The main buffer system of plasma is the CO_2-bicarbonate system, the pH being dependent on the relative proportion of each according to the Henderson-Hasselbalch equation:

$$pH = pK_a + \log \frac{[HCO_3^-]}{[H_2CO_3]}$$

Plasma bicarbonate is maintained within the limits of 24–28 m-equiv./l. by the kidneys and carbonic acid at about 1·3 m-equiv./l. by the lungs. The latter value corresponds to a partial pressure of CO_2 in arterial blood of 40 mm. Hg. The pK_a of carbonic acid in the above equation is 6·1. Changes in acid-base balance are classified as 'metabolic' when the primary change of plasma composition is that of bicarbonate, and 'respiratory' when the primary change is that of CO_2 content. There is, however, almost invariably a compensatory change in the same direction in the other variable, which reduces but does not completely abolish the change in pH. Thus, in respiratory acidosis and alkalosis there is a compensatory change in plasma bicarbonate. Similarly, in metabolic acidosis there is hyperventilation causing reduction of the partial pressure of CO_2 in arterial blood. The one exception is that hypoventilation with increase of P_{CO_2} does not usually occur in a metabolic alkalosis.

The above short discussion of pH changes has only considered alteration in the pH of the extracellular compartment. There is considerable evidence that the intracellular fluid is more acidic than is arterial blood. Estimates of the pH of intracellular fluid of voluntary muscle have recently been reviewed by Irvine *et al.* (1961), most investigators reporting values between 6·90 and 7·05. This necessitates an appreciable gradient of hydrogen ion between the intra- and extracellular compartments, the concentration of hydrogen ion within the intracellular fluid being two to three times that of plasma. Changes in acid-base balance usually cause corresponding alterations in pH in both the extra- and intracellular fluids. Alteration in intracellular pH is rapid in respiratory acidosis and alkalosis (Waddell and Butler, 1959), because of the free diffusibility of CO_2 and carbonic acid across the cell membrane. Conversely, equilibration of intracellular pH is slow in metabolic acidosis or alkalosis because of the much slower diffusion of the bicarbonate ion.

Potassium depletion causes more complex alterations in acid-base balance. As potassium ions leave the muscle cell they are partially replaced by sodium ions in the proportion of from 67–75% (Cooke *et al.*, 1952; Irvine *et al.*, 1961). The resulting cation deficit is partly made up by accumulation of basic aminoacids, especially lysine and arginine (Eckel and Norris, 1955), within the intracellular fluid, and partly by migration of hydrogen ion from the interstitial fluid into the intracellular water. This causes an extracellular alkalosis and an intracellular acidosis, with an increased gradient of hydrogen ion across the cell membrane, sometimes amounting to more than twice the normal value (Irvine *et al.*, 1961). In discussing the effects of changes in acid-base balance on the action of diuretic drugs, the two important parameters are obviously changes in plasma composition and changes in intracellular pH of the renal tubule cell. For technical reasons it is more difficult to analyse changes in the composition and pH of renal tubule cells than of the quantitatively most important body cell, that of voluntary muscle. The available evidence suggests that tubule cells behave similarly to muscle in accumulation of basic aminoacids in potassium deficiency (Iacobellis *et al.*, 1956), and in fall of intracellular pH with potassium loss (Anderson and Mudge, 1955). Renal tubular cells do not, however, lose as much intracellular potassium as voluntary muscle cells (Darrow *et al.*, 1953), except the highly specialized hypertonic cells of the papillary tip.

RENAL MECHANISMS FOR EXCRETION OF WATER AND
ELECTROLYTES

Views on the regulation of water and electrolyte excretion by the kidney have been completely altered in the last decade by the formulation and subsequent elaboration of the counter-current theory of urinary concentration and dilution (Wirz *et al.*, 1951; Wirz, 1960). This theory has given alternative explanations for previous concepts which were difficult to accept on basic thermo-dynamic principles, i.e. active transport of water in a predominantly aqueous medium, and the development and maintenance of high osmotic gradients over an extremely short length of tissue. Transport of water is now regarded as a completely passive physico-chemical process obeying the laws of osmotic equilibrium. Renal tubule cells are considered to be freely permeable to water, with the one important exception of the cells of the collecting tubules which are impermeable to the passage of water in the absence of circulating anti-diuretic hormone but permeable when exposed to anti-diuretic hormone action. Osmotic gradients between urine and plasma are now considered to be developed gradually over at least a centimetre length of renal medullary tissue, instead of the previous view that they occurred across single cells of microscopic dimensions. The theory has also completely altered views of the renal circulation, as it is now thought that only the renal cortex has an unusually generous blood supply. Normally about one-fifth of the blood ejected from the left ventricle under conditions of rest circulates through the kidneys. The figures for an average adult male are 6 l. of blood per minute as the resting cardiac output, and 1·2 l. per minute as the normal renal blood flow. This generous blood supply is necessary to maintain the high glomerular filtration rate of 125 ml./min. in health. About 650 ml. of plasma flows through the kidneys each minute, and about one-fifth of the plasma water is ultra-filtered through the glomeruli, producing a virtually protein-free glomerular filtrate. Obviously the process of glomerular filtration results in a considerably increased concentration of protein in the plasma within the efferent arterioles of the glomerulus. As the renal cortex receives far more blood than is necessary for its metabolic needs, the oxygen content of blood in the renal veins is unusually high and the CO_2 content unusually low. A rapid blood supply within the renal medulla would rapidly disperse osmotic gradients developed by a counter-current system. The actual partitioning of blood flow within the kidney is probably of the order of 88% to the cortex, 10% to the outer medulla, and 2% to the inner medulla including the renal papillae. The low blood supply of the inner medulla, combined with the counter-current arrangement of the medullary capillaries, maintains the unique hyperosmolality of all tissue and body fluids within the renal papillae.

Of the 125 ml. water filtered at the glomerulus, an average of only 1 ml./min. is excreted as urine. This volume can be increased to about 16 ml./min. after ingestion of excess fluid with the production of a water diuresis, and reduced to about 0·3 ml./min. after prolonged fluid deprivation. The urine volume may be still greater, up to 30 ml./min., after production of an osmotic diuresis, when there is an abnormally high quantity of osmotically active solute within the excreted urine. The loading solutes may be carbohydrate, as in uncontrolled diabetes mellitus or after infusions of hypertonic mannitol, electrolytes after diuretic therapy, or urea from a high protein diet or from ingestion of preformed urea. At average urine flow rates, more than 99% of the water filtered at the glomerulus is reabsorbed by the renal tubules. Similarly, 98–99% of the sodium and chloride ions filtered are usually reabsorbed by the tubules, but this can be reduced to only 80% reabsorption under the influence of diuretic drugs.

COUNTER-CURRENT EXCHANGERS AND COUNTER-CURRENT MULTIPLIERS

Counter-current exchangers and multipliers have, until recently, been more familiar to engineers and biologists than to medical men. The principles of counter-current exchange are more easily understood in relation to alterations in temperature than to changes in osmolality as occurs in the mammalian kidney. Fig. 34 shows a simple model of a counter-current exchanger relating to heat. On the left is shown a simple U-tube along which cold water is flowing and dipping into a container filled with hot water. The cold water within the tube only becomes warmed in the portion of the tube within the container, and the hot water in the reservoir rapidly cools because heat is continually being removed by the stream of warmed water within the outgoing limb of the

U-tube. On the right is shown the modification produced by a simple counter-current exchange system. Cold water in the inflow part of the U-tube is warmed by the outflow stream long before the tube enters the hot water in the container and, conversely, water in the outflow tube is cooled by contact with the water in the inflow tube. Heat is only slowly removed from the water in the vessel and, therefore, the rate of cooling is much less than in the case of a simple U-tube system. Similarly, in the renal medulla the counter-current exchange arrangement of the vasa recta maintains the hyperosmolality of the papillary tip and prevents dissipation of the unusually high concentrations of sodium chloride and urea within the tissues.

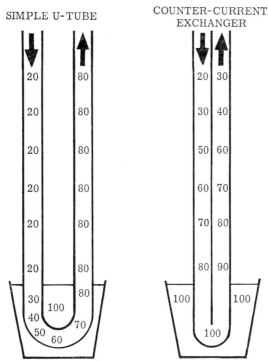

Fig. 34. Diagrammatic representation of a simple counter-current exchange system relating to heat transfer. In the simple U-tube on the left, the fluid in the U-tube remains at room temperature until it reaches the hot water in the vessel. The fluid in the out-going limb remains hot and therefore heat is continually being removed from the vessel contents, which rapidly cool. In the counter-current exchange system on the right, the fluid in the in-going limb is warmed by the fluid in the out-going limb long before it reaches the hot water in the vessel. Conversely the fluid in the out-going limb is progressively cooled by the fluid in the in-going limb. Very little heat is removed by the current of fluid, and consequently the water in the vessel remains hot.

A counter-current exchange mechanism depends on simple physico-chemical processes without external work other than that necessary to maintain the flow of fluid within the system. In a counter-current multiplier, work is continually being done to build up and maintain the gradients, either of heat as in the model, or of osmolality as in the renal medulla. This work in the kidney is dependent on the sodium extrusion mechanism of the cells of the ascending limb of Henle's loop. Sodium, passively followed by chloride, is continuously being transported from the luminal fluid into the cells, and then into the interstitial fluid of the medulla. This produces hyperosmolality of the interstitial fluid which is maintained at the papillary tip by the counter-current system of the vasa recta. In the outer parts of the medulla immediately adjacent to the renal cortex excess solute is removed by the blood flowing from the outgoing capillary limb of the vasa recta. Portions of the medulla intermediate between these two extremes will come to equilibrium states of osmolality dependent on their distance from the cortico-medullary junction (Fig. 35). In this way layers of increasing osmolality within the medulla are built up and maintained by counter-current systems, starting at the outer layer with an osmolality equal to that of the renal cortex, i.e. about 290 mOsm./l., and ending at the papillary tip where the osmolality is maximal, i.e. 1200–1400 mOsm./l. in the healthy adult human subject.

MECHANISMS OF WATER AND SODIUM REABSORPTION

Throughout the length of the nephron, sodium is reabsorbed by the vital activity of the renal tubule cells, reabsorption of water and chloride being passive physico-chemical processes not requiring metabolic energy. Water is reabsorbed by the osmotic gradients produced by sodium transport, and chloride by the electro-chemical potential induced by transport of the positively charged sodium ion. Extrusion of sodium is thought to be a fundamental property of all living cells, but renal tubule cells have the specialized property of removing sodium from the fluid within the tubular lumen and then extruding it into the surrounding interstitial fluid prior to its removal by the renal capillary blood. At least 80% of filtered sodium, chloride and water is reabsorbed isosmotically by the proximal tubule cells within the renal cortex (*A B* in Fig. 36). Obviously, this sodium transport must be against a slight adverse concentration gradient, but this is minimized by the constant transport of water from the tubular lumen to the interstitial fluid. If chloride moved absolutely in step with sodium there would be no electro-chemical gradient. There are, however, potential differences in both the amphibian and mammalian kidney of from 20–40 millivolts, the peritubular fluid being positively charged as compared to the tubular lumen.

In the renal medulla the osmolality of all cells and fluids steadily increases from the outer zone where the osmolality is equal to that of

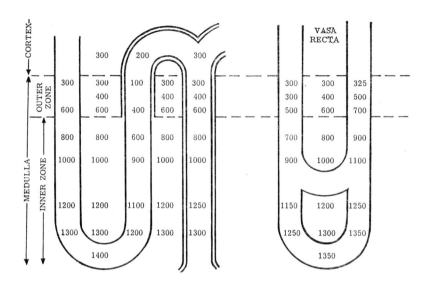

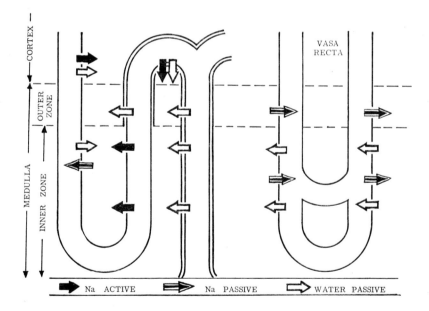

Fig. 35. Diagrammatic representation of the osmolality of the intra-tubular fluid, the interstitial fluid, and the blood within the renal medulla (upper picture). A nephron with a long loop of Henle is shown on the left, and a vasa recta on the right. Active extrusion of sodium by the ascending limb of Henle's loop produces a counter-current multiplier system. Conversely the vasa recta functions as a simple counter-current exchange system (lower picture).

plasma, i.e. 300 mOsm./l., to the inner parts of the renal papilla where the osmolality may be as high as 1200 mOsm./l. in man, and even higher in mammalian species capable of producing a more concentrated urine, e.g. the desert rat. As the fluid in the tubular lumen flows along the descending limb of Henle's loop (*BC* in Fig. 36), there is passive reabsorption of water as the fluid progressively equilibrates with interstitial fluid steadily increasing in osmolality. Presumably the total volume of

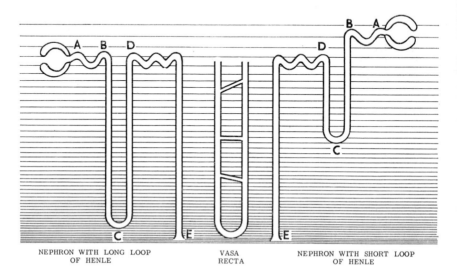

NEPHRON WITH LONG LOOP   VASA   NEPHRON WITH SHORT LOOP
OF HENLE   RECTA   OF HENLE

FIG. 36. Diagrammatic representation of the difference between a nephron with a short loop of Henle (right), and a nephron originating from a juxta-medullary glomerulus with a long loop of Henle (left). The density of shading represents the osmolality of tissue fluids within the kidney. See Fig. 37 and text for explanation lettering.

fluid entering at *B* is about 20% of the glomerular filtration rate, i.e. 24 ml./min., but has been reduced by passive water reabsorption to one quarter this volume, i.e. 6 ml./min. at the loops of Henle. The ascending limb of Henle's loop *CD* acts as a counter-current multiplier, and is responsible for the initiation of the osmotic gradient between the cortex and the papillary tip. Sodium is actively extruded into the interstitial fluid and is closely followed by chloride under the influence of the electro-chemical potential produced. The tubular fluid is now, however, equilibrating with interstitial fluid of gradually diminishing osmolality in its passage from the papilla to the renal cortex, and therefore there is no further reabsorption of water and the volume of tubular fluid remains constant. Extrusion of sodium is, in fact, sufficiently active to reduce the osmolality of the tubular fluid to values less than 300 mOsm./l. in the distal convoluted tubule.

In its passage along the collecting tubules *DE* reabsorption of salt and water varies according to the concentration of circulating anti-diuretic hormone (ADH). In the absence of ADH the collecting tubules are completely impermeable to water, and the already slightly hypotonic fluid in the distal convoluted tubule is still further diluted by continued active extrusion of sodium, passively followed by chloride ions. Again, there is no further reduction in tubular fluid volume, and if all nephrons behaved as described, the maximum urinary volume in water diuresis would obviously be only 6 ml./min., whereas it may be three times this

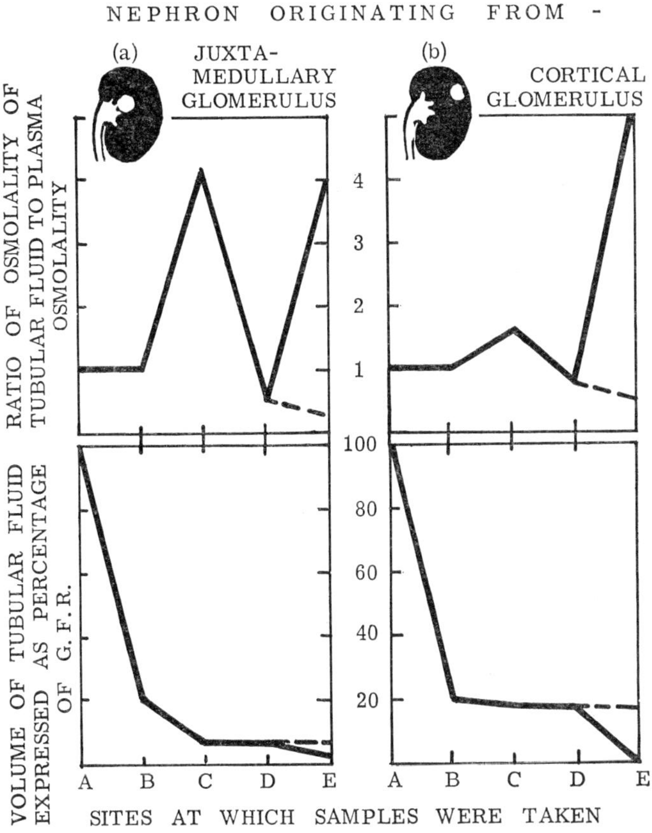

FIG. 37. Graph of the approximate osmolality (expressed as a ratio to the osmolality of plasma), and of the total volume (expressed as a percentage of the volume of the original glomerular filtrate) in a nephron originating from a juxta-medullary glomerulus (left), and in a nephron originating from a glomerulus in the outer renal cortex (right). AB=proximal convoluted tubule, BC=descending limb of loop of Henle, CD=ascending limb of loop of Henle and distal convoluted tubule, and DE=collecting tubule. In the collecting tubule the continuous line represents the conditions under full action of anti-diuretic hormone, and the broken line the conditions in the absence of ADH action.

amount. This apparent discrepancy is explained by the fact that only about one-quarter of all nephrons have a long loop of Henle reaching the papillary tip, and in the remainder there is no loss of volume in the passage of urine down the descending loop of Henle. Only the nephrons with a long Henle's loop act as counter-current multipliers and produce the osmotic gradient between cortex and papilla. The collecting tubules of *all* nephrons, however, pass through the hyperosmotic zone before reaching the papillary tip and discharging urine into the renal pelvis (Figs. 36 and 37). In the presence of circulating ADH the collecting tubules of all nephrons become freely permeable to water, and therefore water is passively reabsorbed by the increasing osmotic gradient from cortex to papillary tip. Under maximal ADH action the final result is a concentrated urine of osmolality only slightly less than that of the interstitial fluid and cells at the papillary tip.

The local hyperosmolality of the inner medulla produced by the counter-current multiplier system of the loops of Henle would be rapidly dissipated by the circulating blood were it not for the peculiar anatomy of the medullary circulation. The blood supply to the inner medulla is itself arranged as a counter-current exchange system, the blood in the descending arterial limb of the vasa recta exchanging with that in the ascending venous limb. In its passage from the renal cortex to the medullary tip the blood steadily accumulates sodium chloride and urea from the blood in the returning ascending limb and therefore becomes hyperosmolar by the time it reaches the capillary tip. The red cells presumably become crenated owing to the high sodium content of the plasma. In addition, the partial pressure of oxygen of the blood and tissues at the papillary tip is unusually low and, conversely, the Pco_2 is unusually high. The counter-current exchanger of the vasa recta would, however, be ineffective if the blood flowed as rapidly in the inner medulla as in the renal cortex, as there would be insufficient time for equilibration. In fact, the blood supply is only from 1% to 2% as rapid as in the renal cortex, allowing sufficient time for counter-current exchange to occur. The low blood supply has the disadvantage of accentuating the reduced partial pressure of oxygen at the papillary tip, explaining the liability to wide-spread papillary necrosis if the medullary circulation is impaired.

REABSORPTION OF BICARBONATE

About 3·25 m-equiv./min. of bicarbonate ion is filtered at the glomeruli, but urine is usually acidic at an average pH of 6·0, and therefore virtually all the filtered bicarbonate is reabsorbed by the tubules. The mechanism is thought to be by ion exchange of hydrogen ion for sodium ion, and occurs throughout the whole length of the nephron. The chemical reactions involved are as follows:

(a) Within the tubule cell: $CO_2 + H_2O \rightleftharpoons H_2CO_3 \rightleftharpoons H^+ + HCO_3^-$
The hydration of CO_2 to carbonic acid is catalysed by the action of the enzyme carbonic anhydrase.

(b) The hydrogen ion formed within the cells now exchanges with sodium of the luminal fluid, the former passing into the tubular lumen and the latter into the tubule cell (Fig. 38).

$$H^+ + NaHCO_3 \longrightarrow Na^+ + H_2CO_3$$

The carbonic acid formed may slowly dissociate to CO_2 and water. The tubule cells are permeable to carbonic acid, CO_2, and water but not to bicarbonate ion, and therefore the net result is tubular reabsorption of both sodium and bicarbonate ions. Carbonic anhydrase is not, therefore, absolutely essential for bicarbonate reabsorption, but considerably increases the rate of reabsorption by facilitation of the reaction producing hydrogen ion for exchange. Total inhibition of renal carbonic anhydrase by diuretics never completely prevents bicarbonate reabsorption, but impedes the process sufficiently to make reabsorption incomplete with production of an alkaline urine containing considerable amounts of bicarbonate.

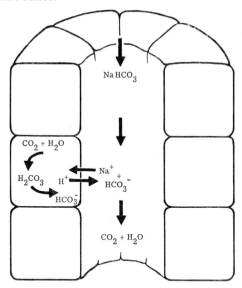

Fig. 38. Diagrammatic representation of bicarbonate reabsorption within the renal tubule. Hydrogen ion is produced from CO_2 and water, partly by the action of carbonic anhydrase which potentiates the hydration of CO_2 to form carbonic acid. The hydrogen ion then exchanges for sodium within the tubular lumen, the net effect being reabsorption of sodium and neutralization of bicarbonate with reduced pH of the intratubular fluid.

Bicarbonate reabsorption is profoundly influenced by changes in acid-base balance. Metabolic acidosis decreases and metabolic alkalosis increases the concentration of bicarbonate in plasma and, therefore, in the glomerular filtrate. Secretion of hydrogen ion by the tubules remains unaffected and in metabolic alkalosis large amounts of bicarbonate are excreted in the urine, whereas in metabolic acidosis, all the filtered bicarbonate is reabsorbed with production of a highly acid urine. Secretion of hydrogen ion in metabolic acidosis is only limited by the high concentration gradient of hydrogen ion between urine and plasma. The kidneys are usually incapable of secreting more hydrogen ion if the gradient has risen to a maximal value of 1000 to 1, equivalent to a minimal urinary pH of 4·4. In respiratory changes in acid-base balance, the ability of the tubule cells to secrete hydrogen ion and reabsorb bicarbonate is increased in respiratory acidosis and decreased in respiratory alkalosis. There is, thus, an acid urine in respiratory acidosis despite an increase in the amount of filtered bicarbonate, and an alkaline urine in respiratory alkalosis despite a decrease in filtered bicarbonate. There is a good correlation between the Pco_2 of arterial blood and the ability of the tubules to reabsorb bicarbonate, but no correlation between reabsorptive capacity and extracellular pH (Relman *et al.*, 1953; Dorman *et al.*, 1954). This does not necessarily prove that the Pco_2 of body fluids is the determining factor in bicarbonate reabsorption. Carbon dioxide rapidly diffuses across cell membranes and, therefore, increase of Pco_2 reduces intracellular pH, including that of the renal tubule cells. The effect of potassium deficiency on bicarbonate reabsorption makes it more likely that the intracellular pH of renal tubule cells, and not the Pco_2 of arterial blood, is the single most important factor involved.

Potassium depletion frequently causes an extracellular alkalosis, with increase of plasma bicarbonate and, therefore, of the amount of bicarbonate filtered at the glomeruli. The urine, however, remains acidic in reaction, indicating complete and consequently increased bicarbonate reabsorption. Depletion of potassium reduces intracellular pH, but has little effect on the Pco_2 of body fluids. The view that bicarbonate reabsorption is primarily dependent on the concentration of hydrogen ion within the renal tubule cells would, therefore, explain the findings both in respiratory changes in acid-base balance and in potassium depletion.

POTASSIUM EXCRETION

Potassium is probably entirely excreted by ion exchange in the distal tubule, the potassium filtered at the glomerulus being completely reabsorbed in the proximal tubule. Potassium ions derived from the distal tubule cells exchange for sodium within the tubular lumen, the net result being an excretion of potassium and a reabsorption of sodium. Potassium and hydrogen ion compete for the available transport system (Berliner *et al.*, 1951), excess of one ion reducing exchange of the other. Thus, intake of neutral potassium salts, e.g. potassium chloride, produce an alkaline urine because hydrogen ion exchange is depressed, and conversely, reduction of hydrogen ion exchange by inhibition of carbonic anhydrase increases potassium output.

Sodium reabsorption at the ion-exchange site of the distal tubule is especially important in relation to diuretic action. There are two mechanisms of reabsorption, which are both potentiated by circulating aldosterone. The first is direct reabsorption of sodium without ion-exchange, which produces an electro-chemical gradient between the tubular lumen and the interstitial tissue. The electro-chemical gradient may rise to values higher than in the proximal tubule, e.g. to 80–90 mVolts, because chloride, which passively follows sodium, is always available in the proximal nephron but may not be present in high concentration in the distal nephron. Direct sodium reabsorption can, therefore, only occur if chloride is available to follow the sodium ions, and partially neutralize the electro-chemical gradient produced. The second mechanism of sodium reabsorption is ion-exchange of potassium or hydrogen ion for sodium within the tubular lumen, a process which does not generate an electro-chemical potential. If sodium is accompanied by a less diffusible anion, e.g. sulphate, bicarbonate or phosphate, direct sodium reabsorption is rapidly impeded by the development of a very high potential difference, and further absorption can only proceed by the ion-exchange mechanism.

Excess potassium loss in the urine, which is an especially important feature of diuretic action is, therefore, facilitated by three separate factors:

(a) There must be an appreciable amount of sodium within the tubular lumen at the ion exchange site. If almost all the filtered sodium has been reabsorbed in more proximal parts of the nephron there will be none available for ion exchange with corresponding reduction of potassium loss.

(b) Potassium loss is increased if the sodium within the tubular lumen is accompanied by a non-diffusible anion rather than by the freely diffusible chloride ion. Sodium can then only be reabsorbed by the ion-exchange mechanism. Bicarbonate is a much less diffusible anion than is chloride, and therefore if sodium is accompanied in the distal nephron chiefly by unabsorbed bicarbonate, potassium loss will be correspondingly high. This occurs after administration of acetazolamide which impedes proximal tubular bicarbonate reabsorption (see p. 242) by inhibition of renal carbonic anhydrase. Potassium loss is always high after this particular drug.

(c) Potassium loss is increased if there is excess of circulating aldosterone which potentiates ion exchange as well as direct sodium reabsorption. Secondary hyperaldosteronism is produced either by severe sodium depletion or by refractory oedema in severe congestive heart failure, the nephrotic syndrome, or cirrhosis of the liver. Potassium loss from diuretics therefore increases after previous doses of the drugs have already produced considerable sodium loss from the body, or if there is severe refractory oedema. In such cases diuretics may be harmful rather than beneficial, as excess potassium and not sodium is excreted in the urine.

ALDOSTERONE IN RELATION TO OEDEMA FORMATION (*see also chapter on Steroids, p. 268*)

Increased secretion of aldosterone occurs in all cases of the nephrotic syndrome and of cirrhosis of the liver with severe peripheral oedema, the daily production being from 1,000–25,000 µg. aldosterone, as compared to the normal secretion of 150–380 µg. per day (Ulick *et al.*, 1958). Hypersecretion of aldosterone is less consistent and less extreme in congestive heart failure, and many cases may show a normal or even a reduced production rate. Transudation of fluid from the vascular to the interstitial compartment from hypoalbuminaemia is more pronounced in the nephrotic syndrome and in cirrhosis of the liver than in heart failure, and the venous pressure is elevated only in cases of heart failure. In congestive cardiac failure there is excess stimulation of right atrial stretch receptors which tends experimentally to diminish aldosterone output. (McCally *et al.*, 1958). The total effective blood volume is better preserved in heart failure than in severe cases of cirrhosis of the liver or of the nephrotic syndrome in relapse. Secondary hyperaldosteronism is probably of more importance in cases of heart failure which have been too energetically treated by diuretics, as shown by evidence of peripheral circulatory failure and a rising blood urea from gross reduction of the renal blood flow.

Aldosterone enhances all varieties of distal tubular sodium reabsorption, including direct absorption together with chloride ion, and exchange of both potassium and of hydrogen ion for sodium within the tubular lumen (Mills *et al.*, 1960). By contrast, hydrocortisol and cortisol do not stimulate hydrogen ion exchange and the urine is therefore less acid. In states of severe secondary hyperaldosteronism the urine is characteristically highly acid, and contains abnormally high amounts of potassium and ammonium together with the relatively nondiffusible anions, phosphate and sulphate, but there is virtually no sodium or chloride as these electrolytes are completely reabsorbed by the tubules. In addition to its action on renal tubular function, aldosterone depresses the Na/K ratio in saliva, sweat, and faeces, and possibly influences the gradient of potassium between interstitial fluid and intra-cellular water. Aldosterone increases magnesium output both in faeces and urine, and prolonged administration may cause magnesium depletion (Hanna and MacIntyre, 1960).

Secondary aldosteronism is obviously of great importance in the genesis of oedema, and bilateral adrenalectomy may cause considerable diuresis in many examples of refractory oedema (Laragh, 1956). Diuresis in the nephrotic syndrome, whether spontaneous or due to therapy, is often associated with a reduction of urinary aldosterone output (Luetscher and Johnson, 1954). Hypersecretion of aldosterone is, however, only one of many factors in oedema formation, and drugs reducing production of aldosterone or inhibiting its effect have only a limited place in modern diuretic therapy.

MERCURIAL DIURETICS

Although mercurial diuretics have been in use for over 40 years, much new information has been made available in the last decade.

PREPARATIONS

The three most widely used organic mercurial diuretics are mersalyl, meralluride (mercuhydrin), and mercaptomerin (thiomerin). Mersalyl and meralluride are somewhat similar compounds containing theophylline in equimolecular proportions. The theophylline has no innate diuretic effect at this dosage, but promotes more rapid absorption from the injection site and reduces local irritation. Mercaptomerin contains mercury combined with a sulphur atom instead of the hydroxyl radicle, and is not in combination with theophylline. It dissociates more slowly than the other compounds and therefore causes less local tissue reaction than the other mercurial diuretics, and can be given by subcutaneous as well as intramuscular injection. However, about one-fifth of patients complain of severe local discomfort after subcutaneous injections of mercaptomerin, and the incidence of sensitivity to repeated injections is greater than is the case with the other mercurials (Gold *et al.*, 1952).

ADMINISTRATION OF MERCURIAL DIURETICS

Mercurial diuretics are usually given by intramuscular injection at two or three day intervals. The dose is from 1–2 ml. of the appropriate solution, containing about 40 mg. mercury in organic combination per ml. As stated above, mercaptomerin may be given by subcutaneous injection. There is now no reason to give mercurial diuretics by intra-venous injection, as there are many safer alternatives for the treatment of refractory oedema. Intravenous mercurials may cause immediate death from ventricular fibrillation. Mercurial diuretics are extensively bound to plasma protein (Lehman *et al.*, 1951), and probably immediate cardiotoxicity is more likely if unbound drug reaches the myocardium.

Toxicity is increased by rapid injection, and by reduction of plasma albumin content. A disproportionately large number of immediate fatalities from intravenous mercurials have occurred in cases of the nephrotic syndrome, where plasma albumin is usually lower than in congestive cardiac failure. There is, in fact, no absolute certainty that mercurial diuretics are more effective when given intravenously than when injected intramuscularly (Modell *et al.*, 1945), and the time of onset of the diuresis may be identical after either route of injection (Grossman *et al.*, 1949).

Oral preparations, e.g. chloromerodrin, are often effective but are complicated by troublesome side-effects especially diarrhoea. The dose has to be comparatively high, from 400–600 mg. mercury per week being necessary to produce the same diuresis as 80–160 mg. mercury per week by injection (Moyer *et al.*, 1952). Oral administration of organic mercurials has now been almost completely replaced by the benzothiadiazine group of diuretics, as these are much less toxic and produce no gastro-intestinal symptoms.

DISTRIBUTION AND DISPOSAL OF MERCURIAL DIURETICS

Mercurial diuretics pass rapidly from the plasma into body tissues, being especially concentrated in the renal cortical cells (Borghgraef *et al.*, 1956; Greif *et al.*, 1956). In the cells they form complexes with monothiol radicles, and the reason for their particular localization within the renal cortex lies in the high content of such groups in renal tubular cells, and the unusually generous renal cortical blood supply. Owing to the very high degree of plasma protein binding of organic mercurials, almost none is filtered at the glomeruli. Urinary excretion therefore depends on renal tubular secretion following concentration within the renal tubular cells. Considerable chemical change occurs in the renal tubule cells, the mercury being excreted as cysteine or acetyl-cysteine complexes (Weiner and Muller, 1955). The excretion rate is rapid, about 50% being eliminated in 4–6 hours, and 60–80% within 24 hours. Cumulative toxicity is, therefore, unlikely provided excretion rates are normally rapid. Excretion in the urine is reduced and delayed in any patient with a reduced glomerular filtration rate with rise of the blood urea, as this is always associated with reduction of renal blood flow and consequent lowered secretion of the mercurial, in cases of oliguria, and in cases with a poor diuretic response. Some of the mercury is eliminated in the faeces even after parenteral administration, most of the drug reaching the gut in the bile. Less than a third of the dose is eliminated in the faeces after injection, but a much higher proportion after administration by mouth, as all organic mercurial diuretics, including those recommended to be given by the oral route, are poorly absorbed by the gut.

MODE OF ACTION OF MERCURIAL DIURETICS

Mercurials in high dosage inhibit many important intracellular enzymes, especially dehydrogenases containing sulphydryl radicles. Histopathological changes are produced in proximal tubule cells (Edwards, 1942), and there is inhibition of succinic dehydrogenase (Rennels and Ruskin, 1954; Wachstein and Meisel, 1954) by high but not by therapeutic doses of mercurial diuretics. The number of active sulphydryl groups is reduced in many renal cells, including the proximal tubular cells, and those of the loops of Henle and of the collecting ducts (Cafruny *et al.*, 1955). The ability of the proximal tubular cells to reabsorb glucose and to secrete *p*-aminohippurate is reduced by therapeutic doses of mercurials in man (Berliner *et al.*, 1948; Brun *et al.*, 1947; Grossman *et al.*, 1949), but not in the dog (Berliner *et al.*, 1948; Kessler *et al.*, 1958). Mercurials in therapeutic doses have no influence on renal acidification mechanisms or on the synthesis or diffusion of ammonia into the distal tubular lumen.

These diverse effects on renal tubular function suggest that mercurials exert a diffuse and rather non-specific inhibitory effect on many intracellular enzymes concerned with the generation of the cellular energy mediating active transport processes. Although the effect is generalized throughout the whole length of the nephron, it is most marked in the proximal convoluted tubule. Stop-flow analysis strongly suggests that mercurials act by reduction of tubular reabsorption of sodium in the proximal tubule (Kessler *et al.*, 1958). The ratio of sodium to creatinine clearance in the proximal segments is doubled by mercurials, but the corresponding clearance ratio of the distal segments is unaffected. Reduction of proximal tubular transport of sodium would be expected to lower the electro-chemical potential gradient across the wall of the tubule, and this in fact has been shown to occur. Under the influence of mercurials, therefore, the volume of isotonic fluid passing from the proximal tubules to the loops of Henle is increased from the normal value of about 24 ml./min. to about twice that amount, and contains double the normal total quantity of sodium and chloride. An abnormally large amount of sodium is therefore available for exchange at the cation exchange site of the distal nephron, with resultant increase of both potassium and hydrogen ion exchange and excretion. Chloride is unaffected by distal ion exchange and therefore chloride excretion under the influence of mercurial diuretics exceeds the output of sodium. Loss of potassium and of hydrogen ions from the body result in a mild potassium deficit and a metabolic alkalosis, two familiar complications of mercurial therapy. Excretion of excess water, after mercurials, with consequent increase of the urinary volume, is entirely secondary to the rise in electrolyte excretion. Urine flow has been shown to be directly correlated with the urinary osmolal clearance whether the osmotic diuresis is produced by mercurial injections increasing electrolyte output, or more directly by infusion of mannitol which is excreted unchanged (Brodsky and Graubarth, 1953; Spritz *et al.*, 1959).

The modern view of mercurial action is that these diuretics primarily inhibit proximal tubular reabsorption and transport of sodium; the effects on water, chloride, potassium and hydrogen ion being regarded as secondary effects. The fact that more chloride than sodium is excreted after mercurial injection has been cited to prove a direct effect on chloride transport (Schwartz and Wallace, 1951; Milne, 1956). This view is contrary to modern principles of electrolyte physiology, as sodium transport is regarded as a fundamental property of all living cells, with chloride having a more passive role as a freely diffusible anion, and with a distribution entirely governed by osmotic and electro-chemical physical processes unrelated to cellular energy. The fact that sodium and not chloride is involved in the ion exchange mechanism of the distal tubule fully explains excess chloride output in the urine after mercurials. In addition, mercurial action is not invariably potentiated by mechanisms increasing the plasma chloride, and consequently the amount of chloride in the glomerular filtrate.

FACTORS POTENTIATING AND INHIBITING THE ACTION OF MERCURIALS

The action of both mercurials and of pure carbonic anhydrase inhibitors is greatly influenced by reaction changes within the body.

The subject of acid-base balance has been confused in the past by the adoption by clinicians of an inexact nomenclature unfamiliar to pure scientists. There is now no longer any need to retain the view that changes in acid-base balance are conditioned by so-called 'fixed anions' and 'fixed cations', and in this section the scientific nomenclature of Brönsted (1923) and Lowry (1923) will be used. Definitions of the terms 'acid' and 'base' are given in the glossary. An acidosis is caused by retention of hydrogen ion or of an acid, or loss of a base. Conversely an alkalosis is produced if there is loss of hydrogen ion or of an acid, or gain of a base. The most important buffer systems in acid-base balance are:

$$H_2CO_3 \leftrightharpoons H^+ + HCO_3^-$$
$$NH_4^+ \leftrightharpoons H^+ + NH_3$$
$$H_2PO_4^- \leftrightharpoons H^+ + HPO_4^=$$

The substances on the left side of the equations are hydrogen ion donators and are therefore acids, whereas those on the right are hydrogen ion acceptors and are therefore bases. In the following equations:

$$HCl \leftrightharpoons H^+ + Cl^-$$
$$H_2SO_4 \leftrightharpoons H^+ + HSO_4^- \leftrightharpoons 2H^+ + SO_4^=$$

hydrochloric and sulphuric acids are hydrogen ion donators and therefore their administration (in suitable dilution) would cause an acidosis, but the chloride and sulphate ions are not hydrogen ion acceptors within the pH range compatible with life as free HCl and H_2SO_4 can only exist in any detectable amount at an extremely low pH.

Respiratory acidosis is caused by excess of carbonic acid within the body due to CO_2 retention. Metabolic acidosis may be produced experimentally by administration of dilute hydrochloric or sulphuric acids, ammonium chloride or ammonium sulphate, the hydrochlorides of dibasic aminoacids or of calcium chloride or potassium chloride. The ammonium salts cause an acidosis because the ammonium ion is an hydrogen ion donator and is therefore an acid. The aminoacid hydrochlorides are a means by which hydrochloric acid may be taken without the undesirable local effects in the upper gastro-intestinal tract produced by ingestion of the uncombined acid. Calcium chloride causes an acidosis because basic phosphate ($HPO_4^=$) is lost to the body as calcium phosphate in the faeces. Potassium chloride has a more indirect effect. Increased exchange of potassium within the renal tubules reduces hydrogen ion exchange, and therefore bicarbonate, which is a base, is lost in the urine.

Mercurials have a self-limiting action by causing preferential excretion of chloride over sodium, and of increasing the output of hydrogen ion in the urine with production of a metabolic alkalosis. This causes a fall of plasma chloride and a rise of plasma bicarbonate and arterial blood pH. Fortunately, this self-limiting action can be overcome by the use of acidifying salts, including ammonium chloride, calcium chloride, the hydrochlorides of dibasic aminoacids, e.g. lysine or arginine monohydrochloride, and, to a lesser extent, potassium chloride. Conversely, agents producing an alkalosis, such as the ingestion of sodium bicarbonate or removal of hydrogen ion in acid vomit, as in pyloric stenosis, reduce the diuretic action of mercurials. These effects of metabolic acidosis and alkalosis have been explained in the past as either due to a redistribution of anions within the body, or as due to change in the pH of body fluids. Increase of plasma chloride or reduction of plasma pH was thought to potentiate mercurial diuretic action. Similar biochemical changes, however, occur after the production of a respiratory acidosis by inhalation of 10% CO_2, and this stimulus does not potentiate mercurial action (Axelrod and Pitts, 1952). Hypokalaemic alkalosis associated with reduction of plasma chloride and rise of arterial blood pH has no effect on the diuretic action of mercurials (Mudge and Hardin, 1956). There is, at present, no single satisfactory explanation for the variable effects of stimuli influencing acid-base balance on mercurial diuretic action. Mudge and Weiner (1958) think that the single most important factor is the intracellular pH of renal tubular cells. They consider that organic mercurials are unstable in acid pH and liberate mecrury in a more active form within the cell. This view would fit all the facts with the one exception of the lack of potentiation of the action by 10% CO_2, which is an agent especially effective in reduction of intracellular pH. Possibly some change produced by hypercapnia inhibits the effect of the increase of hydrogen ion concentration within the tubule cells.

In the past the production of hyperchloraemia by acidifying agents has been thought to be the chief factor in the potentiation of mercurial action. Modern views of the greater importance of sodium than of chloride transport by the renal tubules are consistent with this opinion. In patients with an extremely low plasma chloride proximal tubular reabsorption of sodium, with secondary chloride transport by the electro-chemical potential gradient produced, may result in a fluid containing sodium but no unabsorbed chloride being delivered to the distal nephron. The sodium in such cases is accompanied by relatively non-diffusible anions, e.g. phosphate, sulphate and bicarbonate. Further reabsorption of sodium in the distal tubule can only be by ion exchange of potassium and hydrogen ion for the sodium within the tubular fluid. This will result in an undesirable and potentially dangerous loss of potassium from the body. By contrast, if there is hyperchloraemia, distal tubular reabsorption of sodium is accompanied by secondary diffusion of excess chloride from the tubular lumen to the interstitial fluid without there being unduly high potassium exchange. The presence of sufficient chloride is best shown by excretion of chloride before the mercurial is given. In practice the patient may be expected to respond adequately to mercurials if the urinary chloride before the injection has been increased to values of about 60 m-equiv. Cl per day by administration of ammonium chloride or other suitable adjuvant drug.

Reduction of the glomerular filtration rate proportionately reduces the efficacy of mercurial diuretics. About 20% of the sodium filtered at the glomerulus is excreted in the urine at the time of maximal diuresis. The proportion remains approximately the same as the glomerular filtration rate falls, either from temporary causes such as reduction of the renal blood flow, or permanent causes from progressive destruction of nephrons by chronic bilateral renal disease. The reduction of glomerular filtration rate in severe congestive heart failure is one of the many factors leading to mercurial resistance. Hyponatraemia is a further cause of mercurial resistance. This reduces the amount of sodium within the glomerular filtrate, but in addition most cases of hyponatraemia with oedema occur in severely ill, and often moribund, patients in whom both the glomerular filtration rate and the renal blood flow are reduced below normal values. Intravenous aminophylline potentiates the action of mercurials by production of a temporary increase of the glomerular filtration rate. A dose of 0·5 g. intravenously should be given two hours after the intramuscular injection of the mercurial (Weston and Escher, 1948). In this way the rapid effect of the intravenous aminophylline on the glomerular filtration rate is timed to coincide with the maximal effect of the mercurial diuretic on tubular function. The small amount of aminophylline included in many mercurial preparations reduces the local reaction to the injection, increases the speed of absorption, and reduces cardiotoxicity, but is in too small a dose to have any effect on the glomerular filtration rate.

The simultaneous administration of mercurials and acetazolamide produces a similar or slightly less diuresis than the same dose of the mercurial alone. The benzothiadiazine diuretics have an effect on sodium reabsorption which is completely different and additive to that of mercurials (Pitts, 1959). The two groups of drugs, therefore, have a synergistic action, the diuresis produced by the two drugs together being greater than that from the same dose of either drug alone. Administration of many mercaptan compounds, e.g. dimercaprol (*BAL*), prevents mercurial action by binding the mercury produced and therefore protecting organic sulphydryl groups from the action of the drug (Farah and Maresh, 1948).

THE CHOICE OF POTENTIATING AGENT

Ammonium chloride is by far the most useful and generally used method of potentiating mercurial diuretics. It is cheap and relatively free from toxic effects, but in some patients ammonium chloride produces severe nausea or vomiting. It is contra-indicated if there is a reduced power of excretion of hydrogen ion from renal acidosis either of the glomerular or tubular failure type. In severe uraemia ammonium chloride may produce severe acidosis, and should not be used, as diuretics are ineffective in patients with a considerable reduction of the glomerular filtration rate. Patients with renal tubular acidosis are unlikely to have oedema, as there is a tendency to lose sodium in the urine. In cases of cirrhosis of the liver complicated by ascites and peripheral oedema, ammonium chloride has proved to be of great use as an adjuvant to mercurials (Atkinson *et al.*, 1954), but in severe hepatocellular failure it may cause a considerable increase of blood ammonia with the production of porto-systemic encephalopathy and hepatic pre-coma.

Enteric-coated preparations are of doubtful value as the absorption of the salt is completely unpredictable. Ammonium chloride is best given in solution of less concentration than 2·5% to avoid gastric irritation, and at a dosage of 2 g. two, three or four times daily in adults. Each gram of ammonium chloride is equivalent to 18·7 m-equiv. of chloride and of hydrogen ion. Severe acidosis is to be avoided, and the plasma bicarbonate should not be allowed to fall below 18 m-equiv./l.

Potassium chloride is a less efficient adjuvant to mercurial action than ammonium chloride, but is especially indicated if there is potassium deficiency from previous diuretic action, with increase of distal tubular potassium exchange. This salt causes a mild extracellular acidosis from loss of bicarbonate in the urine, with some hyperchloraemia and fall of plasma bicarbonate and arterial blood pH. It is contra-indicated if there is severe oliguria, as in such cases excess potassium cannot be adequately excreted in the urine. Potassium chloride is best combined with ammonium chloride as an adjuvant to mercurials, the average dosage in an adult being KCl 2–3 g. daily, and NH_4Cl 4–6 g. daily. Calcium chloride has rarely been used as an adjuvant, as the effective dose produces too much gastric irritation and nausea.

There have been several recent reports of the use of the dibasic aminoacid hydrochlorides as adjuvants to mercurials (Brailovsky, Silva, del Campo and Marusic, 1959; Rubin, Spritz, Mead, Herrmann, Braveman and Luckey, 1960; Lasser, Schoenfeld and Friedberg, 1960), L-lysine monohydrochloride by mouth and L-arginine monohydrochloride by intravenous injection being the two compounds used. Ornithine hydrochloride by mouth is unsuitable as it is both more expensive and more toxic than lysine hydrochloride (Milne *et al.*, 1961). Lysine hydrochloride has been given by mouth at a dosage of 10 g. four times daily, each gram. being equivalent to 5·5 m-equiv. chloride and hydrogen ion. A full daily dose of 40 g. is therefore equal in potency to 11·7 g. ammonium chloride. Many patients are able to take this amount of the aminoacid hydrochloride although unable to take an equivalent dose of ammonium chloride. Toxic effects are mainly gastrointestinal, nausea and vomiting occurring in some patients, and diarrhoea from the passage of unabsorbed lysine in the stools (Milne *et al.*, 1961). After absorption the aminoacid is metabolized, the free hydrogen ion and chloride produced being the active agents. Unabsorbed lysine in the colon may be converted to cadaverine by intestinal bacteria. This is then absorbed and excreted in the urine after oxidation to piperidine (Milne *et al.*, 1961). A little of the absorbed lysine is excreted in the urine, and can easily be detected by paper chromatography. The proximal tubular reabsorption mechanism for dibasic aminoacids (Robson and Rose, 1957) is partly saturated by the large intake of lysine, and there is an appreciable excretion of both cystine and arginine in addition to lysine (Milne, unpublished observations). This amount (40 g.) of aminoacid contains over 6 g. of nitrogen and is, therefore, unsuitable in either renal or hepatic failure. Cases of hepatic pre-coma have rapidly deteriorated when treated with lysine monohydrochloride, but arginine hydrochloride intravenously is claimed to be less toxic (Gidekel *et al.*,

1960). Infusions of arginine monohydrochloride cause a great increase of plasma ornithine (Webber, Brown and Pitts, 1961) with rise of blood urea and fall of blood ammonia (Najarian and Harper, 1956) due to stimulation of the Krebs-Henseleit cycle of urea synthesis.

It is too early to assess the importance of dibasic aminoacid therapy as mercurial adjuvants. They have the disadvantage of expense, lysine monohydrochloride costing 1/– per g., and arginine monohydrochloride 1/6 per g. Such large doses of a single aminoacid would probably prove to be toxic if given over long periods. Probably this method of adjuvant therapy has a limited application in refractory cases of oedema who are intolerant to ammonium chloride by mouth, and in cases of hepatic cirrhosis in whom ammonium chloride produces symptoms and signs of hepatic pre-coma. The benzothiadiazine group of diuretics are also toxic in patients with cirrhosis (Read *et al.*, 1959), and in such cases intravenous arginine monohydrochloride may prove to be the adjuvant of choice.

STRUCTURE ACTIVITY RELATIONSHIPS OF MERCURIALS

All mercurial diuretic drugs have the same basic structure: $R.CH_2.CH(OCH_3)CH_2.Hg$—. The radicle R varies from compound to compound, being $NaOOC.C_8H_{14}.CO.NH$ in the case of mercaptomerin, $NaOOC.CH_2O.C_6H_4.CO.NH$ in the case of mersalyl, and $NaOOC.C_2H_4.CO.NH.CO.NH$ in the case of meralluride. In each case R is a polar hydrophyllic radicle and is separated from the mercury atom by a chain of three carbon atoms. Kessler *et al.* (1957) suggest that diuretic activity is dependent on a two-point attachment of the molecule to a receptor site within the proximal tubule cell, the radicle R and the mercury atom being the two sites of attachment. Compounds are known, e.g. *p*-chloro-mercuri-benzoate, which are potent inhibitors of sulphydryl containing enzymes, are concentrated into the tissue of the renal cortex, and are secreted into urine, and yet have no appreciable diuretic action. Mudge and Weiner (1958) have compared in states of varying acid-base balance, the efficacy as a diuretic of meralluride and of mercuric chloride complexed with cysteine, one of the compounds by which organic mercurials are excreted in the urine. The potency of meralluride was found to be much more dependent on body pH than was the compound of smaller molecular weight. The results support the view that diuretic activity is dependent on acid lability of organic mercurials, active breakdown products being liberated in acid media. The lack of potentiation of diuretic effect by respiratory acidosis does not support this attractive and simple explanation of mercurial action. The two separate explanations of steric configuration of the molecule and acid lability are not, however, mutually exclusive and both are probably partially correct. The complex of mercury with cysteine is unlikely to be the actual active agent, because 10–15% of the total mercury is often excreted as this compound before there is significant diuretic effect.

CONTRA-INDICATIONS TO THE USE OF MERCURIAL DIURETICS

Mercurial diuretics are best avoided in cases of severe primary renal disease, especially if this has caused nitrogen retention or oliguria. Both uraemia and oliguria reduce the rate of elimination of mercury from the body, and there may be progressive accumulation of the metal within the renal cortex and further renal injury. There is increased production of casts and accentuation of uraemia and oliguria. All diuretics are ineffective and are more toxic in uraemic patients with gross reduction of the glomerular filtration rate. There is no proof that mercurials can cause a nephrotic syndrome, as claimed by Munck and Nissen (1956). In cases of nephrotic syndrome secondary to congestive heart failure, Burack *et al.* (1958) have reported progressive improvement with reduction of urinary protein loss, after effective therapy of the heart failure with digitalis and mercurial diuretics. There is still, however, some difference of opinion as to the use of mercurials in cases of the nephrotic syndrome due to glomerulo-nephritis, lupus erythematosus, or secondary amyloidosis. Probably the benzothiadiazine diuretics are safer drugs in these conditions, and mercurials are better reserved for cases in which there is still severe oedema after use of other methods of therapy.

CARBONIC ANHYDRASE INHIBITORS

As previously described, sodium bicarbonate is reabsorbed by the tubule cells by a process of ion exchange of hydrogen ion formed within the cells for sodium within the tubular lumen. In order that this should be a continous process, hydrogen ion must be constantly re-formed within the cells from free carbon dioxide derived from the renal capillary blood and from the metabolism of the tubule cells themselves. Hydration of CO_2 to form cabonic acid is slow without carbonic anhydrase activity, but rapid in the presence of the enzyme. Shortly after the introduction of sulphanilamide as an anti-bacterial drug it was found to cause a metabolic acidosis associated with an inappropriately alkaline urine. This was later shown to be due to inhibition of renal carbonic anhydrase (Southworth, 1937; Mann and Keilin, 1940).

Most compounds with a free SO_2NH_2 group are active carbonic anhydrase inhibitors, but substitution of one or two of the hydrogen atoms in the NH_2 group, as in the more modern anti-bacterial sulphonamide drugs, e.g. sulphadimidine and sulphathiazole, make the compound inactive as an enzyme inhibitor. This led to the hypothesis (Sprague,

1958) that the free SO_2NH_2 group competed with carbonic acid for active sites on the enzyme surface, the two groupings being sterically similar:

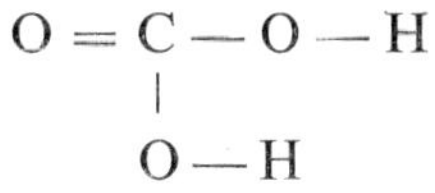

$$O = C - O - H$$
$$|$$
$$O - H$$

Carbonic acid

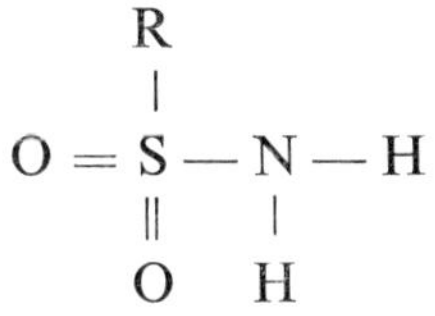

$$\overset{\textstyle R}{\overset{\textstyle |}{O = S - N - H}}$$
$$\overset{||}{O} \quad \overset{|}{H}$$

Carbonic anhydrase inhibitor

Doubt has, however, been recently passed on this attractive hypothesis, as acetazolamide does not behave as a competitive inhibitor of carbonic anhydrase (Leibman *et al.*, 1961), the enzyme kinetics being more suggestive of non-competitive inhibition. All active diuretics of the carbonic anhydrase group or of the benzothiadiazine group either possess a free SO_2NH_2 radicle or such a grouping is formed from the compound by metabolic processes within the body. In the latter case, the drug as administered has no carbonic anhydrase inhibiting potency, but urine containing excreted metabolites of the drug inhibits the enzyme.

Roblin and Clapp (1950) found that, in compounds with the sulphonamide radicle attached to a hetero-cyclic ring, the carbonic anhydrase inhibition was often 300–800 times as much as that of sulphanilamide.

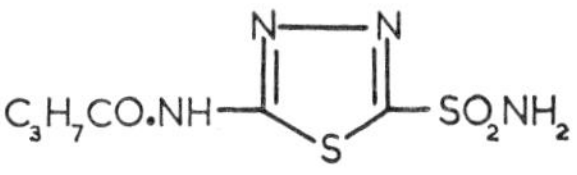

butamide

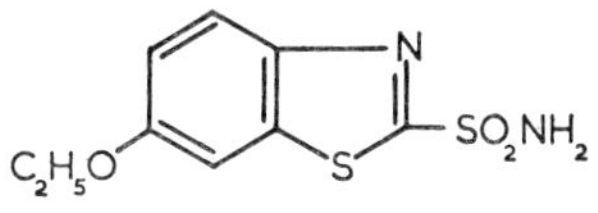

ethoxzolamide

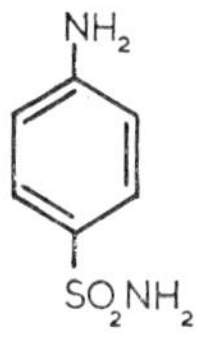

sulphanilamide

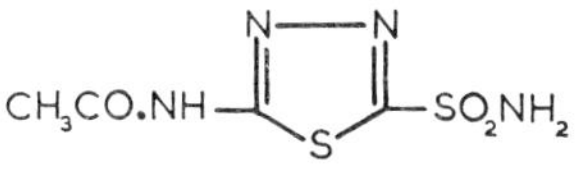

acetazolamide

The most widely used compound of this type is acetazolamide: 2-acetylamino-1, 3, 4-thiadiazole-5-sulphonamide. Other compounds of this type, including ethoxzolamide and butamide are of about equal potency as carbonic anhydrase inhibitors, but are more lipoid-soluble and, therefore, are in higher concentration within the ciliary body of the eye and within the cerebral cortex, making them more active in the treatment of glaucoma and of epilepsy.

ACTION AS DIURETICS

Acetazolamide and related drugs are specific inhibitors of carbonic anhydrase and their diuretic action is entirely dependent on this property. Reabsorption of bicarbonate by hydrogen ion exchange is depressed throughout the whole nephron causing an increased excretion of bicarbonate and of sodium, but no increase of chloride output. Potassium exchange at the distal ion exchange site is increased both by the large amount of sodium reaching the distal tubule and by the reduction of hydrogen ion exchange. This causes considerable loss of potassium in the urine (see p. 229), which is always an undesirable feature in the action of pure carbonic anhydrase inhibitors. The highly alkaline fluid within the tubular lumen diminishes diffusion of ammonia from the distal tubule cells and, therefore, ammonia output is always greatly reduced. Acetazolamide produces an almost immediate alkalinization of the urine when given intravenously, and this occurs within 30 minutes when ordinary therapeutic doses of the drug are taken by mouth. The maximum activity is present about 2 hours after taking the drug and the effect passes off from 12–18 hours after ingestion. Acetazolamide is rapidly and completely absorbed from the gut, and the highest plasma concentrations coincide with the maximal diuretic activity two hours after ingestion. Elimination by the kidneys is fairly rapid, 80% of an oral dose being excreted within 8–12 hours, and there is complete excretion within 24 hours, preventing any cumulative action of the drug. Acetazolamide is secreted by the proximal tubules and competes for excretion with other acids, including diodrast, *p*-aminohippurate, and 5-hydroxyindolylacetic acid. The excretion of these acids is uninfluenced by changes of acid-base balance, and therefore their excretion is depressed by large doses of acetazolamide because of inhibition of their proximal tubular secretion. The effects of the drug on acids excreted by a diffusion mechanism (Milne *et al.*, 1958), e.g. salicylic and indolylacetic acids, is more complex. Acetazolamide competitively depresses proximal tubular secretion of these acids (Weiner *et al.*, 1959) which reduces their excretion rate, but in addition the alkalinization of the urine from carbonic anhydrase inhibition prevents back-diffusion of the acids in the distal nephron. The net effect is usually an increase of salicylate and indolylacetate output, but to a considerably less amount than after alkalinization of the urine by sodium bicarbonate.

The urinary excretion of bicarbonate removes base from the body and, therefore, metabolic acidosis is produced with reduction of plasma bicarbonate and pH, and increase of plasma chloride. Metabolic acidosis, whether produced by acetazolamide itself or by prior administration of ammonium chloride reduces the activity of the drug in removing both bicarbonate and sodium from the body. This inhibition by metabolic acidosis was originally thought to be directly due to the fall in plasma bicarbonate with a corresponding reduction in the amount of bicarbonate filtered at the glomerulus (Counihan *et al.*, 1954). Diuretic potency is, however, unaffected by respiratory alkalosis where there is considerable reduction of plasma bicarbonate, and is inhibited by respiratory acidosis after breathing CO_2, when the plasma bicarbonate increases (Brodsky and Satran, 1959). Maren *et al.* (1961) have recently shown that potassium depletion, with increase of plasma bicarbonate due to hypokalaemic alkalosis, causes a considerable reduction in the diuresis produced by acetazolamide. The results of these experiments can be reconciled if acetazolamide diuresis is directly influenced by pH changes within the renal tubule cells. Diuretic potency is increased by alkalosis, as after taking sodium bicarbonate or by hyperventilation, and is decreased by intracellular acidosis following a metabolic or respiratory acidosis, or produced by potassium depletion. If the tubule cells are highly acid there is already a considerable excess of hydrogen ion available for exchange and therefore continued renewal by the action of carbonic anhydrase is not so necessary as in the normal state.

CLINICAL USE OF CARBONIC ANHYDRASE INHIBITORS AS
DIURETICS

Pure carbonic anhydrase inhibitors are not efficient diuretics for two important reasons. The concentration of bicarbonate in plasma is relatively low, being only about 25 m-equiv./l. Therefore, with a normal glomerular filtration rate, only 3·25 m-equiv. of bicarbonate appear in the glomerular filtrate per minute. In addition, the maximum excretion rate of bicarbonate after ingestion of a therapeutic dose of acetazolamide is only 25% of the amount filtered, the remainder still being reabsorbed by the tubules despite inhibition of carbonic anhydrase. Thus, the maximum excess amount of anion excreted per minute after acetazolamide is only 0·8 m-equiv. per minute, which compares unfavourably with the maximum effect of a mercurial, amounting to three times this amount (Milne, 1956). An even greater disadvantage is the self-inhibiting effect of the acidosis produced by continued carbonic anhydrase inhibition. The diuretic effect rapidly wears off with continued dosage and almost completely disappears after two or three days of continued ingestion. Unlike the self-inhibiting action of mercurials, the refractory state cannot be corrected by simultaneous administration of adjuvants. Correction of the metabolic acidosis by ingestion of sodium bicarbonate would obviously defeat the object of diuretic therapy. Potassium bicarbonate is also unsatisfactory because after ingestion of large doses of potassium salts there is increased potassium exchange and the excess electrolyte output is entirely potassium bicarbonate without there being any further sodium loss. Exchange of potassium for sodium is enhanced by delivery of large amounts of sodium to the distal ion exchange site and by the inhibition of hydrogen ion exchange. The additional effects of severe secondary hyperaldosteronism, as in grave congestive heart failure, further increases this exchange, and under these circumstances acetazolamide will produce excess potassium bicarbonate excretion alone without any increase of sodium output (Counihan *et al.*, 1954). For these reasons, pure carbonic anhydrase inhibitors were only used in mild cases of congestive heart failure, and they have now been completely abandoned as more potent drugs of the benzothiadiazine group are available.

In addition, acetazolamide and other related drugs have many undesirable side-effects. Most persons taking these drugs experience paraesthesiae of the hands and feet, and drowsiness from inhibition of carbonic anhydrase in extrarenal sites. Less frequent complications include the formation of renal calculi and bone-marrow depression. Carbonic anhydrase inhibitors, because they produce a metabolic acidosis, reduce urinary citrate output (Harrison, 1954; Evans *et al.*, 1957). Urinary citrate forms a soluble unionized chelate complex with calcium and prevents precipitation of calcium phosphate, despite an alkaline urine. After acetazolamide, a urine of high alkalinity containing little or no citrate is excreted, and calcium phosphate is easily precipitated. Calcium phosphate calculi may, therefore, be formed or there may be strangury from the passage of urine containing large angular crystals of calcium phosphate (Crawford *et al.*, 1959).

COMPOUNDS INTERMEDIATE IN ACTION BETWEEN PURE CAR-
BONIC ANHYDRASE INHIBITORS AND THE BENZOTHIADIAZINE
DIURETICS

The introduction of two separate sulphamido groups into a benzene ring increases the carbonic anhydrase inhibiting activity, e.g. the drugs dichlorphenamide, 1, 3 disulphamyl-4, 5-dichlorobenzene, and disamide, disulphamido-chlorotoluene. These drugs differ from pure carbonic

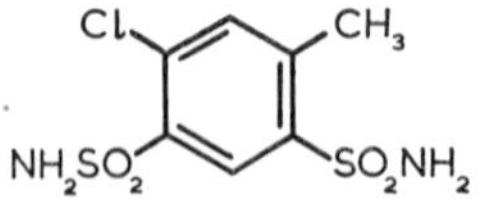

disamide

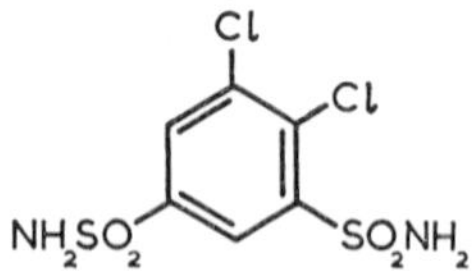

dichlorphenamide

anhydrase inhibitors as they cause a considerable increase of urinary chloride and therefore are more active diuretic agents. They are not as effective as the benzothiadiazine group as increase of urinary chloride is not so great. In addition, they suffer from the disadvantage of the pure carbonic anhydrase inhibitors in producing excessive potassium loss which always occurs in a drug causing a considerable increase of urinary bicarbonate. They have similar toxic side-effects to acetazolamide and other pure carbonic anhydrase inhibiting drugs. Acetazolamide (Nadell, 1953) and more recently dichlorphenamide (Thomson *et al.*, 1958) have also been used in the treatment of carbon dioxide retention in chronic bronchitis and emphysema. As in other patients a metabolic acidosis is produced with reduction of plasma bicarbonate due to bicarbonate loss in the urine. If this was the only effect of the drug deterioration would occur as there would be further fall of arterial blood pH. In many cases, however, there is a fall of P_{CO_2} and a rise of P_{O_2} of arterial blood (Naimark *et al.*, 1960). As there is no fall of CO_2 production, this must be due to increased alveolar ventilation. There is no change in the sensitivity of the respiratory centre to inhaled CO_2 either in emphysematous patients or in normal subjects (Fishman *et al.*, 1955; Cranston *et al.*, 1955). The net effect on arterial blood pH is usually insignificant, clinical improvement being presumably chiefly due to reduction of P_{CO_2}. In a recent controlled clinical trial of dichlorphenamide McNichol and Pride (1961) report a significant reduction of P_{CO_2} in 9 out of 17 patients, with a slight increase of the forced expiratory volume. At present there is no certain way of prediction of response to therapy without a clinical trial of dichlorphenamide at a dosage of 50 mg. four times daily.

THE BENZOTHIADIAZINE GROUP OF DIURETICS

The benzothiadiazine group of diuretics were discovered during a systematic study of the diuretic activity of drugs of the benzene-1, 3-disulphonamide series (Novello and Sprague, 1957; Sprague, 1958). The substance 6-chloro-disulphamyl-aniline was found to cyclize with

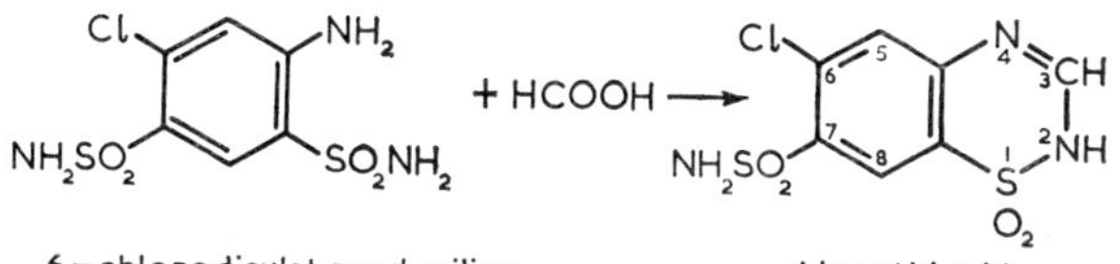

6-chlorodisulphamylaniline   chlorothiazide

formic acid to form the potent diuretic 6-chloro-7-sulphamyl-1, 2, 4-benzothiadiazine-1, 1-dioxide or chlorothiazide. The basic chlorothiazide molecule has since been modified in four separate ways to produce more active compounds:

(a) By exchange of a tri-fluoro-methyl radicle CF_3 for the Cl. in the 6 position.

(b) Reduction by addition of two hydrogen atoms at the unsaturated 3, 4 linkage.

9

Table 15

Benzothiadiazine Diuretics

Drug (approved name)	Alteration of basic chlorothiazide formula				Average daily dose	Average cost per daily dose	Average cost per 100 mg. drug
	Exchange of CF_3 for Cl in 6 position	Reduction of unsaturated double bond at 3:4 position	Substitution by an organic radicle in 3 position	Substitution by a methyl radicle in 2 position			
Chlorothiazide	–	–	–	–	1000 mg.	10d.	1d.
Flumethiazide	+	–	–	–	1000 mg.	Not now available	
Hydrochlorothiazide	–	+	–	–	100 mg.	10d.	10d.
Hydroflumethiazide	+	+	–	–	100 mg.	6d.	6d.
Benzthiazide	–	–	+ Benzylthiomethyl $CH_2.S.CH_2C_6H_5$	–	100 mg.	1/2	1/2
Trichlormethiazide	–	+	+ Dichloromethyl $CHCl_2$	–	10 mg.	Not priced in Gt. Britain	
Bendrofluazide	+	+	+ Benzyl $CH_2.C_6H_5$	–	10 mg.	5d.	4/2
Methyclothiazide	–	+	+ Dichloromethyl $CHCl_2$	+	5 mg.	2d.	3/3
Cyclopenthiazide	–	+	+ Cyclopentylmethyl $CH_2.C_5H_9$	–	1 mg.	4d.	30/–
Polythiazide	–	+	+ Trifluoroethyl-thiomethyl	+	1 mg.	Not yet commercially available	

(c) Substitution of a hydrogen at the 3 position by various organic radicles.

(d) Substitution of a methyl group at the 2 position of the molecule.

Commercially available benzothiadiazine diuretics are listed in Table 15.

These drugs exert two separate effects on renal tubular function. At low dosage there is a depression of proximal tubular reabsorption of sodium and chloride from the glomerular filtrate, whilst at high dosage there is an effect due to the activity of the drugs as inhibitors of carbonic anhydrase. As with acetazolamide, the urine becomes alkaline and there is increased excretion of bicarbonate. In order to obtain maximum effect on sodium and chloride reabsorption, the dose must be high enough to produce significant carbonic anhydrase inhibition. The benzothiadiazine drugs, therefore, combine the action of mercurials on proximal sodium reabsorption with that of the pure carbonic anhydrase inhibitors on bicarbonate reabsorption, but the former action is by far the more important. The free SO_2NH_2 grouping which makes these drugs active in carbonic anhydrase inhibition also appears to be necessary in the action on sodium and chloride reabsorption. No active drug of this configuration is known which is not either an active inhibitor of carbonic anhydrase or is converted into such a compound by metabolic processes within body cells. The effect on proximal tubular reabsorption of sodium and chloride is, in fact, different from the action of mercurial diuretics. The effect is additive and therefore simultaneous administration of the two drugs produces a greater increase of sodium and chloride output than either of the two drugs alone. Obviously, if the effect on proximal tubular function was identical, this summation of action would not occur. In addition, the action of the benzothiadiazine diuretics is unaffected by dimercaprol and is much less dependent than that of mercurials or of pure carbonic anhydrase inhibitors on changes of acid-base balance within the body. Their activity remains unaffected under conditions of metabolic acidosis or metabolic alkalosis, whereas the activity of mercurials is prevented by alkalosis and that of pure carbonic anhydrase inhibitors by acidosis. When acetazolamide and chlorothiazide are administered simultaneously, the effect of the latter drug on proximal sodium and chloride reabsorption is unaffected, but the weaker carbonic anhydrase inhibiting potency of chlorothiazide is swamped by the more powerful action of acetazolamide and there is, therefore, considerably increased excretion of bicarbonate than with chlorothiazide alone. Stop-flow experiments in the dog (Kessler *et al.*, 1959) localize the effect of the benzothiadiazine diuretics to the proximal tubule in relation to sodium and chloride reabsorption and to the distal tubule in their action on inhibition of hydrogen ion exchange and decreased ammonium excretion. The separate action on sodium reabsorption of mercurial diuretics and the benzothiadiazine diuretics allows sodium reabsorption by the tubules to be divided into three separate fractions, i.e. about 20% which is inhibited by mercurials, about 15–20% which is inhibited by the benzothiadiazine diuretics and, finally, from 60–65% which is unaffected by full dosage of either type of drug.

The inhibition of proximal tubular reabsorption of sodium allows a greater quantity of sodium to be delivered to the ion exchange site in the distal tubule and some is accompanied by the relatively non-diffusible anion bicarbonate, owing to inhibition of carbonic anhydrase. This dual effect accentuates potassium exchange for sodium more than after administration of mercurial diuretics, and thus, there is a considerably increased urinary loss of potassium. Unless potassium supplements are given, this increased urinary loss causes some potassium depletion with reduction of plasma potassium. The hypokalaemic alkalosis (see p. 218) due to potassium loss is greater than the effect on acid-base balance produced by carbonic anhydrase inhibition, which would cause a metabolic acidosis. The net effect is an increased concentration of bicarbonate in plasma and extracellular fluid with a mild extracellular alkalosis. This does not inhibit the effect of benzothiadiazine diuretics on continued dosage as it would that of mercurials.

ABSORPTION, DISTRIBUTION AND EXCRETION

Chlorothiazide is poorly absorbed from the gut in man, an average of 80–90% being lost in the faeces (Young *et al.*, 1959). This poor absorption in man has been independently confirmed for both chlorothiazide and flumethiazide (Milne, unpublished observations). This opinion is contrary to the views reported in many recent American reviews based on the experiments of Baer and Bayer (1959) in the dog. In this species, chlorothiazide is rapidly and completely absorbed, being detectable in plasma within 15 minutes of ingestion of an oral dose and reaching maximum concentration within 45 minutes. At least 50% of the dose is excreted within 6 hours, whereas almost all of an intravenous dose is excreted in this period. By contrast, the other benzothiadiazine drugs listed in Table 15 are rapidly and completely absorbed by the gut in man and this difference partly explains the considerably higher effective dosage of chlorothiazide and flumethiazide in man. However, this is probably not the whole explanation of the difference in potency, because hydrochlorothiazide is considerably more active than equal doses of chlorothiazide when injected intravenously in the dog. The difference in action may partly be explained by the differences in distribution within the body. Chlorothiazide and flumethiazide are chiefly distributed within the extracellular fluid and do not easily enter body cells. The other members of the benzothiadiazine group are more lipoid-soluble and their volumes of distribution become greater as their activity per unit weight increases. Chlorothiazide and flumethiazide are, in fact, only present in high concentration within the cells of the kidney and the liver. The drugs are concentrated within the cells of these two organs before being excreted, both in the bile and the urine. Excretion in the bile causes considerable prolongation of the effects of the drug. The fraction of the drug excreted back into the intestinal lumen is then again reabsorbed further down the gut. In the kidney, the drugs are excreted by the proximal tubular secretory mechanism for weak organic acids, similar to that described for acetazolamide. The drugs are, therefore, first concentrated within renal tubule cells and secreted into the proximal tubular lumen with a clearance considerably higher than that of the glomerular filtration rate and approximating to that of *p*-amino-hippurate. Hydrochlorothiazide and hydroflumethiazide are rapidly and completely absorbed from the gut in man, and then excreted similarly to chlorothiazide.

Introduction of an organic radicle into the molecule at the 3 position as shown in Table 15 makes the compound more unstable in solution, there being spontaneous hydrolysis within body fluids. After adminis-

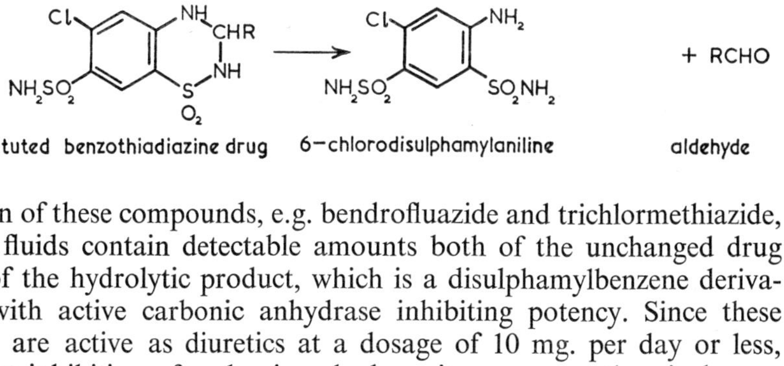

substituted benzothiadiazine drug   6—chlorodisulphamylaniline   aldehyde

tration of these compounds, e.g. bendrofluazide and trichlormethiazide, body fluids contain detectable amounts both of the unchanged drug and of the hydrolytic product, which is a disulphamylbenzene derivative with active carbonic anhydrase inhibiting potency. Since these drugs are active as diuretics at a dosage of 10 mg. per day or less, the net inhibition of carbonic anhydrase is no greater than in benzo-thiadiazine drugs given at higher dosage, e.g. chlorothiazide and hydrochlorothiazide. The more active substituted benzothiadiazine drugs are excreted slowly over a full 24 hours after administration, both as the unchanged drug and as the disulphamyl-benzene hydrolytic product (Milne, unpublished observations). Like chlorothiazide and flumethiazide they are also excreted in the bile, entry being entirely by the unchanged drug, as the disulphamyl-benzene derivative produced by hydrolysis does not appreciably enter the bile after injection (Milne, unpublished observations). The organic radicle *R* has been carefully selected to produce a non-toxic product after hydrolysis, e.g. in the case of bendrofluazide, phenylacetaldehyde is formed which is oxidized to the non-toxic phenylacetic acid and rapidly excreted as phenylacetyl-glutamine, and in the case of trichlormethiazide dichloracetic acid is the end metabolic product. This acid is very much less toxic than either monochlor or trichloracetic acid. In summary, the benzothiadiazine diuretics can be divided into four groups, according to their dosage and physical properties.

Group A: chlorothiazide and flumethiazide are predominantly water-soluble and are poorly absorbed from the gut in man. This is the main reason for their relatively low potency, the dosage being about 1 g. per day.

Group B: Hydrochlorothiazide and hydroflumethiazide are slightly more lipoid-soluble and are rapidly and completely absorbed from the gut but are otherwise similar to group A. The increased absorption and the greater penetration of cells increases their potency so that the average dose is 100 mg. per day.

Group C: Trichlormethiazide, bendrofluazide and methylchlothiazide are much more unstable and more lipoid-soluble drugs. They are partly broken down in the body and the average dose is 10 mg. daily.

Group D: Cyclopenthiazide and polythiazide (Scriabine *et al.*, 1961) are similar drugs with still greater potency, the average dose being only 1 mg. daily. The reason for this increased activity over group C has not yet been explained. These compounds are the most potent diuretics on a weight basis so far described.

Other drugs without the typical benzothiadiazine ring structure have been found to be potent diuretics and to act in a similar manner on renal tubular function. One such group has a benzophenone ring structure with a chlorine atom and a sulphamyl group substituted in adjacent carbon atoms, as occurs in chlorothiazide and its derivatives.

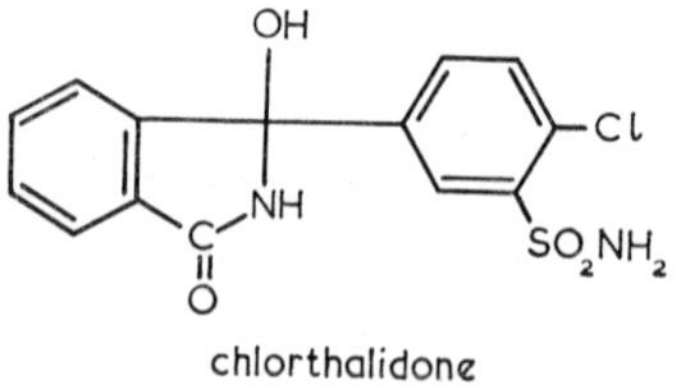

chlorthalidone

The most active compound is chlorthalidone ('Hygroton'), and is chemically 3-(4-chloro-3-sulphamylphenyl)-3-hydroxy-1-oxoisoindoline The drug does not appear to differ in any important pharmacological respect from the compounds of the benzothiadiazine series. It is slowly absorbed from the gut, and therefore the diuretic action may persist for 48 hours after ingestion (Stewart and Constable, 1961; Scobie, 1961).

The production of more potent diuretics has so far been of greater theoretical than practical interest. These newer drugs are the products of research of various pharmaceutical manufacturers who have made intensive study of structure-activity relationship of the benzothiadiazine group of drugs. The most detailed and informative research of this type has been published by Lund and Kobinger (1960). In the future the discovery of more potent drugs of the benzothiadiazine series will allow the commercial production of diuretics at a less expense to the consumer. To date, however, the average cost per daily dose of the various members of the benzothiadiazine group is remarkably similar and, thus, there has not been any great practical use in the large number of commercially available drugs of this type. The hypotensive action of benzothiadiazine drugs is discussed on p. 317.

CLINICAL USE

The benzothiadiazine group of drugs are active diuretic agents producing comparatively few toxic side-effects and having the great advantage of being active when taken by mouth. They have proved especially useful in controlling the oedema of congestive heart failure and, to a lesser extent, that of the nephrotic syndrome. These drugs are less useful in oedema and ascites complicating cirrhosis of the liver, because in these patients potassium depletion is especially toxic and precipitates hepatic pre-coma or actual coma (Reid *et al.*, 1959). It is too early to state which is the best drug in clinical practice. Hydrochlorothiazide and hydroflumethiazide are probably better drugs than the original chlorothiazide because they produce less potassium loss in the urine, and in man a large proportion of the amount of chlorothiazide taken by mouth is inactive and is lost in the faeces. The newer, more potent, drugs of the benzothiadiazine class have not yet been used long enough to be certain that they will be as useful as hydrochlorothiazide and hydroflumethiazide in clinical practice. Besides their use as diuretics, these drugs are now extremely popular as potentiating agents for ganglion-blocking drugs and the more specific sympathetic-blocking drugs in the treatment of hypertension.

Most of this synergistic action is due to reduction of blood volume secondary to their diuretic action (Dollery *et al.*, 1959). The benzothiadiazine drugs are also useful in treatment of cases of nephrogenic diabetes insipidus (Kennedy and Crawford, 1959), where they cause a considerable reduction of urinary output and of the secondary polydipsia of the condition. This effect may partly be due to reduction of the glomerular filtration rate, and partly to an ill-understood effect on renal tubular function. Because of their popularity in the treatment of the two common clinical conditions of oedema and hypertension, the benzo-thiadiazine group of drugs are amongst the most widely prescribed drugs in pharmacology today.

TOXIC SIDE-EFFECTS

The most important toxic side-effect of this group of drugs is potassium depletion secondary to their effect in increasing potassium exchange for sodium in the distal tubule. Unless potassium supplements are given there is severe hypokalaemia after administration of this type of drug. Probably chlorothiazide and flumethiazide are the worst offenders, the more potent drugs causing less potassium loss. The severity of the hypokalaemia produced by the benzothiadiazine drugs seems excessive when compared with the relatively slight degree of potassium loss they produce. Recent work has shown that they have no action in altering potassium gradients from the extracellular to the intracellular compartments, especially in relation to voluntary muscle. They produce no change in plasma electrolyte content when given intravenously to the nephrectomized dog (Blackmore, 1961). The toxic effects of potassium depletion are more closely related to the gradient between intra- and extracellular fluids rather than to the magnitude of the potassium loss. The hypokalaemia may cause muscular weakness and apathy, and may precipitate hepatic coma in cases of severe hepatic cirrhosis. The effect on heart muscle in congestive heart failure is even more important. Potassium depletion sensitizes the myocardium to the toxic effects of digitalis with production of abnormal rhythms such as pulsus bigeminus, auriculoventricular dissociation, ventricular tachycardia or even fatal ventricular fibrillation.

The benzothiadiazine diuretics may cause increase of plasma uric acid without an associated increase of urea, creatinine or any other fraction of plasma non-protein nitrogen. Uric acid is now known to be excreted by the kidney by a triple process involving glomerular filtration and both tubular reabsorption and secretion (Gutman et al., 1959). Organic acids excreted by proximal tubular secretion, e.g. probenecid and the chlorothiazide group of drugs, prevent the uptake of uric acid by the proximal tubular epithelium prior to secretion into the tubular lumen (Platts and Mudge, 1961). There is, thus, actual retention of uric acid within the body and this may cause attacks of clinical gout in patients with a hereditary predisposition to the disease (Laragh et al., 1958; Oren et al., 1958). The drugs sometimes reduce glucose tolerance and may precipitate diabetes mellitus in pre-diabetic subjects or increase insulin requirements in previously well-controlled diabetics. This side-effect is the direct opposite of the action of the sulphonamide derivatives used in mild cases of diabetes. The effects on uric acid and glucose metabolism are usually reversible and disappear within 2 or 3 days of the cessation of diuretic therapy.

Some patients exhibit gastro-intestinal intolerance to the benzothiadiazine group of drugs, as shown by epigastric pain, vomiting or diarrhoea. Occasionally there may be purpura with thrombocytopaenia, but agranulocytosis or aplastic anaemia is very uncommon (Jaffe and Kierland, 1958; Zuckerman and Chasan, 1958; Nordquist *et al.*, 1959).

DIURETICS INHIBITING ALDOSTERONE SECRETION

These drugs which inhibit steroid synthesis in the adrenal cortex were discovered by the chance observation of Nelson and Woodard, 1949, that the insecticide DDD (2, 2-di-*p*-chlorophenyl-1, 1-dichloro-ethane) produced atrophy of the adrenal cortex in the dog. More recently the

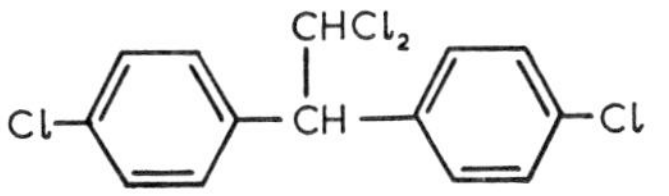

DDD

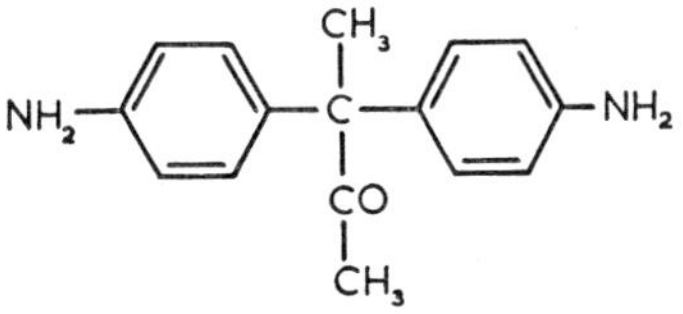

amphenone–B

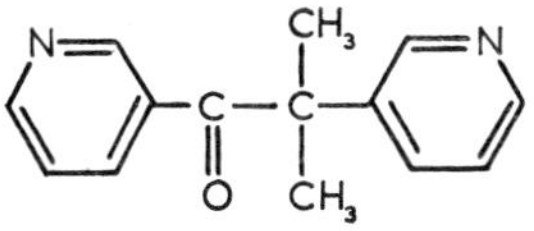

methyl–dipyridyl–propanone
(SU 4885)

derivatives amphenone-B and the drug methyldipyridyl-propanone (SU4885; Metopyrome) have been studied in detail. Amphenone-B is too toxic to be used in practical therapeutics and causes methaemoglobinaemia, liver injury, gastric disturbances and drowsiness, but the newer drug SU4885 is much less toxic and has a more selective action on the adrenal cortex. These drugs inhibit the enzyme concerned with 11-hydroxylation in the steroid nucleus. There is, thus, reduced secretion of the adrenal steroids cortisol, corticosterone and aldosterone, with increased production of 11-deoxy-steroids including 11-deoxycortisol (substance S), and 11-deoxycorticosterone. Secretion of these 11-deoxy-steroids progressively rises with continued dosage of SU4885 because inhibition of cortisol production increases pituitary production of adrenocorticotrophic hormone with stimulus of abnormal steroid production. As deoxycorticosterone has effects on sodium reabsorption similar to those of aldosterone, the desired diuretic effect is reduced on continued dosage unless A.C.T.H. production is inhibited by simultaneous administration of prednisone or prednisolone (Coppage *et al.*, 1959). In addition, this prevents the undesirable effects of reduced cortisol production. This drug is still in the experimental stage and its use as a diuretic is only indicated in exceptional circumstances of severe refractory oedema associated with clear evidence of secondary hyperaldosteronism.

ALDOSTERONE ANTAGONISTS

Drugs of the type of SU4885 have too general an action on adrenal cortical function and it is obviously preferable to use a drug which has a more specific effect on aldosterone action. Various steroid lactones have been found to antagonize the action of aldosterone on distal tubular function (Kagawa *et al.*, 1957; see also chapter 8). The drug which has been most used is the spironolactone SC9420, now commercially available as aldactone. The drug presumably acts by competitive displacement of aldosterone from receptor sites in the distal tubule. It is inactive in untreated Addisons disease (Liddle, 1957), and has little effect when there is only mild oedema with slight excess of aldosterone production. Inhibition of the effects of aldosterone causes increased sodium and chloride output and by reduction of cation exchange there is decreased excretion of potassium, hydrogen ion and ammonium. This combination of effects on electrolyte output is unusual as most other diuretics enhance the excretion both of sodium and potassium. The drug has usually been more effective in severe cases of the nephrotic syndrome (Liddle, 1958) and in hepatic cirrhosis (Shaldon *et al.*, 1960) than in congestive heart failure. The effect of the drug is reduced on continued dosage because the increased sodium loss stimulates further aldosterone production (Bolte *et al.*, 1958).

This drug is, perhaps, most useful to counteract excessive potassium loss from other diuretics, e.g. those of the benzothiadiazine group, in cases of refractory oedema with severe secondary hyperaldosteronism. The simultaneous use of spironolactone allows maximal diuretic action without potassium loss by inhibition of distal tubular potassium exchange.

NON-SPECIFIC AND GENERAL SIDE-EFFECTS OF DIURETIC THERAPY

There are now a large number of available diuretics, all with different and usually additive actions on sodium reabsorption by the kidney. Even the most refractory cases of oedema can be made to have a satisfactory diuresis with a combination of available active agents. Sometimes, however, there is the danger that therapy may be too enthusiastic.

For example, I have seen a patient treated with the following formidable combination of drugs: (a) an almost salt-free diet; (b) cation exchange resins by mouth reducing sodium absorption from the gut; (c) frequent injections of mercurial diuretics; (d) the use of maximum dosage of lysine-hydrochloride as an adjuvant to mercurial therapy; (e) oral hydrochlorothiazide in full dosage; (f) the production of an osmotic diuresis by mannitol infusions; (g) the use of full doses of aldactone as an aldosterone antagonist. Vigorous therapy of this type may often result in severe salt depletion with reduction of plasma volume, fall in blood pressure, peripheral circulatory failure, and fall in glomerular filtration rate with rise of blood urea. In very ill patients with severe secondary hyperaldosteronism and refractory oedema these undesirable side-effects may occur at a stage when the patient still shows overt clinical oedema. Periodical estimation of the blood urea is particularly useful in the control of therapy. It is often wise to leave the patient with a mild degree of oedema rather than to produce severe salt depletion with peripheral circulatory failure and uraemia. At this stage the use of plasma expanders, particularly salt-free human albumin, may be useful in preventing signs and symptoms of reduced blood volume. Excessive haemo-concentration may easily lead to arterial or venous thromboses including cerebral thrombosis, coronary thrombosis or thrombosis of leg veins with secondary pulmonary embolism. Progressive reduction of plasma sodium is a particularly unfavourable effect of prolonged diuretic therapy. Hyponatraemia is a bad prognostic sign and often indicates that the patient has severe and irreversible general disease. The decrease in osmolality of plasma and extracellular fluid is secondary to severe metabolic effects within the cell, often associated with loss of intracellular potassium and gain of intracellular sodium. The wise clinician should avoid a state of severe salt depletion where he is forced suddenly to reverse the aims of therapy, and give the patient saline infusions in order to maintain circulatory efficiency. Cases of hepatic cirrhosis with ascites and oedema are often the most difficult of all oedematous patients to manage. Too vigorous therapy, especially if associated with excess potassium loss, may easily precipitate severe and often fatal hepatic coma.

GLOSSARY

ACID: A substance capable of donating a proton or hydrogen ion. Hydrochloric and sulphuric acids are strong acids, and carbonic acid is a weak acid. At the pH range of body fluids the ammonium ion and the monobasic phosphate ion ($H_2PO_4^-$) are capable of donating a proton and therefore behave as weak acids.

ACIDOSIS: This may be defined in two different ways: (a) a condition in which there has been gain of an acid or of hydrogen ion or in which there has been loss of a base; or (b) a state in which the pH of arterial blood is below the normal value. The two definitions agree except in potassium depletion where there is dissociation of pH changes in the extra- and intracellular fluids.

ALKALOSIS: This may be defined in two different ways: (a) a condition in which there has been loss of an acid or of hydrogen ion or in which there has been gain of a base; or (b) a state in which the pH of arterial blood is above the normal value. The two definitions agree except in potassium depletion where there is dissociation of pH changes in the extra- and intracellular fluids.

ANION: The negatively charged ion of an electrolyte, e.g. Cl^-, $SO_4^=$, $H_2PO_4^-$, $HPO_4^=$, HCO_3^-. Some anions are capable of accepting a proton and forming an acid and are therefore bases, e.g. HCO_3^- and $HPO_4^=$; others are capable of proton donation and are therefore acids, e.g. $H_2PO_4^-$; whilst others at the pH of body fluids can neither donate nor accept a proton and are therefore neither acids nor bases, e.g. Cl^- and $SO_4^=$.

BASE: A substance capable of accepting a proton or hydrogen ion. Important bases in physiology are the bicarbonate ion, dibasic phosphate ($HPO_4^=$), and ammonia. Many clinicians refer to the cations Na^+, K^+, Ca^{++}, and Mg^{++}, as 'fixed bases'. This is an incorrect nomenclature, as these substances are cations and are neither acids nor bases.

CATION: The positively charged ion of an electrolyte, e.g. Na^+, K^+, Ca^{++}, and Mg^{++}.

COUNTER CURRENT EXCHANGER: An arrangement by which a current of fluid maintains a gradient of heat, gas tension, concentration, or osmolality without the performance of external work except that necessary to maintain the flow of fluid.

COUNTER CURRENT MULTIPLIER: An arrangement by which, with the assistance of external work, a current of fluid is enabled to build up a gradient of heat, gas tension, concentration or osmolality. The ascending loop of Henle performs this function by active extrusion of sodium from the cells into the interstitial fluid of the renal medulla.

ELECTRO-CHEMICAL POTENTIAL: A difference in electrical charge produced by the active movement of an electrolyte. The cells of the renal tubules take up sodium from the luminal fluid, and extrude this cation into the interstitial fluid of the kidney. An electrochemical potential gradient is thereby produced, the interstitial fluid being positively charged in relation to the charge of the fluid within the tubular lumen. This gradient results in transfer of the negatively charged and diffusible chloride ion from the tubular lumen to the interstitial fluid.

METABOLIC CHANGE IN ACID-BASE BALANCE: A state of acidosis or alkalosis produced by a primary change in the bicarbonate concentration of body fluids, with a secondary corresponding change in P_{CO_2} which reduces, but does not completely prevent, alteration in the pH of body fluids. Alkalosis is produced by bicarbonate ingestion which adds base to the body, by vomiting or by the excretion of an inappropriately acidic urine which removes hydrogen ion from the body. Acidosis is produced by ingestion of NH_4Cl, $CaCl_2$, free HCl, or HCl combined with dibasic aminoacids, e.g. lysine or arginine.

MILLIEQUIVALENT: A unit mass of either a cation or an anion. This unit is defined as the atomic or molecular weight of the electrolyte in milligrams, divided by its valency. The advantage of this system of recording the mass of an electrolyte in body fluids is that a single unit of a cation has exactly the same positive charge as a unit of an anion has negative charge.

MILLIMOLE: A unit mass of a non-electrolyte or of an undissociated salt. A millimole is equal to the molecular weight of the substance in milligrams, and is equivalent to a single milliosmole of the substance.

OSMOLALITY: The total concentration of solute within a fluid. The unit of osmolality used in physiology is the milliosmole. A millimole of a non-electrolyte, e.g. urea or glucose, or of an undissociated salt is equivalent to a single milliosmole. In the case of univalent electrolytes a milliequivalent is equal to a milliosmole, but in the case of polyvalent electrolytes, a milliosmole is equal to two or more milliequivalents according to the valency of the electrolyte. The concentration of fluids expressed as mOsm./l. is measured by the depression of freezing point produced by the solute. In aqueous solution a concentration of 1000 mOsm./Kg. of water will depress the freezing point by $1.86°C$. All body fluids have an identical osmolality, averaging 290 mOsm./l. in man, except for the hyperosmolality of the fluid within the renal medulla produced by the counter-current multiplier system of the loops of Henle.

OSMOTIC PRESSURE: The pressure difference on two sides of a membrane produced by inequality of concentration of a solute to which the membrane is impermeable. The capillary walls are impermeable to plasma proteins, and the difference of protein concentration between plasma and interstitial fluid produces an osmotic pressure equivalent to 30 mm. Hg. This would tend to cause a transfer of water from the interstitial compartment to the vascular compartment, but is balanced by the hydrostatic pressure of the blood within the capillaries tending to force water in the opposite direction.

RESPIRATORY CHANGE IN ACID-BASE BALANCE: A state of acidosis or alkalosis produced by a primary change in the CO_2 content of body fluids, with a secondary corresponding change in bicarbonate concentration which reduces, but does not completely prevent, alteration in the pH of body fluids. Acidosis is produced by inhalation of excess CO_2, or by lung disease, e.g. emphysema, which reduces the capacity of the lungs to remove CO_2 from the body. Alkalosis is produced by hyperventilation, whether produced by voluntary effort or by abnormal stimulation of the respiratory centre, e.g. after salicylate ingestion.

REFERENCES

*Denotes review

ANDERSON, H. M. and MUDGE, G. H. (1955). *J. clin. Invest.* **34,** 1691

ATKINSON, M., PATON, A. and SHERLOCK, S. (1954). *Lancet,* **1,** 128

AXELROD, D. R. and PITTS, R. F. (1952). *J. clin. Invest.* **31,** 171

BAER, J. E. and BAYER, K. H. (1959). *Int. Rec. Med.* **172,** 413

BERLINER, R. W., KENNEDY, T. J., JR. and HILTON, J. G. (1948). *Amer. J. Physiol.* **154,** 539

BERLINER, R. W., KENNEDY, T. J., JR. and ORLOFF, J. (1951). *Amer. J. Med.* **11,** 274

BLACKMORE, W. P. (1961). *Proc. Soc. exp. Biol. (N.Y.)* **106,** 681

BOLTE, E., VERDY, M., MARC-AURELE, J., BROUILLET, J., BEAUREGARDE, P. and GENEST, J. (1958). *Canad. med. Ass. J.* **79,** 881

BORGHGRAEF, R. R., KESSLER, R. H. and PITTS, R. F. (1956). *J. clin. Invest.* **35,** 1055

BRAILOVSKY, D., SILVA, S., DEL CAMPO, E. and MARUSIC, E. (1959). *Amer. J. med. Sci.* **238,** 287

BRODSKY, W. A. and GRAUBARTH, H. N. (1953). *Amer. J. Physiol.* **172,** 67

BRODSKY, W. A. and SATRAN, R. (1959). *Amer. J. Physiol.* **197,** 585

BRÖNSTED, J. N. (1923). *Rec. Trav. chim. Pays-Bas,* **42,** 718

BRUN, C., HILDEN, T. and RAASCHOU, F. (1947). *Acta pharmacol. (Kbh.)* **3,** 1

BURACK, W. R., PRYCE, J. and GOODWIN, J. F. (1958). *Circulation,* **18,** 562

CAFRUNY, E. J., FARAH, Q. and DI STEFANO, H. S. (1955). *J. Pharmacol. exp. Ther.* **115,** 390

COOKE, R. E., SEGAR, W. E., CHEEK, D. B., COVILLE, F. E. and DARROW, D. C. (1952). *J. clin. Invest.* **31,** 798

COPPAGE, W. S., JR., ISLAND, D., SMITH, M. and LIDDLE, G. W. (1959). *J. clin. Invest.* **38,** 2101

COUNIHAN, T. B., EVANS, B. M. and MILNE, M. D. (1954). *Clin. Sci.* **13,** 583

CRANSTON, W. I., SANDERSON, P. H. and STAPLETON, P. (1955). *J. Physiol. (Lond.),* **129,** 71P

CRAWFORD, M. A., LOUGHRIDGE, L., MILNE, M. D. and SCRIBNER, B. H. (1959). *J. clin. Path.* **12,** 524

DARROW, D. C., COOKE, R. E. and COVILLE, F. E. (1953). *Amer. J. Physiol.* **172,** 55

DOLLERY, C. T., HARINGTON, M. and KAUFMANN, G. (1959). *Lancet,* **1,** 1215

DORMAN, P. J., SULLIVAN, W. J. and PITTS, R. F. (1954). *J. clin. Invest.* **33,** 82

ECKEL, R. E. and NORRIS, J. E. C. (1955). *J. clin. Invest.* **34,** 931

EDWARDS, J. G. (1942). *Amer. J. Path.* **18,** 1011

EVANS, B. M., MACINTYRE, I., MACPHERSON, C. R. and MILNE, M. D. (1957). *Clin. Sci.* **16,** 53

FARAH, A. and MARESH, G. (1948). *J. Pharmacol. exp. Ther.* **92,** 73

FISHMAN, A. P., SAMET, P. and COURNAND, A. (1955). *Amer. J. Med.* **19,** 533

GIDEKEL, L. I., SHERLOCK, P., PETERSON, A. S. and VANAMEE, P. (1960). *New Engl. J. Med.* **263,** 221

GOLD, H., GREINER, T. H., MATHES, S. B., MARAH, R. R., WARSHAW, L. J., MODELL, W., KWIT, N. T., OTTO, H. L., GARB, S., BAKST, H. and KRAMER, M. L. (1952). *Amer. J. med. Sci.* **223**, 618

GREIF, R. L., SULLIVAN, W. J., JACOBS, G. S. and PITTS, R. F. (1956). *J. clin. Invest.* **35**, 38

GROSSMAN, J., WESTON, R. E., EDELMAN, I. S. and LEITER, L. (1949). *Fed. Proc.* **8**, 62

GUTMAN, A. B., YÜ T. F. and BERGER, L. (1959). *J. clin. Invest.* **38**, 1778

HANNA, S. and MACINTYRE, I. (1960). *Lancet*, **2**, 348

HARRISON, H. E. (1954). *Pediatrics*, **14**, 285

IACOBELLIS, M., MUNTWYLER, E. and DODGEN, C. L. (1956). *Amer. J. Physiol.* **185**, 275

IRVINE, R. O. H., SAUNDERS, S. J., MILNE, M. D. and CRAWFORD, M. A. (1961). *Clin. Sci.* **20**, 1

JAFFE, M. O. and KIERLAND, R. R. (1958). *J. Amer. med. Ass.* **168**, 2264

KAGAWA, C. M., CELLA, J. A. and VAN ARMAN, C. G. (1957). *Science*, **126**, 1015

KENNEDY, G. C. and CRAWFORD, J. D. (1959). *Lancet*, **1**, 866

KESSLER, R. H., HIERHOLZER, K., GURD, R. S. and PITTS, R. F. (1958). *Amer. J. Physiol.* **194**, 540

KESSLER, R. H., HIERHOLZER, K., GURD, R. S. and PITTS, R. F. (1959). *Amer. J. Physiol.* **196**, 1346

KESSLER, R. H., LOZANO, R. and PITTS, R. F. (1957). *J. Pharmacol. exp. Ther.* **121**, 432

LARAGH, J. H. (1956). *Amer. J. Med.* **21**, 423

LARAGH, J. H. (1958). *Ann. N.Y. Acad. Sci.* **71**, 409

LASSER, R. P., SCHOENFELD, M. R. and FRIEDBERG, C. K. (1960). *New Engl. J. Med.* **263**, 728

LEHMAN, J. F., BARRACK, L. P. and LEHMAN, R. A. (1951). *Science*, **113**, 410

LEIBMAN, K. C., ALFORD, D. and BOUDET, R. A. (1961). *J. Pharmacol. exp. Ther.* **131**, 271

LIDDLE, G. W. (1957). *Science*, **126**, 1016

LIDDLE, G. W. (1958). *Arch. intern. Med.* **102**, 998

LOWRY, T. M. (1923). *Chem. and Ind.* **42**, 43

LUETSCHER, J. A., JR. and JOHNSON, B. B. (1954). *J. clin. Invest.* **23**, 1441

LUND, F. J. and KOBINGER, W. (1960). *Acta pharmacol.* (*Kbh.*) **16**, 297

MCCALLY, M., ANDERSON, C. H. and FARRELL, G. L. (1958). The Endocrine Society. Programme of the 40th meeting. Springfield. Ill. C. T. Thomas

MCNICHOL, F. C. and PRIDE, N. B. (1961). *Lancet*, **1**, 906

MAFFLY, L. H. and LEAF, A. (1959). *J. gen. Physiol.* **42**, 1257

MANN, T. and KEILIN, D. (1940). *Nature* (*Lond.*), **146**, 164

MAREN, T. H., SORSDAHL, O. A. and DICKHAUS, A. J. (1961). *Amer. J. Physiol.* **200**, 170

MILLS, J. N., THOMAS, S. and WILLIAMSON, K. S. (1960). *J. Physiol.* (*Lond.*), **151**, 312

MILNE, M. D. (1956). *Proc. roy. Soc. Med.* **49**, 624

MILNE, M. D., ASATOOR, A. M., EDWARDS, K. D. G. and LOUGHRIDGE, L. W. (1961). *Gut*, **2**, 323

MILNE, M. D., SCRIBNER, B. H. and CRAWFORD, M. A. (1958). *Amer. J. Med.* **24**, 709

MODELL, W., GOLD, H. and CLARKE, D. A. (1945). *J. Pharmacol. exp. Ther.* **84**, 284

MOYER, J. H., HANDLEY, C. A. and WILFORD, I. (1952). *Amer. Heart. J.* **44**, 608

MUDGE, G. H. and HARDIN, B. (1956). *J. clin. Invest.* **35**, 155

MUDGE, G. H. and WEINER, I. M. (1958). *Ann. N.Y. Acad. Sci.* **71**, 344

MUNCK, O. and NISSEN, N. I. (1956). *Acta med. scand.* **153**, 307

NADELL, J. (1953). *J. clin. Invest.* **32**, 622

NAIMARK, A., BRODOVSKY, D. M. and CHERNIACK, R. M. (1960). *Amer. J. Med.* **28**, 368

NAJARIAN, J. S. and HARPER, H. A. (1956). *Amer. J. Med.* **21**, 832

NELSON, A. A. and WOODARD, G. (1949). *Arch. Path.* (*Chicago*), **48**, 387

NORDQUIST, P., CRAMER, G. and BJORNTROP, P. (1959). *Lancet*, **1**, 271
NOVELLO, F. C. and SPRAGUE, J. M. (1957). *J. Amer. chem. Soc.* **79**, 2028
OREN, B. G., RICH, M. and BELLE, M. S. (1958). *J. Amer. med. Ass.* **168**, 2128
*PITTS, R. F. (1959). The Physiological Basis of Diuretic Therapy. Springfield. Ill.
    C. T. Thomas ·
PLATTS, M. M. and MUDGE, G. H. (1961). *Amer. J. Physiol.* **200**, 387
READ, A. E., LAIDLAW, J., HASLAM, R. M. and SHERLOCK, S. (1959). *Clin. Sci.* **18**,
    409
RELMAN, A. S., ETSTEN, B. and SCHWARTZ, W. B. (1953). *J. clin. Invest.* **32**, 972
RENNELS, E. G. and RUSKIN, A. (1954). *Proc. Soc. exp. Biol.* (*N.Y.*) **85**, 309
ROBINSON, J. R. and MCCANCE, R. A. (1952). *Ann. Rev. Physiol.* **14**, 115
ROBLIN, R. O., JR. and CLAPP, J. W. (1950). *J. Amer. chem. Soc.* **72**, 4890
ROBSON, E. B. and ROSE, G. A. (1957). *Clin. Sci.* **16**, 75
RUBIN, A. L., SPRITZ, N., MEAD, A. W., HERRMANN, R. A., BRAVEMAN, W. S. and
    LUCKEY, E. H. (1960). *Circulation*, **21**, 332
SCHWARTZ, W. B. and WALLACE, W. M. (1951). *J. clin. Invest.* **30**, 1089
SCOBIE, B. A. (1961). *N.Z. med. J.* **60**, 105
SCRIABINE, A., P'AN, S. Y., ROWLAND, D. and BERTRAND, C. (1961). *J. Pharmacol.*
    exp. Therap. **133**, 351
SCRIABINE, A., KOROL, B., KONDRATAS, B., YU M, P'AN, S. Y. and SCHNEIDER,
    J. A. (1961). *Proc. Soc. exp. Biol.* (*N.Y.*) **107**, 864
SHALDON, S., MCLAREN, J. R. and SHERLOCK, S. (1960). *Lancet*, **1**, 609
SOUTHWORTH, H. (1937). *Proc. Soc. exp. Biol.* (*N.Y.*) **36**, 58
SPRAGUE, J. M. (1958). *Ann. N.Y. Acad. Sci.* **71**, 321
SPRITZ, N., FRIMPTER, G. W., BRAVEMAN, W. S. and RUBIN, A. L. (1959). *Circu-*
    lation, **19**, 600
STEWART, W. K. and CONSTABLE, L. W. (1961). *Brit. med. J.* **1**, 523
THOMSON, W. T., JR., RICHARDSON, D. W. and WINGO, C. F. (1958). *Amer. J. med.*
    Sci. **236**, 603
ULICK, S., LARAGH, J. H. and LIEBERMAN, S. (1958). *Trans. Ass. Amer. Phys.* **71**, 225
WACHSTEIN, M. and MEISEL, E. (1954). *Science*, **119**, 100
WADDELL, W. J. and BUTLER, T. C. (1959). *J. clin. Invest.* **38**, 720
WEBBER, W. A., BROWN, J. L. and PITTS, R. F. (1961). *Amer. J. Physiol.* **200**, 380
WEINER, I. M. and MULLER, O. H. (1955). *J. Pharmacol. exp. Ther.* **113**, 241
WEINER, I. M., WASHINGTON, J. A. and MUDGE, G. H. (1959). *Bull. Johns Hopk.*
    Hosp. **105**, 274
WESTON, R. E. and ESCHER, D. J. (1948). *J. clin. Invest.* **27**, 561
*WIRZ, H. (1960). Water and Electrolyte Metabolism. p. 100. Amsterdam: Elsevier
WIRZ, H., HARGITAY, B. and KUHN, W. (1951). *Helv. phsyiol. pharmacol. Acta*, **9**,
    196
YOUNG, D. S., FORRESTER, T. M. and MORGAN, T. N. (1959). *Lancet*, **2**, 765
ZUCKERMAN, A. J. and CHASAN, A. A. (1958). *Brit. med. J.* **2**, 1338

CHAPTER 8

NEW STEROIDS

This chapter deals essentially with new steroids but other related material has been included when it seemed relevant. For example, in connection with the anti-fertility steroids other substances with an effect on fertility have been discussed.

NEWER CORTICOSTEROIDS

Corticosteroids have now been used for a number of years and there is no doubt that they represent valuable and in some cases life-saving therapeutic agents. Cortisone was introduced into clinical practice by Hench and his co-workers in 1948 and shortly afterwards hydrocortisone became available. Since then a number of chemical changes have been made in these compounds in the hope of increasing their clinical usefulness. In addition, new corticosteroids have been isolated from biological material of which the most important is aldosterone. It is worth noting that these compounds are used for three main purposes, namely:

(1). To replace the secretion of the adrenal glands when this is deficient, either as the result of disease or following surgical removal.

(2). To produce a level of corticosteroids well above the normal in order to induce certain changes in the tissues which may be of therapeutic value. These effects are often due to an anti-inflammatory or to an anti-allergic effect, e.g. in rheumatoid arthritis and in status asthmaticus respectively. The level of corticosteroid may be raised either by the administration of cortisone or one of its derivatives or, occasionally, by stimulating the patient's own adrenal by giving adrenocorticotrophic hormone (corticotrophin, ACTH).

(3). To depress the secretory activity of the adrenal cortex in conditions in which this is abnormally high, e.g. in patients with adrenogenital syndrome.

Furthermore steroid derivatives have recently been made (e.g. spironolactone) which are believed to antagonize the action of aldosterone and which are of value in the treatment of certain types of oedema when employed either alone or in association with diuretics. Another steroid which is interesting in this connection is one which tends to increase sodium excretion. The existence of this substance was suspected for some years because of certain clinical findings (see Annotation, 1959). It was isolated from the urine of a patient with congenital adrenal hyperplasia and subsequently from hog adrenals and found to be 3-β-16-α-dehydroxy-allopregnan-20-one which has also been synthesized (Neher *et al.*, 1958). The presence of a hydroxyl group in the 16 position is interesting, since this has already been shown to have a marked effect on electrolyte regulating activity of synthetic steroids, e.g. triamcinolone. The pharmacology and possible therapeutic use of this new compound remain to be worked out.

Although cortisone was the corticosteroid originally introduced and is still being used, it has certain important disadvantages and this has led to an intensive search for derivatives of cortisone (or hydrocortisone) which might retain the value of the original compound and not have some of its drawbacks. The main deleterious effects of cortisone, when used in large doses to produce a pharmacological effect, are as follows:

(1) Action due essentially to excessive mineralocorticoid activity, i.e. sodium retention, potassium loss, oedema and also hypertension.

(2) Action associated with excessive metabolic effects, i.e. osteoporosis and nitrogen depletion; development and accentuation of diabetes.

(3) Effect on tissue repair and healing, notably peptic ulceration and its complication, increased liability to infection.

(4) Complications due to inhibition of the anterior pituitary, and notably of corticotrophin secretion; these occur on cessation of treatment. The capacity of the adrenal cortex to respond to corticotrophin stimulation may be deferred for many weeks after cessation of prolonged steroid therapy, and normal function appears to be more rapidly returned by repeated treatment with corticotrophin (Krusius and Oak, 1958).

The synthesis of new steroids has overcome some of these difficulties, but has, unfortunately, in some cases, led to the appearance of new toxic effects.

METHODS OF MEASURING ANTI-INFLAMMATORY ACTIVITY

Anti-inflammatory agents are used essentially (1) to control the abnormality in various rheumatic conditions, (2) to decrease general bodily reactions to infection when these are deleterious, e.g. acute febrile condition, some types of tuberculosis, and (3) applied locally, to decrease local inflammatory reactions—the main uses are for application to the skin and to the eye. Menkin (1960) reviews the biochemical mechanisms of inflammation and suggests that anti-inflammatory substances act by suppressing the cellular activity of injured cells at the site of inflammation, so that these cells are incapable of 'forming the chemical factors that essentially constitute inflammation'.

Salicylates have been used for many years to relieve the signs and symptoms of rheumatic fever and, increasingly, of rheumatoid arthritis. The pharmacology of salicylates (and of phenylbutazone) is discussed by Robson and Keele (1956). With the introduction of the corticosteroids, which are potent anti-inflammatory agents, there has been an increased impetus to the elaboration of methods for the measurement of anti-inflammatory activity. These can be used to try and discover new substances having such effects and to compare the activities of various known substances; also to try and study the mechanisms by which such effects may be produced. It may be said in general that such methods frequently measure different aspects of inflammation, e.g. oedema, cellular exudate, erythema, so that the interpretation of the result obtained in terms of possible therapeutic use presents great difficulties. Nevertheless, these methods have provided valuable results.

Roskam (1958 and 1959) has reviewed the methods used in testing anti-inflammatory substances and divided them under four headings, namely (1) effect on erythema or rise in temperature due to inflammation, (2) effect on permeability as measured by the passage of dye through a membrane (e.g. synovial membrane) or into a tissue (e.g. skin) (3) effect on the volume of an organ, e.g. the rat's foot, subjected to some irritant which will increase exudation. Formalin, dextran and egg white are some of the irritants that have been used. (4) More severe and complex inflammatory reactions leading to exudation, granulation tissue formation and necrosis. A granuloma found around a non-absorbable foreign body, e.g. cotton wool, or around an irritant put into an air pouch, e.g. croton oil can be excised and weighed, and the effect of anti-inflammatory substances on such a reaction can thus be measured.

The references already quoted, as well as Kellett (1959) and Selye and Gaétan (1956) should be consulted for details of the tests used. Three tests commonly used at present are the *formalin foot test* in which the animal is injected with formalin beneath the plantar aponeurosis of one foot; the *cotton pellet test* in which weighed sterile cotton wool pellets are implanted subcutaneously in rats; and the *granuloma pouch method* in which a pocket of air is produced subcutaneously in the rat, and a solution of croton oil in arachis oil injected into the pouch. These examples emphasize how varied the experimental inflammatory reactions are and thus the difficulty of evaluating results obtained with such tests in terms of possible clinical use of the substances investigated.

PREDNISOLONE AND PREDNISONE (Fig. 39)

These are derivatives of hydrocortisone and cortisone respectively, in which there is a double bond between the first and second carbon atoms in the A ring of the steroid molecule. At the present time they probably represent the compounds of first choice in the treatment of conditions in which large pharmacological doses of glucocorticoid are required. These compounds are about 4 to 5 times as active as cortisone for glucocorticoid and anti-inflammatory action, without any enhancement

of the mineralocorticoid activity. Thus the side effect of sodium retention and potassium depletion are to some extent eliminated. However,
as the study of Ward *et al.* (1958) has shown, these new steroids can still
produce other undesirable effects, such as obesity, supraclavicular fat
pads, hypertrichosis, acne, psychic changes, striae, purpura, hypertension and particularly osteoporosis and peptic ulceration with its complications. The use of these substances thus requires the same general
precautions as that of cortisone.

Prednisolone trimethylacetate has a low solubility and a microcrystalline suspension has been used by intra-articular injection, for the
local treatment of rheumatoid arthritis (Annotation, 1959).

TRIAMCINOLONE (Fig. 39)

This is a prednisolone which is fluorinated in the 9α position (this
enhances mineralocorticoid activity), but also hydroxylated in the 16
position, by which the mineralocorticoid action is lost. It is a potent
antiphlogistic substance made with the hope that the side effects would
be reduced; this has unfortunately not been realized. The compound is
only slightly more active than prednisolone and has produced quite a
variety of side effects, some typically seen in cortisone therapy and others
not commonly seen with other corticosteroids. Thus Neustadt (1959)
found that patients on triamcinolone were liable to suffer from hot
flushes, erythema of the face and increased perspiration but, more
important still, could develop muscular weakness, sometimes associated
with marked loss of weight. These side effects usually subsided after
patients were transferred to another steroid. Williams (1959) has performed muscle biopsies on patients on triamcinolone and thus demonstrated widespread muscle damage; there was also electromyographic
evidence of primary muscle-fibre lesions. It is to be noted that a similar,
though less severe, myopathy was observed by Harman (1959) in two
patients treated with prednisolone and that Ellis (1956) produced widespread necrosis of skeletal muscle in rabbits treated with large doses of
cortisone. Wells (1958) has noted the appearance of arthritis in patients
with no previous history of joint symptoms, following triamcinolone
administration. Golding (1960) reviews the literature on triamcinolone
and concludes that the drug has advantages over cortisone and prednisone if the patient is oedematous or in heart failure, but against this
must be set the side effects outlined above. He emphasizes that every
patient is a law unto himself and it is very difficult to generalize about
which particular steroid will suit an individual best.

DEXAMETHASONE (9-α-fluoro-16-α-methyl-prednisolone) (Fig. 39)

This has the same structure as triamcinolone, except that the hydroxyl
group at C16 is replaced by a methyl group, which more than neutralizes

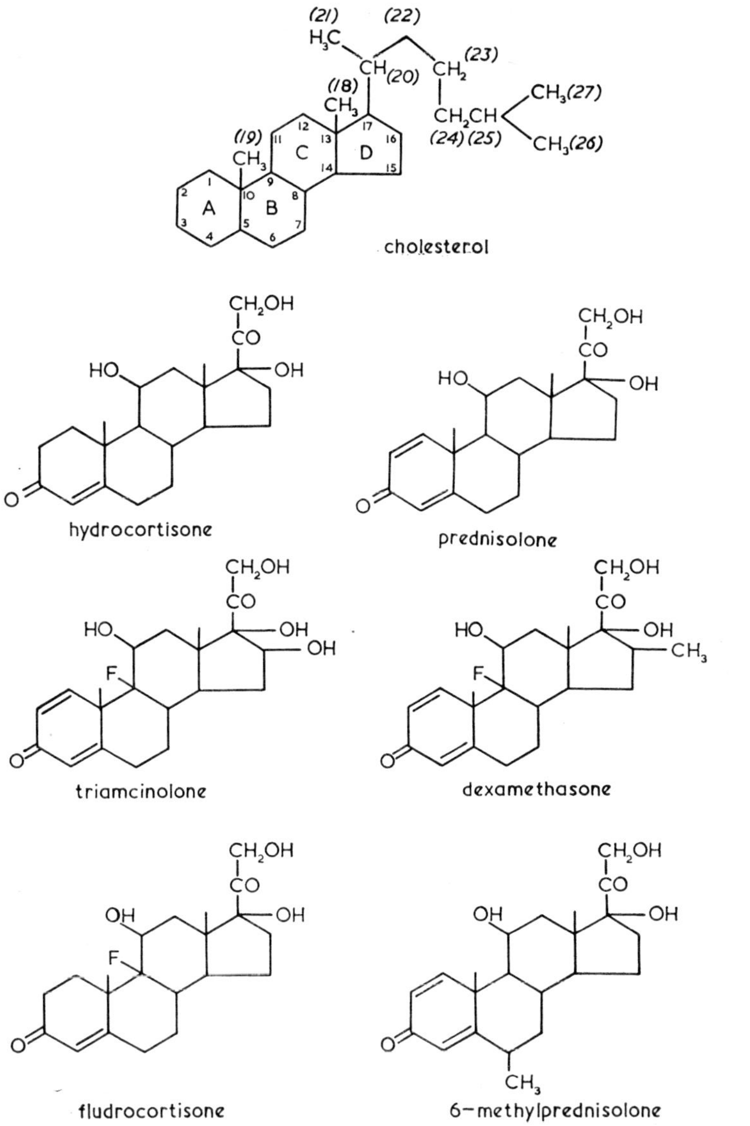

FIG. 39. Structure of some anti-inflammatory corticosteroids and their relation to cholesterol.

the sodium-retaining effect of the fluorine at C9, and also enhances the glucocorticoid effect of the compound. It is the most potent of these steroids being about 5 times as active as prednisone in this respect. Since dexamethasone and triamcinolone have no mineralocorticoid activity, they are not suitable for the treatment of Addisonian patients or after adrenalectomy, where the parent substances are still the drugs of choice. In fact, patients with Addison's disease satisfactorily maintained on cortisone, rapidly develop signs and symptoms of sodium depletion when switched to dexamethasone (Bayliss, 1959).

Dudley Hart (1960) concludes from his review of the evidence that dexamethasone has no advantages over prednisone or prednisolone since side effects are equally common with appropriate doses. The symptoms peculiar to triamcinolone, and described above under that heading, are not apparently seen with dexamethasone but on the other hand increased appetite, gain in weight and abdominal distention occur (Boland, 1959; Neustadt, 1959). Dexamethasone is a potent inhibitor of adrenocortical function and may prove useful in this respect to control adrenogenital syndrome and perhaps some cases of metastatic malignant disease (Dudley Hart, 1960). Bunim *et al.* (1958) have performed various metabolic studies with dexamethasone and found that it may produce a significant and sustained negative calcium balance chiefly as a result of increased faecal loss. This effect is virtually unique among the corticoids.

Betamethasone has the same structure as dexamethasone, except that the methyl group is in the β position. It is a potent anti-inflammatory agent, but there is at present no evidence that it possesses any particular advantages over prednisone (*Brit. med. J.* 1961. **2,** 825).

6α-METHYL PREDNISOLONE (Fig. 39)

The preliminary animal studies suggested that this compound might be of value therapeutically (Liddle, 1958), but clinical tests do not suggest that it offers any advantages over prednisolone though it is appreciably more expensive (Lewis, 1960; Boland, 1959). It is slightly more active so that 4 mg. of methyl prednisolone has an antiphlogistic activity equivalent to 5 mg. of prednisolone (Bayliss, 1959).

FLUDROCORTISONE (Fig. 39)

This is hydrocortisone fluorinated at C9, which increases the anti-inflammatory effect and even more so the sodium retaining properties of the compound, so that the relative mineralocorticoid action of fludrocortisone is much higher than that of cortisone. Fludrocortisone is thus unsuitable for systemic administration as an antiphlogistic agent, but has proved useful in the local treatment of dermatological and ophthalmological disease. Its main use is as a substitute for parenteral deoxycortone in the treatment of adrenal insufficiency. Some of these patients are well maintained on cortisone alone, but others require an additional mineralocorticoid effect, and this is well supplied by the administration of fludrocortisone in doses of 0·1 mg. per day or on alternate days, though the exact amount has to be determined by clinical experience for every patient (Bayliss, 1959). Fludrocortisone is slow in producing its effect and long lasting, so that adjustments in dosage should be made gradually and carefully.

Fluprednisolone (6α-fluoroprednisolone) has received a preliminary trial in patients with rheumatoid arthritis. It is about $2\frac{1}{2}$ times as active as prednisolone and at therapeutic doses of 2–7 mg. per day has not so far produced any salt or water retention. It requires further investigation (Boland, 1960).

A number of other glucocorticoids have recently been described, some of which are several hundred times more active than prednisolone, according to Wettstein (1960) but details of their actions are not yet available.

OTHER ANTI-INFLAMMATORY AGENTS

A number of other substances have recently been investigated in animals and also used clinically for their anti-inflammatory activity.

Antimalarial drugs

Domenjoz and Theobald (1958) found that mepacrine, primaquine and proguanil had anti-inflammatory activity of the order of cortisone when tested on the rat formalin induced oedema and this has essentially been confirmed by Kellett (1959). This supports the conclusion from a number of clinical observations, suggesting that certain antimalarials are of value in the treatment of rheumatic disorders. This work was started by a chance observation (Page, 1951) that mepacrine produced improvement of a rheumatic polyarthritis in a patient who was being treated for lupus erythematosus. Chloroquine is the drug which has been mainly used (see p. 359), though mepacrine, hydroxychloroquine and amodiaquine have also been tried. Side effects are not uncommon and include dyspepsia, vomiting, giddiness, headache and visual disturbances and corneal opacities which appear to be reversible after cessation of treatment (Kersley and Palin, 1959). The literature up to 1958 is reviewed by Fuld and Horwich (1958). Young (1959) presents the results of a study with chloroquine phosphate, extending over several years, and claims that the treatment was followed by a return of the sedimentation rate to normal in a much higher percentage of patients than has occurred in series treated solely with steroids, phenylbutazone and aspirin; in order to obtain the full benefit of chloroquine treatment, its administration must be continued for more than 18 months.

Glycyrrhetinic Acid

Liquorice has been used medicinally for many years and it has recently been discovered that it contains one or more active principles with anti-inflammatory action. The main water soluble constituent of liquorice is 'glycyrrhizin' from which the aglycone 'glycyrrhetinic acid' may be obtained by hydrolysis (Finney and Somers, 1958). Crude glycyrrhetinic acid contains chiefly the 18β form and has a structure and

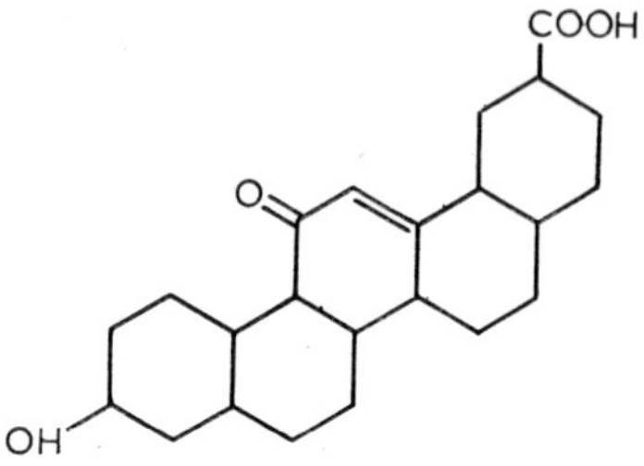

glycyrrhetinic acid

configuration reminiscent of hydrocortisone, though it has no gluco-corticoid activity. Finney and Somers (1958) have shown that glycyrrhetinic acid has an anti-inflammatory action by the three main tests described above (p. 262). The disodium salt of glycyrrhetinic acid hydrogen succinate is soluble in water (unlike the parent compound) and may thus be more suitable for clinical use. It has some effect on the water and mineral metabolism in rats but not in cats (Finney and Tarnoky, 1960). There are reports on the use of glycyrrhetinic acid in the treatment of various skin conditions (Colin-Jones and Somers, 1957; Quentin Evans, 1958). When administered systemically in man it can produce water retention and oedema.

Iproniazid

Experimental tests in rats show that iproniazid has a definite anti-inflammatory action which does not occur in adrenalectomized animals (Setnikar, Salvaterra and Temelcov, 1959). There are preliminary reports of the action of this drug in rheumatic conditions, but more evidence is needed.

ALDOSTERONE

A large amount of work has been done on this in the last few years; it has been reviewed by Ross (1959) and in the Ciba Symposium on Aldosterone (1958) and only some of the main findings will be discussed here. This steroid appears to be specifically secreted by the zona glomerulosa of the adrenal cortex and its production, unlike that of the other adrenal steroids, is to a large extent not under the control of the anterior pituitary and of corticotrophin. The zona glomerulosa may thus be considered as a separate endocrine structure, functionally as well as anatomically distinct from the inner zones of the adrenal cortex (Farrell, 1959).

The biological actions of aldosterone cause a rise in Na and a fall in K in the extracellular fluid. There is a retention of Na and excretion of K by the kidney and a fall in the Na^+/K^+ ratio of saliva and faeces. In acute experiments it has been reported to cause a rise in the K^+ (intra-cellular fluid)/K^+ (extracellular fluid) ratios in muscle and brain, though

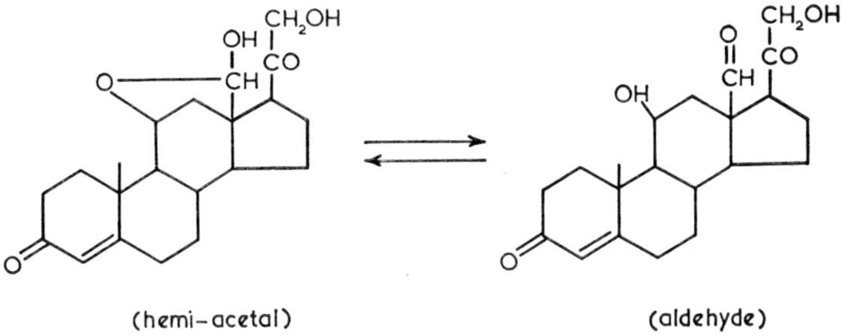

(hemi–acetal)   (aldehyde)

aldosterone

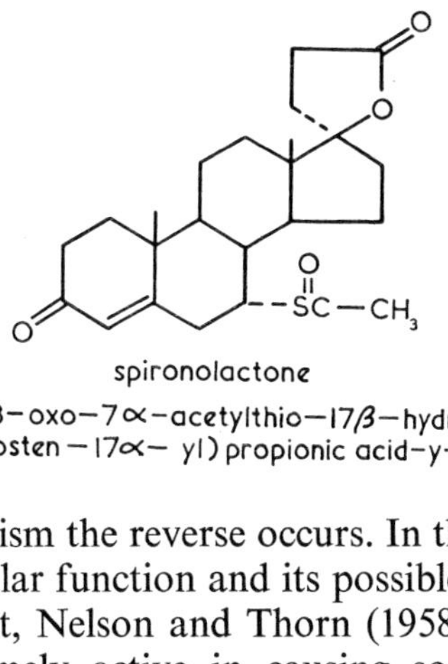

spironolactone
3—(3—oxo—7α—acetylthio—17β—hydroxy—4—
androsten—17α— yl) propionic acid—y—lactone

in primary aldosteronism the reverse occurs. In the kidney, aldosterone appears to affect tubular function and its possible mechanism of action is reviewed by August, Nelson and Thorn (1958) (see also chapter 7). Aldosterone is extremely active in causing sodium retention. Thus Wright and his co-workers (Coglan et al., 1960) in their review on aldo-sterone, refer to the finding of Desaulles who showed that aldosterone was 2,000 times as effective as corticosterone in causing urinary sodium retention and to their own work demonstrating that, when given intra-muscularly, aldosterone is 40 times as active as deoxycorticosterone acetate.

In doses of the order of 250 µg. per day aldosterone will maintain patients with Addison's disease. It is best given by the intramuscular route though effects have also been observed when it is given orally and intravenously. In doses of 1 mg. per day it has very little glucocorticoid activity (Hetzel *et al.*, 1956; Ledingham *et al.*, 1961).

CONTROL OF ALDOSTERONE SECRETION

There is good evidence that the secretion of aldosterone is in some ways regulated by the volume of the body fluids, possibly the extra-cellular fluid volume. According to Farrell (1958), however, the most important stimulus to aldosterone production appears to be sodium intake. Bartter *et al.* (1959) have also provided evidence that potassium concentration may affect aldosterone secretion, independently of the effect on intravascular volume. Thus potassium loading constantly leads to increase of aldosterone secretion and potassium deprivation to decrease. The problem of the relative importance of body fluid and electrolytes in controlling aldosterone secretion remains to be settled. The possible mechanism by which fluid volume controls aldosterone secretion is discussed by Farrell (1958, 1959). He describes experiments in which, in open chest surgery in dogs, sutures were placed on the right atrium and gentle traction was applied to the atrial wall. The secretion of aldosterone was thereby depressed to about one half within an hour. Stretching of the left atrium was without effect. These results suggest that stretch receptors located in the right atrium reflexly inhibit aldo-sterone output, although the participation of similar receptors in the neighbouring veins cannot be excluded; reduced atrium volume, on the other hand, would reduce aldosterone output as a result of removal of this tonic inhibition. Thus changes in body fluid volume or in the volume of extracellular fluid could be detected as changes in right atrial volume. The observations of Davis (1957) that constriction of the inferior vena cava leads to increased aldosterone secretion may be explained, at least in part, by the effect of caval constriction on venous return and atrial volume.

Receptors for the control of aldosterone secretion are also present in the common carotid artery, since it has been shown (Bartter *et al.*, 1959) that constriction of the common carotid artery leads to increase of aldosterone secretion, but does not do so after the carotid arteries have been partially deprived of their nerve supply.

Farrell has also produced evidence which suggests that aldosterone output is controlled by an area of the brain stem which acts by releasing a specific trophic hormone. It was first shown that removal of the head of an experimental animal, the trunk being maintained normal with respect to respiration, temperature and blood pressure, rapidly leads to a decline of aldosterone output to very low values. Next, by producing lesions in various parts of the brain, it was shown that the central grey substance of the anterior midbrain probably contains centres important in regulating aldosterone secretion and that destruction of this area markedly decreases aldosterone output. There was thus presumptive evidence that a humoral factor is concerned in aldosterone secretion and Farrell has named this *glomerulotropin*, implying that the zona glomerulosa of the adrenal cortex is the target organ. The name corticotrophin (or ACTH) is reserved for the substance which stimulates the inner zones of the adrenal to secrete cortisol and related substances (though some of these substances are probably also secreted in the zona glomerulosa). Neutral saline extracts of diencephalic tissue, prepared in the cold, are entirely free of corticotrophin activity but are quite active in stimulating aldosterone output. Further investigations showed that glomerulotropin is essentially present in the pineal-posterior commisure area, which contains about 10 times as much activity as the remaining posterior diencephalon. Corticotrophin does increase aldosterone secretion in man but the effect is self limiting, even if the administration of corticotrophin is continued (Bartter *et al.*, 1959). There is, in addition, evidence that an aldosterone-stimulating hormone is produced by the kidney (Davis *et al.*, 1961).

ALDOSTERONISM
This has been divided into primary (Conn's disease) where there is adenoma, carcinoma or hyperplasia of the adrenal cortex, and secondary, where the mechanisms affecting aldosterone secretion are abnormal (Ayres *et al.*, 1958; Ross, 1959). In both conditions there is probably an abnormally high secretion of aldosterone, though this varies greatly from case to case.

In primary aldosteronism, first described by Conn in 1955 there are recurrent episodes of muscular weakness associated with hypochloraemia, hypokalaemia and alkalosis, hypertension, polyuria resistant to vasopressin and in some cases tetany in the presence of normal serum calcium and phosphorus. The absence of oedema is noteworthy. An interesting feature is that aldosterone secretion by the non-tumorous adrenal tissue is markedly inhibited by an aldosterone-secreting tumour, an effect which may persist for a long time after removal of the tumour. Hence it is important that the capacity of these surgically treated cases to withstand sodium depletion should be determined.

Secondary aldosteronism can be associated with various oedematous states (e.g. congestive heart failure, nephrosis, cirrhosis) or induced by excessive fluid loss (e.g. untreated diabetes, salt losing nephritis, excessive diuretic action). In this condition there is much less displacement of intracellular potassium by sodium and the plasma potassium is usually normal. It is possible, as Ayres *et al.* (1958) suggest, that secondary aldosteronism is merely the result of sodium retention and not essential for the actual production of oedema.

Hypoaldosteronism has been described as a condition in which there is deficient secretion of aldosterone, with normal secretion of other adrenocortical hormones (Hudson *et al.*, 1957).

RELATION OF ALDOSTERONE TO OEDEMA (see also chapter 7, p. 230)

This was reviewed by Robson and Keele (1956) and it was then stressed that though there is increased aldosterone excretion in oedema

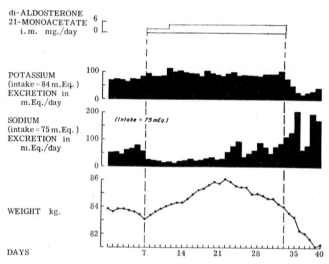

FIG. 40. Effect of aldosterone on weight and sodium and potassium excretion in normal subject receiving a constant diet. An escape from sodium retention occurred on the 16th day of aldosterone administration. (August *et al.*, 1958.)

associated with nephrosis, cardiac failure and cirrhosis, these changes in excretion are not aetiological factors, but are merely secondary phenomena. This is supported by the finding that in patients with primary aldosteronism there is no oedema, unless other factors are present, e.g. an adrenal tumour (see Goldsmith *et al.*, 1958). Moreover it has been shown that the administration of large doses of aldosterone (up to 6 mg. per day) in normal subjects does not produce oedema. There is initially a period of weight gain and sodium retention, but these then return to the normal level despite the continued administration of aldosterone; increased potassium excretion occurs throughout the period of therapy (August, Nelson and Thorn, 1958; see Fig. 40). The injection of large doses of aldosterone into adrenalectomized dogs (1 mg. per day which is 20 times the maintenance dose) similarly does not lead to the development of oedema (Gross and Lichtlen, 1958). The subject is well reviewed by Lieberman (1958) who points out that enhanced tubular reabsorption appears to be primarily responsible for the sodium retention in oedematous patients with disease of the heart, liver and kidney and that such patients appear to be more sensitive than normal subjects to the sodium retaining effect of adrenal hormones. For example, Nelson and August (1959) found that when aldosterone was administered to oedematous patients the sodium retention was more complete—there was moreover no secondary 'escape' from the renal sodium-retaining effect of the steroid as there is in normal subjects. Though the reason for this is unknown, it does suggest that aldosterone is one of the factors responsible for the maintenance of oedema; moreover, it is also not clear why increased secretion of this hormone should be evoked in diseases of the heart, liver and kidney. At the same time it is obvious that other mechanisms besides aldosterone must contribute to the formation of oedema in such patients and they require further study. One point of practical interest mentioned in Lieberman's review is that change from the recumbent to the standing position in a normal subject is followed by increased output of aldosterone and that the oedematous subject appears to be more sensitive to a similar alteration in position (see Fig. 41). This must contribute markedly to the value of bed rest in the treatment of oedema. The mechanisms and management of oedema are extensively discussed in a book on the subject (Moyer and Fuchs, 1960).

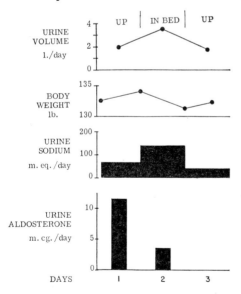

FIG. 41. Effect of position on aldosterone excretion in a patient with idiopathic hypoproteinemia and oedema. Note decrease in aldosterone output associated with increase of output of sodium and water when the patient was put to bed (Lieberman, 1958).

ALDOSTERONE IN FAMILIAL PARALYSIS

The evidence is reviewed by Ross (1959). According to Conn and his co-workers an attack is initiated by a tremendous increase in the excretion of aldosterone in the urine, resulting in a retention of sodium lasting throughout the period of paralysis. This retention of sodium is followed by sequestration of potassium within the cells, both serum and urinary potassium concentration dropping abruptly. The urinary excretion of sodium then increases, the serum potassium concentration rises and the attack subsides. Conn thus considers that retention of sodium is the primary factor which sets into motion the characteristic chain of events in the attack of paralysis and that an abnormally high concentration of sodium within the muscle cell is partly responsible for the disturbance of muscle function. A more recent study by Jones *et al.* (1959) has shown that sodium retention and increased excretion of aldosterone do not necessarily precede attacks of periodic paralysis in all cases, and the question thus remains open.

Spironolactone (formula p. 269)

It has been suggested that aldosterone may be aetiologically significant in salt and water retention in congestive heart failure, nephrosis, liver cirrhosis and toxaemia of pregnancy (Gaunt *et al.*, 1955). Hence aldosterone antagonists might be of value in the treatment of such conditions. In 1955 Landau *et al.* (1955) demonstrated that large doses of progesterone increased the excretion of sodium in man, presumably due to antagonism of aldosterone. Subsequently Landau and Lugibihl (1958) demonstrated the naturetic effect of progesterone in a woman with Addison's disease treated with aldosterone and cortisone. After the aldosterone had been discontinued, progesterone no longer had any effect on sodium excretion. More interesting still were the results with spirolactosteroids first described by Kagawa *et al.* (1957) and by Liddle (1957) on the diuretic effect of such compounds in animals and man. They are believed to antagonize the action of aldosterone, of deoxycorticosterone and of related compounds by promoting the excretion of salt and water by the renal tubules.

The most active of these compounds has been given the generic name of spironolactone and is chemically 3-(3-oxo-7α-acetylthio-17β-hydroxy-4-androsten-17α-yl) propionic acid-7-lactone (see p. 269). Its pharmacological properties are described by Kagawa *et al.* (1959) and by Streeten (1961). The drug has no cortisone-like, androgenic, anabolic or oestrogenic activity. Its use in the treatment of oedema and ascites is described in chapter 7, p. 254.

METABOLISM OF CORTICOSTEROIDS

This is an extensive subject which will be dealt with briefly with particular reference to diagnosis and treatment. Of the many steroids isolated from the adrenal cortex, two are of chief importance in man, i.e. hydrocortisone (cortisol) and aldosterone; corticosterone is the main glucocorticoid produced in some other species, e.g. rodents, but only small quantities are produced in humans. Many of the findings described here are taken from the excellent review by Peterson (1959).

In normal subjects the plasma level of cortisol varies within the limits of 5–25 µg. % and of aldosterone between the limits of 0·03–0·08 µg. % More than 95% of the cortisol circulates bound to plasma protein (called 'transcortin') which appears to be part of the α-globulin fraction. At physiological concentrations of cortisol this protein appears to be almost completely saturated, and at concentrations above the normal there is binding to serum albumin with which 70–80% of the steroid is protein bound. The protein binding affects the distribution, transport and excretion of the cortisol and it has been found that its concentration in the extracellular fluids is lower than in the plasma. Aldosterone appears to be bound by serum albumin, and 70–80% of this steroid is bound. Plasma binding probably plays a part in limiting the metabolism and excretion of the steroids.

Table 16 gives some indication of the rate of elimination of the main steroids produced by the adrenal cortex and used clinically and shows that there are quite marked differences between these various substances. There appears to be no significant localization of the steroids in the

Table 16

Biological half times of plasma steroids
(Peterson, 1959.)

	Normal	Cirrhosis	Thyrotoxicosis
Cortisol	110 (80)	300	60
Cortisone	30	35	12
Aldosterone	(50)	(80)	—
Prednisone	60	—	—
Prednisolone	200	240	—
9α-Fluorocortisol	90	95	—
9α-Fluoroprednisolone	100	100	—
Dexamethasone	200	—	—

All figures are in minutes and refer to therapeutic doses, except those in brackets which were obtained after the infusion of a trace dose. Figures within each group (normal, cirrhosis, thyrotoxicosis) represent the results of studies on a single subject.

tissues or storage depots (other than the plasma proteins) and thus they are not well protected from rapid metabolic transformation by the liver. It is obvious from the figures in Table 16 that the much higher activity of the newer corticosteroids is not due to a much slower elimination from the plasma, a conclusion also arrived at by Nugent *et al.* (1959) from their study of the elimination of hydrocortisone and prednisolone in man.

The rate of metabolism of cortisol is delayed in liver disease, myxoedema, pregnancy, old age and starvation. Oestrogen and prolonged salicylate therapy also produce a delay in the disappearance of infused cortisol (Peterson *et al.*, 1960). The metabolism of cortisol is increased in thyrotoxicosis and in some patients with spontaneous hypoglycemia. The role of the liver in the metabolism of corticosteroids is discussed by Streeten (1959). The rate of cortisol and corticosterone secretion has also been found to be decreased in patients with myxoedema and cirrhosis and after oestrogen and long term salicylate therapy, and increased in patients with thyrotoxicosis. The use of drugs which inhibit aldosterone secretion is described in chapter 7, p. 253. (See also Peterson *et al.*, 1957; Jenkins *et al.*, 1959.)

NEW PROGESTOGENS

Progesterone is the hormone produced by the corpus luteum and, during pregnancy, by the human placenta and has been used clinically for a number of years. The only other progestogen given in the British Pharmacopoeia (1958) is ethisterone which is active by oral administration, though not very potent. A large number of new compounds have been made recently, some of which are more active than the natural hormone even when given orally. Clinical results with progesterone (and ethisterone) have, on the whole, been disappointing and it may be that the newer compounds will be better. They are reviewed in the Annals of the New York Academy of Sciences (1958, **71,** 479) and by Drill (1959).

Two main groups of compounds have been made, namely (1) derivatives of progesterone itself, and (2) derivatives of 19-nortestosterone (so called since it lacks the angular methyl group at carbon-19). A list of the newer progestogens is given by Pincus (1959). It is to be noted that some of the new compounds also possess oestrogenic, androgenic and anabolic activities and that the suitability of a substance as a progestogen depends not only on its activity as such, but also on the other actions it may have. Some of the compounds are potent inhibitors of the pituitary and will inhibit ovulation. They have thus been used in the control of fertility and this will be considered separately.

A further point needs consideration, and has important clinical implications. Progestogens are usually assayed by their ability to produce a typical reaction (progestational proliferation) in the endometrium of the rabbit and also by their ability to increase the carbonic anhydrase content of the endometrium (Adams and Ludwak-Mann, 1955). Yet a compound may be highly active by the progestational test and nevertheless not be able to maintain pregnancy in the ovariectomized rabbit. This is illustrated in Table 17, obtained from the data of Saunders and Drill (1958).

PROGESTOGENS

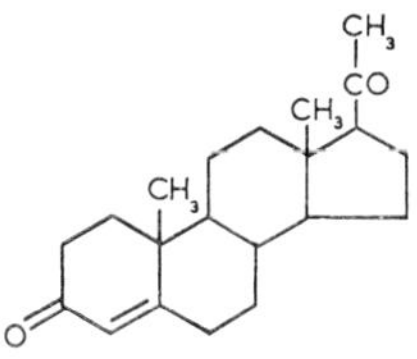

progesterone

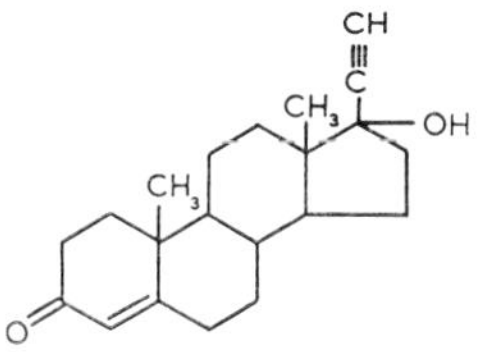

ethisterone

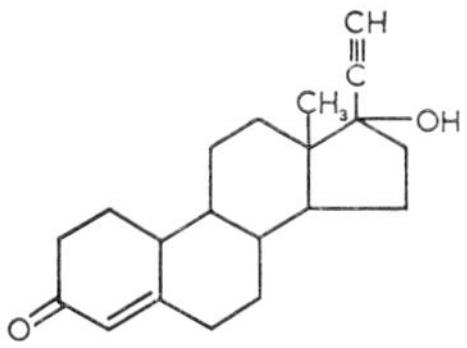

17∝–ethinyl–19–nortestosterone
(norethindrone, Norlutin)

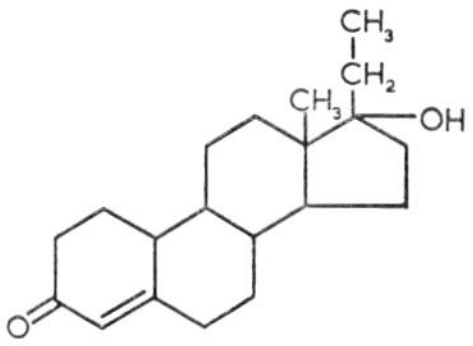

17∝–ethyl–19–nortestosterone
(norethandrolone, Nilevar)

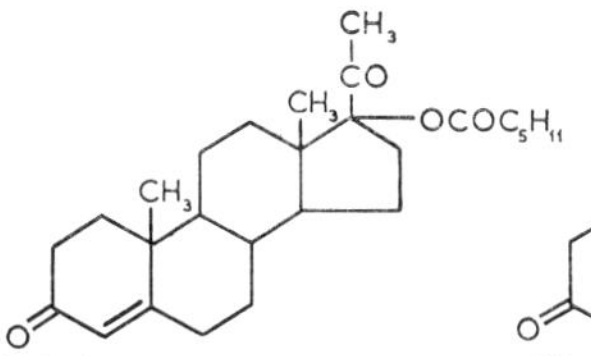

17∝–hydroxyprogesterone
(Delalutin) caproate

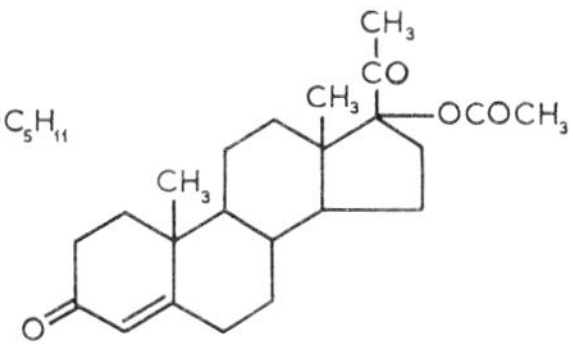

17∝–hydroxyprogesterone acetate
(Prodox)

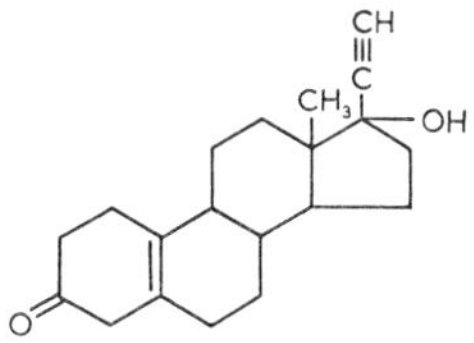

17∝–ethinyl–5 (10)–oestraenolone
(norethynodrel)

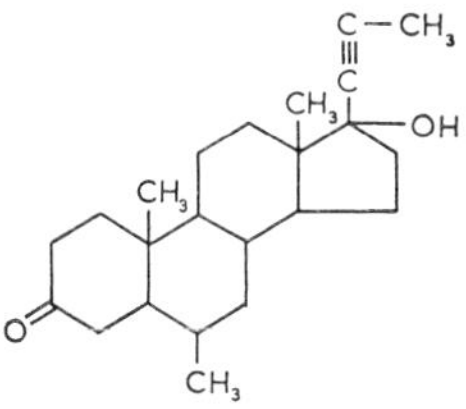

6∝ : 21–dimethylethisterone
(dimethisterone, Secrosteron)

The formulae of the main compounds, together with those of progesterone and ethisterone, are given above. The main derivatives of
progesterone are esters, i.e. the caproate ('Delalutin') and the acetate
('Prodox') of hydroxyprogesterone; the acetate and caproate of hydroxyprogesterone with a methyl group in the 6α position (medroxyprogesterone) are also being investigated, as is 6α:21-dimethylethisterone
(Dimethisterone, 'Secrosteron') (David *et al.*, 1959). Of the 19-nortesto-
sterones, that with an ethinyl group in the 17α position (norethisterone,

10

Table 17

Maintenance of pregnancy in rabbits

Compound	Number of rabbits in which pregnancy was maintained
None	0/10
Progesterone	16/18
19-Nortestosterone	0/6
17-Ethyl-19-nortestosterone	9/14
17-Ethyl-19-nortestosterone (oral)	0/5
Norethynodrel	0/7
Norethynodrel (oral)	0/9

Rabbits were ovariectomized on the 10th day of pregnancy and treated with 1 mg. steroid/kg./day (by injection unless otherwise stated) until necropsy 7 days later (data from Saunders and Drill, 1958).

norethindrone, 'Norlutin') is the most interesting. It has a low oestrogenic activity when given orally, and practically no androgenic action (McGinty and Djerassi, 1958). The enanthoate of ethyl nortestosterone is also being investigated. Norethandrolone (i.e. ethyl nortestosterone, 'Nilevar') is used essentially as an anabolic agent (see later).

Lastly norethynodrel must be mentioned since it has been used extensively in the control of fertility but not essentially as a progestogen. It can be regarded as an oestrane derivative (17α-ethinyl-5(10)-oestraenolone) and has indeed some oestrogenic activity, which may account for its failure to maintain pregnancy in ovariectomized rabbits. 'Enavid' is norethynodrel fortified with 1·5% of ethinyloestradiol-3-methyl ether, to enhance its pituitary inhibiting activity. Pincus *et al.* (1956) have studied the activity of some of these compounds in animals and some of their results are given in Table 18. It is noteworthy that ethinyl (and methyl) nortestosterone is about 10 times as active as progesterone when the typical progestational change in the rabbit's endometrium is taken as criterion; its relative activity to progesterone is much

Table 18

Relation between the capacity of various progestogens to produce endometrial proliferation and to sustain implantation in the rabbit

(Pincus *et al.*, 1956)

	Progestational proliferation	Implantation sustaining dose
	mg.	mg.
Progesterone	1–2	0·5–1·5
Ethinyl nortestosterone	0·1–0·2	0·25*
Norethynodrel	2–4	>2·0
Methylnortestosterone	0·1+	Not studied

*Less active at higher doses.

less striking when the capacity to maintain pregnancy is measured; moreover, increasing the dose of ethinyl nortestosterone makes it even less effective in this respect. Pincus (1959) has found that two compounds, namely medroxyprogesterone and 17a-(2-methallyl)-19-nortestosterone, are more than 10 times as active as norethisterone on the rabbit's endometrium. The latter compound is particularly interesting, since it is highly active when applied locally to the rabbit endometrium (i.e. it is a true progestogen) and will also maintain pregnancy in the ovariectomized rabbit (Elton and Edgren, 1958). Nevertheless, neither of these compounds has apparently any progestational effect on the human endometrium (Pincus, 1959). This may be due to species differences, as previously observed in relation to progestational effects by Robson and Sharaf (1951).

Hydroxyprogesterone caproate has to be given by intramuscular injection and is then a long acting potent progestogen. The latent period between injection of this preparation (250–500 mg.) and withdrawal bleeding is 10–14 days, i.e. 2–3 times longer than after injection of progesterone (Gold and Cohen, 1958). The other compounds are given orally. Hydroxyprogesterone acetate is several times more active than ethisterone when given orally, and a daily dose of the acetate of 100 mg. will produce a secretory endometrium (Wied and Davis, 1958). Swyer et al. (1960) have tried to determine the relative oral activity of some of these compounds in women, by their ability to delay normal menstruation. They found that norethisterone and 'Enavid' were about equally active, while dimethisterone and methallyl-19-nortestosterone had a very low activity by this criterion.

Effects in the male
Heller et al. (1958) investigated the effect of four progestogens in man (19 subjects), namely progesterone, norethisterone, ethyl nortestosterone and 'Enavid' (which contains some oestrogen). All four produced a reversible stage of azoospermia. Testicular biopsy at this stage showed damage compatible with azoospermia in the norethisterone and 'Enavid' groups, but in the other two there was, inexplicably, moderately active spermatogenesis. All subjects suffered complete loss of libido. Norethynodrel (i.e. 'Enavid' without the added ethinyloestradiol-3-methyl ether) also produced azoospermia with the appropriate testicular morphology (Heller et al., 1959).

Clinical use
Three of the new progestogens are given in New and Nonofficial Drugs for 1961, namely hydroxyprogesterone caproate ('Delalutin') for intramuscular administration, and medroxyprogesterone acetate ('Provera') and norethindrone (norethisterone 'Norlutin') for oral

administration. Dimethisterone ('Secrosteron') and hydroxyprogesterone acetate ('Prodox') probably also deserves to be put in the same
group of progestogens suitable for clinical use.

It is much too early to try to assess the clinical value of these compounds in the treatment of various menstrual disorders and in pregnancy. A preliminary assessment is made by Rakoff (1959) whilst Bishop
and Cabral de Almeida (1960) give some results with dimethisterone.
There has been some evidence that the administration of progestogens
during pregnancy may produce masculinizing effects on the foetus
(Rakoff, 1959; Grumbach *et al.*, 1959) and presumably the more active
new compounds will be more liable to produce this effect. It has indeed
been suggested that any new progestogen should be tested experimentally in pregnant animals for this action, before being used in therapeutics
(Revesz *et al.*, 1960; Schöler and Wachter, 1961). Prolonged administration of norethindrone and of 'Enavid' may also lead to extreme stromal
hypertrophy of the endometrium (Dockerty *et al.*, 1959). It is obvious
that patients on the new potent substances will have to be carefully
observed for possible deleterious effects.

THE CONTROL OF FERTILITY BY DRUGS

There has been much interest in recent years in the possibility of
controlling fertility by using drugs administered systemically. Since the
most spectacular results have been achieved by the use of steroids, this
is a suitable place in which to review recent work on the subject. Detailed
discussions are given by Jackson (1959) and Pincus (1959), while Baker
(1960) reviews the effects of drugs on the foetus.

Fertility can be modified by treatment either of the male or the
female, but the results in the former have, until recently, not been
encouraging. In fact, Jackson (1959) concluded that 'control of human
male fertility offers little prospect of success at the present time.' It is a
measure of the rate of progress in pharmacological research, that striking
results on the control of spermatogenesis were published the following
year.

CONTROL IN THE MALE

Coulston, Beyler and Drobeck (1960) have investigated the biological
effects of a new series of bis (dichloracetyl) diamines, which have been
prepared by Surrey and his co-workers. Three compounds in particular
have been studied, namely Win 13,099, Win 17,416 and Win 18,446 (see
formulae on p. 281) and all three have a low toxicity in animal studies.

All three compounds produce remarkably specific effects on the testes
(rats, dogs and monkeys) characterized by arrest of spermatogenesis,
which is completely reversible within a few weeks of withdrawal of the
drug. The Leydig, Sertoli and spermatogonal cells appear to be normal

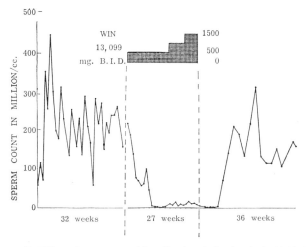

even under the full influence of these drugs. Win 18,446 is the most active and Win 17,416 the least active of the three. There is strong evidence that neither pituitary nor testicular hormonal functions are modified by these drugs (Beyler *et al.*, 1961) and hence that the effect is exerted directly on the testicular cells. It is interesting that the ovaries and uterus of female rats receiving large doses of Win 13,099 for many weeks were normal, as were the sex accessory glands of male rats so treated. Of further interest is the finding that Win 13,099 and Win 17,416 are potent amoebicidal agents, whereas Win 18,446 is devoid of such action.

These drugs were also administered to human volunteers and produced striking inhibition of spermatogenesis as shown by examination of the semen and by testicular biopsies; sperm motility was depressed and sperm morphology was altered to an extraordinary degree (Heller, Moore and Paulsen, 1961, see Fig. 42); again Win 17,416 was less active than the other two compounds. There is evidence too that the effect on spermatogenesis is reversible after discontinuation of the drugs.

FIG. 42. Effect of treatment with a diamine derivative (Win 13,099) on spermatogenesis in man (Heller *et al.*, 1961).

The drugs did not affect sexual libido or potency and there was no decrease in the excretion of gonadotrophin. Two of the compounds (Win 13,099 and Win 18,446) produced some gastric disturbances and one (Win 18,446) produced some effect on the blood and on the sedimentation rate which requires further investigation.

CONTROL IN THE FEMALE

It is in the female that the most striking results have been obtained and there appears to be the prospect that even better methods will be developed in the next decade. This applies particularly to the inhibition of fertility. This can theoretically be achieved in a number of ways, namely:

  (a) Inhibition of ovogenesis and particularly ovulation.
  (b) Effects on the sperm in the female genital tract before fertilization, including inhibition of fertilization.
  (c) (i) Toxic effects on the fertilized ovum at or before implantation.
      (ii) Inhibition of implantation.
  (d) Interruption of established pregnancy.

The inhibition of ovulation

It has long been known that ovulation does not usually occur during pregnancy and that progesterone is concerned in this effect. Progesterone can inhibit ovulation in many species of animals (Jackson, 1959). Pincus first showed in 1956 that oral administration of large doses of progesterone (300 mg. per day) from the 5th to the 28th day of the cycle inhibited ovulation in a high proportion of women and no pregnancies occurred, although sexual intercourse was practised freely. Progesterone, however, is unsatisfactory because of the large doses necessary and of the high frequency of premature menstruation, even when oestrogen is also given (see Pincus, 1959). The discovery of new and potent oral progestogens has made it possible to investigate this approach with a greater possibility of success.

Pincus and his co-workers (see Pincus, 1959) studied the effects of three new compounds on the menstrual cycle of regularly ovulating women, namely norethindrone, norethynodrel and norethandrolone. All three compounds at the level of 10 mg. per day were highly effective. In a series of laparotomies performed on patients receiving norethindrone, no newly formed corpora lutea were found. Pincus (1959) quotes similar results obtained at laparotomy by Matsumoto on women who received cyclical treatment with norethynodrel. Bleeding during treatment was infrequent with norethindrone and norethynodrel, but not unusual with norethandrolone. If oestrogen was added to the progestogen treatment, bleeding during treatment became much less common and of three oestrogens studied, ethinyloestradiol-3-methyl ether was more effective than either stilboestrol or allenolic acid. Pincus and his co-workers also carefully studied endometrial biopsies in these experimental subjects and found that all three compounds rapidly stimulate a progestational response but that after 7–9 days of medication the response of the endometrial glands fails whilst the stromal cells continue to be stimulated so that by the last day of treatment a predecidual state is usually attained.

Contraceptive trials

In view of these results it seemed likely that contraception could be achieved through the inhibition of ovulation by these steroids, though it is not clear yet whether the effect on the endometrium contributes to the prevention of conception. It should be noted that during such treatment the basic ovogenetic processes appear to continue unhindered, only the formation of large follicles and corpora lutea being inhibited (see Pincus, 1959). To maintain menstrual cycles of normal length it is necessary to supplement the progestogen treatment with a small amount of oestrogen. Trials were therefore initiated in Puerto Rico with 'Enavid' (i.e. norethynodrel with addition of ethinyloestradiol methyl ether), and subsequently in other places. The drug (10 mg. per day) is usually given from the 5th day after menstruation for 20 days. A combination of 5 mg. norethynodrel with 0·075 mg. ethinyl oestradiol methyl ether, i.e. half the doses present in 'Enavid' is also available under the name 'Conovid'. There is no doubt that such medication is highly effective in preventing conception though if the dose is further decreased the contraceptive effect fails (Eckstein *et al.*, 1961; Mears, 1961). According to Pincus (1959) 'faithful daily tablet-taking according to the prescribed regime gives a 99·8% chance of protection against conception.' Tyler and Olson (1959) have obtained similar results both with 'Enavid' and with norethindrone. What still remains to be decided accurately is the liability to side effects and the possible long-term effects of such medication.

Among the side effects observed are menstrual bleeding during treatment, nausea, vomiting and dizziness. According to Tyler and Olson (1959) 37% of a large group of patients discontinued the treatment because of the side effects. In the studies of Pincus and his co-workers side effects were much less common and were often psychogenic in origin, being frequently reported in patients receiving a placebo. Banks *et al.* (1959) report that all their patients on 'Enavid' complained of some tenderness of the breasts. There have been a few reports of toxic effects on the liver (transient jaundice) with high doses of nor steroids, but Pincus (1959) performed liver function tests on patients receiving steroids for contraception and did not observe any abnormalities. There is general agreement that quite a high proportion of patients discontinue this type of contraception and in fact Pincus *et al.* (1959) emphasize this and also that alternative methods of oral contraception are desirable.

The other important question is whether prolonged cyclical medication with these steroids will produce any delayed effects. Prolongation of cycles and amenorrhoea do occur after cessation of treatment (Tyler and Olson, 1959) but Pincus (1959) states that regular menstruation can usually be re-established by a further 20-day course of medication. He has also found no pathological changes in the reproductive tract on pelvic examination, in endometrial biopsies or in vaginal smears taken from time to time during the course of medication over a 30 month period. Nevertheless, the possibility that long term toxic effects of steroid contraception may occur must be borne in mind, and carefully investigated.

Increasing fertility with the newer progestogens

The ovum becomes implanted in a secretory endometrium under the influence of the corpus luteum hormone. It is a possibility that infertility may be due to insufficient progestogen secretion and that it may be cured by progestogen therapy administered during the postovulatory phase of the cycle to supplement intrinsic hormone production. Such experiments are described by Tyler and Olson (1959) and by Banks *et al.* (1959) but their significance is difficult to evaluate and much more work will have to be done before it will be possible to decide whether such therapy can promote fertility.

OTHER SYSTEMIC METHODS OF PREVENTING FERTILITY IN THE FEMALE

These are essentially in the experimental stage and none have been investigated clinically on the scale of the newer steroids. Nevertheless, very interesting results have been obtained in animals and these will be briefly discussed.

A substance acting on the fertilized ovum

This substance was investigated in the Merrell Laboratories in Cincinnati and called MER-25 (ethamoxytriphetol). It is a triphenyl ethanol derivative, namely 1-(p-2-diethylaminoethoxyphenyl)-1-phenyl-2-p-methoxyphenyl ethanol, and was shown to antagonize various actions of oestrogens (Lerner *et al.*, 1958). Subsequently Segal and Nelson (1958) showed that it could prevent pregnancy when administered orally to female rats during the first four days after mating, i.e. during the period when the ova are passing through the oviduct. The compound does not act by preventing decidual development or by interfering with the maintenance of luteal function, but there is evidence that it produces degradation of the developing ova after extrusion of the second polar body, either by a direct cytotoxic action or possibly by producing an effect on the maternal duct system which will prevent it supporting normal zygotic development. Chang (1959) confirmed these results both in rats and rabbits. The therapeutic index of the compound in the rabbit was, however, low since 25 mg./kg. gave an inconsistent effect on the ovum and 50 mg./kg. for four days killed some of the treated animals.

A further interesting compound now being investigated is chlorami-phene (1-[p-(β-diethylamino-ethoxy)phenyl]-1,2-diphenyl-2-chloroethy-lene), which can interrupt the oestrous cycle and produce loss of fecundity when administered to female rats (Holtkamp et al., 1960). The last effect is still produced by doses which do not prevent ovulation and fertilization (Segal and Nelson, 1961).

It is remarkable that both chloramiphene and ethanoxytriphetol can *induce ovulation* in women, according to preliminary reports by Greenblatt et al. (1961) and Kistner and Smith (1961). Further investigation of this unexpected finding is required.

Antimetabolites and nucleotoxic substances

A large number of these have been investigated and are discussed in the review by Jackson (1959). A number of these substances are also discussed by Thiersch (1956) who has done very interesting work in this field. The problem of using these substances is rather similar to that involved in cancer chemotherapy, with two important differences, namely (1) that in malignant disease all the cells have to be destroyed whereas in the control of conception a lethal effect on a small percentage of the cells may be adequate to prevent subsequent development of the foetus, (2) on the other hand, toxic effects on the conceptus may lead to developmental abnormalities if death of the foetus does not occur, which is thus a serious hazard. It is indeed this possibility which led to the abandonment of clinical work with aminopterin (Thiersch, 1952). Another difficulty with many of these drugs is that even though they will destroy the foetus, the placenta frequently survives. Robson (1959) has divided these drugs under three headings, namely (1) spindle poisons, (2) chromosomal poisons, and (3) antimetabolites, which include some drugs the mechanism of whose action has not been particularly well studied.

The *spindle poisons* were first studied because of their known effect on tumour growth. This suggests that they will also have an effect on the rapidly growing conceptus (Didcock et al., 1952, 1956). These drugs are most effective in established pregnancy (in mice and rabbits) and seem to have little effect before implantation. Of the substances tested, viz. podophyllotoxin, colchicine, trimethyl colchicinic acid methyl ether and colcemid, the last one seems to be most effective. Thiersch (1958) found that repeated destruction of the litter in rats with N-desacetyl thio colchicine did not impair fertility or reproduction in these animals, nor cause abnormalities in subsequent offspring.

The *chromosomal poisons* investigated include mustine (nitrogen mustard), chlorambucil, triethylene melamine, triethylene phosphoramide and busulphan (Myleran). On the whole these drugs are not highly effective, though they will act at various stages of pregnancy. Thus for example, Robson (1959) found that busulphan was equally effective at all stages of pregnancy in mice, though the effective dose was nearly half the L.D.50.

Among the large number of *antimetabolites* investigated, the most interesting results have been obtained with DON (6-diazo-5-oxo-L-norleucine) and with azaserine (O-diazoacetyl-L-serine) (Murphy and Karnofsky, 1956). The effects of DON have been investigated in mice, rats and rabbits (Thiersch, 1957; Jackson *et al.*, 1959). In the mouse the drug will interrupt pregnancy at all stages, the effective dose being only a small fraction of the L.D.50; rabbits were rather more resistant and required a dose of 20 mg./kg. as compared with 2 mg./kg. in mice. Large doses of adenine sulphate tend to inhibit the effect of DON on the rat embryo, thus suggesting that DON produces its effect by inhibiting the synthesis of purine bases. The intra-amniotic injection of DON into pregnant rabbits kills the foetus but leaves the placenta intact and the evidence suggests that the drug acts directly on the developing embryo. It has not been established, however, whether this is also the site of action when DON is administered before implantation.

Miscellaneous Compounds

It is well known that *methyl cholanthrene* produces inhibition of growth (Haddow and Robinson, 1937) and this led to its investigation in pregnancy. It is highly effective when given at the time of implantation in mice but less active in the later stages of pregnancy. A large dose is needed to interrupt gestation when the drug is injected directly into the amniotic fluid in rabbits; the placenta as usual remains unaffected (Jackson and Robson, 1958).

The nitrofuran derivative *furazolidone* has a depressant effect on normal and malignant growth and has been used in the treatment of testicular tumours. This drug too proved more effective in preventing or interrupting gestation at or before conception than at later periods and was also effective when injected directly into the amniotic fluid in rabbits (Jackson and Robson, 1957). Further work on nitrofuran derivatives seems desirable.

There have been a number of claims, particularly by Sanyal, that *2,6-dimethylhydroquinone* (m-xylohydroquinone), which is naturally present in an oil extracted from the field pea (*Pisum sativum*), can cause sterility in animals and in women, but other workers have failed to confirm this (see review by Jackson, 1959). For example, Thiersch (1956) gave this substance to mature female rats and completely failed to prevent implantation or affect the foetus. He is also sceptical of the results in women reported by Sanyal.

The very interesting findings of Shelesnyak (1957) may be mentioned here. A single injection of *ergotoxine* ethanesulphonate upsets the hormonal balance in rats in such a way that pregnancy is terminated; it also interferes with implantation and with the formation of the decidua. These effects can be antagonized by the administration of progesterone or of prolactin which presumably stimulates endogenous progesterone secretion in the animals ovaries. Large doses of atropine may also interfere with these actions of ergotoxine. Unfortunately the site and mechanisms of action of ergotoxine have not yet been elucidated. Shelesnyak suggests that ergotoxine produces its effects by interfering with the metabolism of steroids, although his experiments do not exclude the possibility that the action is one on some part of the central nervous system, ultimately involving the pituitary. It has also been found that anti-histamines, applied locally into the uterine lumen, will prevent the development of a decidual reaction and interfere with pregnancy. This effect is not reversed by progesterone. The doses of anti-histamine used are high and systemic administration of these drugs is ineffective. Suppression of deciduoma formation has also been observed following local administration of oxytocin and of adrenaline.

5-Hydroxytryptamine (5HT) and Iproniazid

Reserpine was found to have some effect on pregnancy by Gaunt *et al.* (1954) and this led to the investigation of the effect of 5HT and anti-amine oxidases, since 5HT is known to be released in the body by reserpine. It has been found that 5HT will interrupt pregnancy at all stages in mice and rats and produce marked disorganization and bleeding in the placenta (Poulson *et al.*, 1960; Waugh and Pearl, 1960.) Similar effects during the first half of pregnancy have been obtained with iproniazid and other inhibitors of amine oxidase, but these substances are ineffective during the second half of pregnancy (Poulson *et al.*, 1960). The mechanism of action of these effects remains to be elucidated. It is of interest that they will inhibit sexual development in immature female mice, the effect in male animals being much less (Botros and Robson, 1960). 5HT produces rapid and striking degeneration with haemorrhage of the experimental deciduoma in mice. It is interesting that placental haemorrhage and interruption of pregnancy in mice and rabbits has been observed following the administration of endotoxins from gram negative organisms, though the mechanism by which these effects are produced has not been elucidated (Zahl and Bjerknes, 1943, 1944).

Lastly some mention should be made of the interesting work of Bruce (1959). She mated albino mice and then introduced in their cage other males. The presence of a strange albino male prevented the development of pregnancy in about 25% of the females, but with a strange male of a different strain (wild type) pregnancy was blocked in some 75% of females; this happened even if the male was put in a separate box from the female, i.e. in close proximity without actual physical contact. Later work suggests that this pregnancy block works through an olfactory factor, since the reaction is virtually abolished by the prior removal of the olfactory bulbs of the female (Bruce and Parrott, 1960). The subject is reviewed by Parkes and Bruce (1961).

ANABOLIC AND ANDROGENIC STEROIDS

The anabolic effect of male hormone was first clearly demonstrated by Kochakian and Murlin in 1935. They observed that extracts of male urine not only had an androgenic effect but also caused retention of nitrogen in dogs, and it was subsequently shown that testosterone had a similar effect. Koch and his co-workers (Kenyon *et al.*, 1938) demonstrated that testosterone propionate decreased nitrogen excretion in man. The use of testosterone and its esters as anabolic agents is, however, limited by the occurrence of androgenic side effects and in recent years attempts have been made to dissociate these two effects and thus to obtain compounds which would have a high anabolic and little androgenic activity. The search for such substances was facilitated by the technique developed by Eisenberg and Gordon (1950) in which the increase in weight of the levator ani muscle in castrated rats is used as an index of anabolic activity; a satisfactory result obtained by this method is, unfortunately, no guarantee that a similar dissociation will be observed in man, and any new compound so discovered requires extensive clinical investigation. Another important point is the possibility that these substances may cause mild derangement of hepatic function when large doses are used over long periods. Kory *et al.* (1959) who made this observation using norethandrolone (Nilevar) nevertheless suggest that low doses may be safely used as an anabolic agent, even for long term therapy. In another investigation, severe jaundice, which lasted for 10 weeks, developed in one patient on norethandrolone and histological evidence of cholestasis was found in liver biopsies in 4 out of 27 patients treated with this drug (Schaffner *et al.*, 1959).

Anabolic steroids are still essentially in the experimental stage. They are being tried in a variety of conditions, such as preparation and recovery from surgery, recovery from severe illness, recovery from burns and severe trauma, nutritional care in wasting diseases, such as carcinomatosis and tuberculosis, care of decubitus ulcers in the chronically ill, and care of malnourished and premature infants.

The main compounds which are being investigated as anabolic agents are norethandrolone (ethyl-nortestosterone, Nilevar), 19-nortestosterone phenylpropionate ('Durabolin') and methandienone ('Dianabol'). Fluoxymesterone(9α-fluoro-11β-hydroxy-17α-methyltestosterone, Ultandren) has marked anabolic action but it is also a potent androgen, so that there is no dissociation of two effects in this compound. Similarly stanolone (androstane-17(β)-ol-3-one, 'Anabolex') has both anabolic and androgenic actions. The corresponding methyl compound (Androstalone) appears to be more selectively anabolic (Harris, 1961).

Of all these compounds, *norethandrolone* appears to be the best at present for selective anabolic action. Experimentally it has an effect on the levator ani muscle (used as an index of anabolic activity) equal to testosterone propionate but only about 1/17th the androgenic activity of testosterone (Drill and Riegel, 1958). Clinically, McSwiney and Prunty (1957) gave this compound to a number of patients and found that 50 mg. per day (orally or intramuscularly) produced nitrogen retention, with a fall of urinary calcium and usually a fall in faecal calcium. There was also a gain of weight or an arrest of a fall in weight in all cases. The treatment produced a definite, though not marked, androgenic effect. The effect in four elderly underweight patients was investigated by Woodford Williams and Webster (1958) who also demonstrated a gain in weight associated with a positive nitrogen balance. They observed no androgenic or other unpleasant side effects (see Fig. 43).

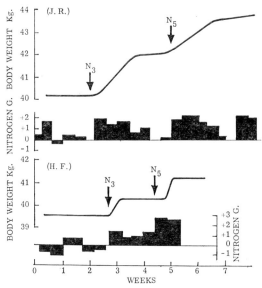

FIG. 43. Effect of treatment with norethandrolone on body weight and nitrogen balance. Both patients began treatment with 30 mg. per day (N_3), which was later increased to 50 mg. per day (Woodford Williams and Webster, 1958).

Fluoxymesterone (Ultandren) is a halogenated derivative of methyl testosterone. The experimental evidence shows that it is a potent androgenic as well as myotrophic (i.e. anabolic) substance (Lyster *et al.*, 1956). It is effective in man when given orally, the dose being up to

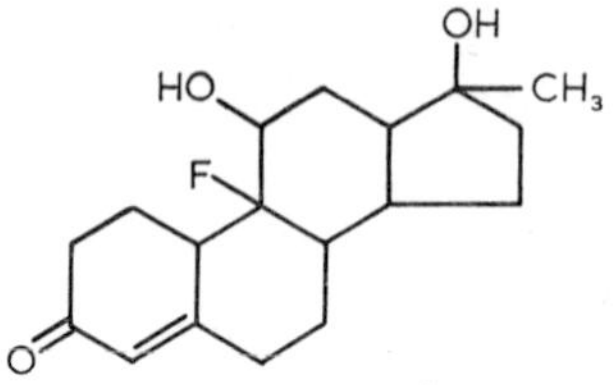

fluoxymesterone
(9 ∝-fluoro-11 β-hydroxy-
17-methyltestosterone)

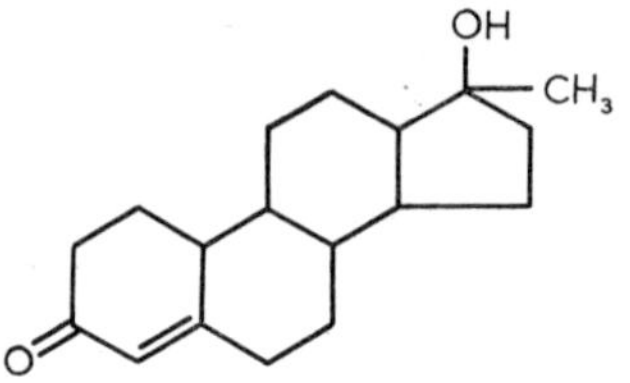

methyl testosterone

5 mg. per day. Bucke (1959) tested it in patients with hypogonadism and found that the maintenance dose varied between 2 and 4 mg. per day in comparison with a daily dose of 20–40 mg. of methyl testosterone needed to produce an equivalent effect.

Effect on histamine excretion

Male rats excrete much less free histamine in the urine than females (Gustafsson *et al.*, 1957); castration of males leads to an increase in histamine excretion while the administration of testosterone to females reduces the histamine excretion (Kim, 1959; Marshall, 1961). It is believed that the effect of the androgen is on the conjugation of histamine. Kim (1961) has shown that an anabolic steroid with weak androgenic action (Durabolin) is much more potent than testosterone in decreasing the histamine excretion in female rats and believes that the effect of these steroids may be related to their anabolic and not to their androgenic activity. This requires further investigation.

Experimental work on steroids in relation to atherosclerosis, hypertension and ganglion blockade is described by Drill and Riegel (1958).

REFERENCES
* Denotes review or symposium.

ADAMS, C. E. and LUDWAK-MANN, C. (1955). *J. Endocr.* **13**, xix
ANNOTATION (1959). *Brit. med. J.* **1**, 492
ANNOTATION (1959). *Brit. med. J.* **2**, 1339
AUGUST, J. T., NELSON, D. H. and THORN, G. W. (1958). *J. clin. Invest.* **37**, 1549
AUGUST, J. T., NELSON, D. H. and THORN, G. W. (1958). *New Engl. J. Med.* **259**, 917
AYRES, P. J., GARROD, O., TAIT, A. S. and TAIT, J. F. (1958). 'Aldosterone', ed. Muller, A. F. and Connor, P. M. London: Churchill
*BAKER, J. B. F. (1960). *Pharmacol. Rev.* **12**, 37

BANKS, A. L., RUTHERFORD, R. N. and COBURN, W. A. (1959). *Northw. med. (Seattle)*, **58**, 1395

BARTTER, F. C., MILLS, I. H., BIGLIERI, E. G. and DELEA, C. (1959). *Recent Progr. Hormone Res.* **15**, 311

BAYLISS, R. I. S. (1959). *Proc. roy. Soc. Med.* **52**, 929

BEYLER, A. L., POTTS, G. O., COULSTON, F. and SURREY, A. R. (1961). *Endocrinology*, **69**, 819

BISHOP, P. M. F. and CABRAL DE ALMEIDA, J. C. (1960). *Brit. med. J.* **1**, 1103

BOLAND, E. W. (1959). *Ann. N.Y. Acad. Sci.* **82**, 887

BOLAND, E. W. (1960). *J. Amer. Med. Ass.* **174**, 835

BOTROS, M. and ROBSON, J. M. (1960). *J. Endocr.* **20**, 10

BRUCE, H. M. (1959). *Nature (Lond.)*, **184**, 105

BRUCE, H. M. and PARROTT, D. M. V. (1960). *Science*, **131**, 1526

BUCKE, R. M. (1959). *Brit. med. J.* **1**, 1379

BUNIM, J. J., BLACK, R. L., LUTWAK, L., PETERSON, R. E. and WHEDON, G. D. (1958). *Arthritis and Rheumatism*, **1**, 313

CHANG, M. C. (1959). *Endocrinology*, **65**, 339

*Ciba Symposium on Aldosterone (1958). Ed. Muller, A. F. and O'Connor, C. M. London: Churchill

COGLAN, J. P., DENTON, D. A., GODING, J. R. and WRIGHT, R. D. (1960). *Postgrad. med. J.* **36**, 76

COLIN-JONES, E. and SOMERS, G. F. (1957). *Med. Press*, **238**, 206

CONN, J. W. (1955). *J. Lab. clin. Med.* **45**, 3 and 661

COULSTON, F., BEYLER, A. L. and DROBECK, H. P. (1960). *Toxicol. appl. Pharmacol.* **2**, 115

DAVID, A. FELLOWES, K. P. and MILLSON, D. R. (1959). *J. Pharm (Lond.)*, **11**, 491

DAVIS, J. O. (1957). *J. nat. Med. Ass.* **49**, 42

DAVIS, J. O., CARPENTER, C. J., AYERS, C. R., HOLMAN, J. E. and CASPER, A. (1961). *J. clin. Invest.* **40**, 684

DIDCOCK, K. A., JACKSON, D. and ROBSON, J. M. (1956). *Brit. J. Pharmacol.* **11**, 437

DIDCOCK, K. A., PICARD, C. W. and ROBSON, J. M. (1952). *J. Physiol, (Lond.)*, **117**, 65P

DOCKERTY, M. B., SMITH, R. A. and SYMMONDS, R. E. (1959). *Proc. Mayo Clin.* **34**, 321

DOMENJOZ, R. and THEOBALD, W. (1958). *Experientia (Basel)*, **14**, 33

DRILL, V. A. (1959). *Fed. Proc.* **18**, 1040

DRILL, V. A. and RIEGEL, B. (1958). *Recent Progr. Hormone Res.* **14**, 29

DUDLEY HART, F. (1960). *Postgrad. med. J.* **36**, 26

ECKSTEIN, P., WATERHOUSE, J. A. H., BOND, G. M., MILLS, W. G., SANDILANDS, D. M. and SHOTTON, D. M. (1961). *Brit. med. J.* **2** , 1172

EISENBERG, E. and GORDON, G. S. (1950). *J. Pharmacol. exp. Ther.* **99**, 38

ELLIS, J. T. (1956). *Amer. J. Path.* **32**, 993

ELTON, R. L. and EDGREN, R. A. (1958). *Endocrinology*, **63**, 646

FARRELL, G. (1958). *Physiol. Rev.* **38**, 709

FARRELL, G. (1959). *Recent Progr. Hormone Res.* **15**, 275

FINNEY, R. S. H. and SOMERS, G. F. (1958). *J. Pharm, (Lond.)*, **10**, 613

FINNEY, R. S. H. and TARNOKY, A. L. (1960). *J. Pharm, (Lond.)*, **12**, 49

FULD, H. and HORWICH, L. (1958). *Brit. med. J.* **2**, 1199

GAUNT, R., RENZI, A. A., ANTONCHAK, N., MILLER, G. J. and GILMAN, M. (1954). *Ann. N.Y. Acad. Sci.* **59**, 22

GAUNT, R., RENZI, A. A. and CHART, J. J. (1955). *J. clin. Endocr.* **15**, 621

GOLD, J. J. and COHEN, M. R. (1958). *Ann. N.Y. Acad. Sci.* **71**, 691

GOLDING, R. J. (1960). *Postgrad. med. J.* **36**, 23

GOLDSMITH, R. S., BARTTER, F. C., ROSCH, P. J., MERONEY, W. H. and HERNDON, E. G. (1958). *J. clin. Endocr.* **18**, 323

GREENBLATT, R. B., BARFIELD, W. E., JUNGCK, E. C. and RAY, A. W. (1961). *J. Amer. med. Ass.* **178**, 101

GROSS, F. and LICHTLEN, P. (1958). In 'Aldosterone', p. 39. Ed. Muller, A. F. and Connor, P. M. London: Churchill

GRUMBACH, M. M., DUCHARME, J. R. and MOLOSHOK, R. E. (1959). *J. clin. Endocr.* **19**, 1369

GUSTAFSSON, B., KAHLSON, G. and ROSENGREN, E. (1957). *Acta physiol. scand.* **41**, 217

HADDOW, A. and ROBINSON, A. M. (1937). *Proc. roy. Soc. B.* **122**, 442

HARMAN, J. B. (1959). *Lancet*, **1**, 887

HARRIS, L. H. (1961). *J. clin. Endocr.* **21**, 1099

HELLER, C. G., LAIDLAW, W. M., HARVEY, H. T. and NELSON, W. O. (1958). *Ann. N.Y. Acad. Sci.* **71**, 649

HELLER, C. G., MOORE, D. J., PAULSEN, C. A., NELSON, W. O. and LAIDLAW, W. M. (1959). *Fed. Proc.* **18**, 1057

HELLER, C. G., MOORE, D. J. and PAULSEN, C. A. (1961). *Toxicol. appl. Pharmacol.* **3**, 1

HETZEL, B. S., McSWINEY, R. R., MILLS, I. H. and PRUNTY, F. T. G. (1956). *J. Endocr.* **13**, 112

HOLTKAMP, D. E., GRESLIN, J. G., ROOT, C. A. and LERNER, L. J. (1960). *Proc. Soc. exp. Biol. (N.Y.)*, **105**, 197

HUDSON, B., BARRETT, A. J. and BORNSTEIN, J. (1957). *Aust. Ann. Med.* **6**, 250

JACKSON, D. and ROBSON, J. M. (1957). *J. Endocr.* **15**, 355

JACKSON, D. and ROBSON, J. M. (1958). *Brit. J. exp. Path.* **39**, 133

JACKSON, D., ROBSON, J. M. and WANDER, A. C. E. (1959). *J. Endocr.* **18**, 204

*JACKSON, H. (1959). *Pharmacol. Rev.* **11**, 135

JENKINS, J. S., MEAKIN, J. W. and NELSON, D. H. (1959). *Endocrinology*, **64**, 572

JENKINS, J. S., POTHIER, L., REDDY, W. J. and THORN, G. W. (1959). *Brit. med. J.* **1**, 398

JONES, R. V., McSWINEY, R. R. and BROOKS, R. V. (1959). *Lancet*, **1**, 177

KAGAWA, C. M., CELLA, J. A. and VAN ARMAN, C. G. (1957). *Science*, **126**, 1015

KAGAWA, C. M., STURTEVANT, F. M. and VAN ARMAN, C. G. (1959). *J. Pharmacol. exp. Ther.* **126**, 123

KELLETT, D. N. (1959). Ph.D. Thesis, University of London

KENYON, A. T., SANDIFORD, I., BRYAN, A. H., KNOWLTON, K. and KOCH, F. C. (1938). *Endocrinology*, **23**, 135

KERSLEY, G. D. and PALIN, A. G. (1959). *Lancet*, **2**, 886

KIM, K. S. (1959). *Amer. J. Physiol.* **197**, 1258

KIM, K. S. (1961). *Nature (Lond.)*, **191**, 1368

KISTNER, R. W. and SMITH, O. W. (1961). *Fertility and Sterility* **12**, 121

KOCHAKIAN, C. D. and MURLIN, J. R. (1935). *J. Nutr.* **10**, 437

KORY, R. C., BRADLEY, M. H., WATSON, R. N., CALLAHAN, R. and PETERS, B. J. (1959). *Amer. J. Med.* **26**, 243

KRUSIUS, F. E. and OKA, M. (1958). *Ann. rheum. Dis.* **17**, 184

LANDAU, R. L., BERGENSTAL, D. M., LUGIBIHL, K. and KOSCHT, M. E. (1955). *J. clin. Endocr.* **15**, 1194

LANDAU, R. L. and LUGIBIHL, K. (1958). *J. clin. Endocr.* **18**, 1237

LEDINGHAM, J. G. G., MARTIN, F. I. R., MOXHAM, A., HURTER, R. and NABARRO, J. D. N. (1961). *Lancet*, **1**, 630

LERNER, L. J., HOLTHAUS, F. J. and THOMPSON, C. R. (1958). *Endocrinology*, **63**, 295

LEWIS, A. A. G. (1960). *Postgrad. med. J.* **36**, 39

LIEBERMAN, A. M. (1958). *Arch. intern. Med.* **102**, 990

LIDDLE, G. W. (1957). *Science*, **126**, 1010

LIDDLE, G. W. (1958). *Metabolism*, **7**, 405

LYSTER, S. C., LUND, G. H. and STAFFORD, R. O. (1956). *Endocrinology*, **58**, 781

MARSHALL, P. B. (1961). *Brit. J. Pharmacol.* **16**, 50

McGINTY, D. A. and DJERASSI, C. (1958). *Ann. N.Y. Acad. Sci.* **71**, 500

McSWINEY, R. R. and PRUNTY, F. T. G. (1957). *J. Endocr.* **16**, 28

MEARS, E. (1961). *Brit. med. J.* **2**, 1179

MENKIN, V. (1960). *Brit. med. J.* **1**, 1521

MOYER, J. H. and FUCHS, M. (1960). 'Edema.' Philadelphia and London: Saunders

MURPHY, M. L. and KARNOFSKY, D. A. (1956). *Cancer*, **9**, 962

NEHER, R., DESAULLES, P., VISCHER, E., WIELAND, P. and WETTSTEIN, A. (1958). *Helv. chim. Acta*, **41**, 1667
NELSON, D. H. and AUGUST, J. T. (1959). *Lancet*, **2**, 883
NEUSTADT, D. H. (1959). *J. Amer. med. Ass.* **170**, 1253
NUGENT, C. A., EIK-NES, K. and TYLER, F. H. (1959). *J. clin. Endocr.* **19**, 526
PAGE, F. (1951). *Lancet*, **2**, 755
PARKES, A. S. and BRUCE, H. M. (1961). *Science*, **134**, 1049
PETERSON, R. E. (1959). *Ann. N. Y. Acad. Sci.* **82**, 846
PETERSON, R. E., HERTZ, R. and LUBS, H. A. (1957). *Proc. Soc. exp. Biol. (N. Y.)*, **94**, 421
PETERSON, R. E., NOKES, G., CHEN, P. S. and BLACK, R. L. (1960). *J. clin. Endocr.* **20**, 495
*PINCUS, G. (1959), *Vitam. and Horm.* **17**, 307
PINCUS, G., CHANG, M. C., ZARROW, M. X., HAFEZ, E. S. E. and MERRILL, A. (1956). *Endocrinology*, **59**, 695
PINCUS, G., ROCK, J., CHANG, M. C. and GARCIA, C. R. (1959). *Fed. Proc.* **18**, 1051
POULSON, E., BOTROS, M. and ROBSON, J. M. (1960). *Science*, **131**, 1101
QUENTIN EVANS, F. (1958). *Brit. J. Clin. Practice*, **12**, 209
RAKOFF, A. E. (1959). *Fed. Proc.* **18**, 1006
REVESZ, C., CHAPPEL, C. I. and GAUDRY, R. (1960). *Endocrinology*, **66**, 140
ROBSON, J. M. (1959). *Mem. Soc. Endocr.* **6**, 54
ROBSON, J. M. and KEELE, C. A. (1956). 'Recent Advances in Pharmacology', 2nd ed. London: Churchill
ROBSON, J. M. and SHARAF, A. A. (1951). *J. Physiol, (Lond.)*, **115**, 313
ROSKAM, J. (1958). *Sem. Hôp.* **34**, 971
ROSKAM, J. (1959). *Presse méd.* **67**, 2327
ROSKAM, J., LECOMTE, J., VAN CAUWENBERGE, H. and HUGUES, J. (1959). VI Congress International de Therapeutique, Strasbourg, p. 81
ROSS, E. J. (1959). 'Aldosterone in Clinical and Experimental Medicine.' Oxford: Blackwell
SAUNDERS, F. J. and DRILL, V. A. (1958). *Ann. N. Y. Acad. Sci.* **71**, 516
SCHAFFNER, F., POPPER, H. and CHESROW, E. (1959). *Amer J. Med.* **26**, 249
SCHÖLER, H. F. L. and DE WACHTER, A. M. (1961). *Acta endocr. (Kbh.)*, **38**, 128
SEGAL, S. J. and NELSON, W. O. (1958). *Proc. Soc. exp. Biol. (N. Y.)*, **98**, 431
SEGAL, S. J. and NELSON, W. O. (1961). *Anat. Rec.* **139**, 273
SELYE, H. and GAÉTAN, J. (1956). *Ann. N. Y. Acad. Sci.* **64**, 481
SETNIKAR, I., SALVATERRA, M. and TEMELCOV, O. (1959). *Brit. J. Pharmacol.* **14**, 484
SHELESNYAK, M. C. (1957). *Recent Progr. Hormone Res.* **13**, 269
STREETEN, H. P. (1959). *Gastroenterology*, **37**, 643
STREETEN, H. P. (1961). *Clin. Pharm. Therap.* **2**, 359
SWYER, G. I. M., SEBOK, L. and BARNS, D. F. (1960). *Proc. roy. Soc. Med.* **53**, 435
THIERSCH, J. B. (1952). *Amer. J. Obstet. Gynec.* **63**, 1928
THIERSCH, J. B. (1956). *Acta endocr. (Kbh.), Suppl.* **28**, 37
THIERSCH, J. B. (1956). *Acta endocr. (Kbh.), Suppl.* **28**, 46
THIERSCH, J. B. (1957). *Proc. Soc. exp. Biol. (N. Y.)*, **94**, 33
THIERSCH, J. B. (1958). *Proc. Soc. exp. Biol. (N. Y.)*, **98**, 479
TYLER, E. T. and OLSON, H. J. (1959). *J. Amer. med. Ass.* **196**, 1843
WARD, L. E., POOLEY, H. F., POWER, M H., MASON, H. L., SLOCUMB, C. H. and HENCH, P. S. (1958). *Ann. rheum. Dis.* **17**, 145
WAUGH, D. and PEARL, M. J. (1960). *Amer. J. Path.* **36**, 431
WELLS, R. (1958). *Lancet*, **2**, 498
WETTSTEIN, A. (1960). *Mschr. Kinderheilk.* **108**, 164
WIED, G. L. and DAVIS, M. E. (1958). *Ann. N. Y. Acad. Sci.* **71**, 599
WILLIAMS, R. S. (1959). *Lancet*, **1**, 698
WOODFORD WILLIAMS, E. and WEBSTER, D. (1958). *Brit. med. J.* **2**, 1447
YOUNG, J. P. (1959). *Ann. intern. Med.* **51**, 1159
ZAHL, P. A. and BJERKNES, C. (1943). *Proc. Soc. exp. Biol. (N. Y.)*, **54**, 329
ZAHL, P. A. and BJERKNES, C. (1944). *Proc. Soc. exp. Biol. (N. Y.)*, **56**, 153

CHAPTER 9

CHOLESTEROL .

A large amount of experimental and clinical evidence suggests that there is a relationship between atherosclerosis and an alteration in lipid metabolism, and various methods have therefore been used in an attempt to modify the blood and body lipids, in the hope of preventing or changing the development of cardiovascular disease. No attempt will be made here to discuss the pathology of these conditions or to examine the evidence linking them with abnormal lipid metabolism. In a recent review of the subject, Florey (1960) concludes that 'on the whole the observations do not carry complete conviction that an increased level of blood lipids is the primary cause of atherosclerosis, though it may well be important in the development of the lesions.' Much information on cholesterol and lipoproteins is reviewed in the book edited by Cook (1958). It is emphasized there that the measurement of plasma cholesterol represents merely the algebraic sum of a large number of variables. The plasma cholesterol is synthesized almost exclusively in the liver. The sterol is bound to proteins and discharged into the extracellular fluid. The resultant cholesterol protein complexes permeate the arterial and capillary endothelium and circulate by way of lymphatics and veins back into the blood. This cycle occurs repeatedly for several days until the circulatory sterol is withdrawn from the extracellular fluid for utilization or degradation. Thus any change in the plasma cholesterol could be attributed to many factors, such as an alteration in plasma volume or in capillary permeability, redistribution of existing extracellular cholesterol between interstitial fluid and plasma, an alteration in the rate of hepatic cholesterol synthesis or a change in the rate of tissue utilization or degradation. In addition to all this there is the possibility that the lipid in atherosclerosis is formed by the activity of cells in the vessel wall, possibly to some extent independently of the cycle described above. For example, Field et al. (1960) using ^{14}C labelled cholesterol, showed that a major portion of the cholesterol of the intima in man is derived from plasma through interchange, but that a considerable amount is synthesized in the intima. The significance of the plasma cholesterol level and of factors which modify it must be viewed in the light of all these factors.

The present chapter will be mainly devoted to the effect of dietary measures and drugs on body lipids, i.e. measures undertaken in the hope of influencing vascular disease. No attempt will be made to differentiate between various lipid fractions in the blood since the impression has been gained that these more complex analyses, interesting as they are in their own right, do not at present yield more evidence than simpler analyses relevant to the problems being considered. The physiology of the circulatory cholesterol and lipoprotein is discussed by Boyd and Oliver (1958).

In view of what has been said above, a change in the diet can be expected to have only a limited effect on the serum cholesterol. According to Page (1958), the most effective treatment is a low fat, high protein diet. The total amount of fat *consumed* in such diets should not be greater than 10–15% of the total calories. Most patients at first lose weight on such diets and along with weight loss there is an associated fall in plasma cholesterol. After a few months, however, the weight levels off and the lipids tend to return, but not to reach their original level. If diets contain less than 10% of the total calories as fat, the response may be more dramatic, but the clinical condition of the patient may be unsatisfactory, with marked gastrointestinal disturbances. Hatch *et al.* (1955) on the basis of an experiment on patients with hypertension put on various diets, believe that the total calorie intake is of greater significance in the control of plasma lipid levels than the quantities of cholesterol or fat ingested. As Page has emphasized, there is wide variation in the response of different patients to high and low fat diets. Some, for example, are able to consume very large amounts of fat with little or no effect on the plasma lipids.

There has been a good deal of discussion about the significance of animal and vegetable fat, and of saturated and unsaturated fatty acids on the blood cholesterol level, the suggestion being that animal fats and saturated fats would tend to keep up blood cholesterol. Malmros and Wigand (1957) found in experiments on healthy subjects receiving about 150 g. of fat per day, that certain vegetable fats, particularly corn oil and safflower oil, had a depressing effect on the serum cholesterol, though in some cases this showed a tendency later to increase, possibly because the patients failed to observe their dietary restrictions. Keys *et al.* (1958) conclude from their studies that an excess of saturated fatty acids in the diet seems to explain the high serum cholesterol levels in populations subsisting on 'luxurious American and European diets.' The mere addition to the diet of small amounts of fats very rich in linoleic acid (or other polyethenoids) is of little value. However, the substitution of one type of fat (i.e. unsubstituted) for the other is both effective and acceptable for dietetic purposes.

Turpeinen *et al.* (1960) investigated the effect of replacing dietary milk fat by soy bean oil (containing much more unsaturated fatty acids) on the cholesterol level of subjects in a mental hospital. They observed a small but highly significant decrease in the cholesterol level, i.e. from 236 to 216 mg. per 100 ml. serum. There were large individual variations in the response to the dietary change, but on the whole, the subjects with higher initial serum cholesterol levels also tended to show greater decreases.

Lastly there are some interesting observations made by Ruthstein *et al.* (1958), the significance of which it is difficult to evaluate at present. They found that in tissue cultures of human aortic cells, deposition of lipoid can be induced by cholesterol, is reversible, can be inhibited by an unsaturated fatty acid (linoleic acid) and can be potentiated by the corresponding saturated fatty acid (stearic acid).

EFFECTS OF DRUGS ON BLOOD CHOLESTEROL

Drugs can affect the blood cholesterol in three main ways, namely:

1. By decreasing the intestinal absorption; this can be of only very limited value since the main source of blood cholesterol is from liver synthesis.
2. By depressing the biosynthesis of cholesterol in the liver; this could potentially produce a marked effect. The main steps in the biosynthesis of cholesterol are shown in Fig. 44 (Popják *et al.*, 1960) and the biosynthesis of cholesterol is reviewed by Popják and Cornforth (1960).
3. By increasing the rate of degradation of cholesterol.

In addition, certain drugs have been used of which the mechanism of action is not really understood.

3-acetyl-coenzyme A
↓
acetoacetyl-coenzyme A + acetyl-coenzyme A
↓
3-hydroxy-3-methylglutaryl-coenzyme A
↓
mevalonic acid
↓
5-phosphomevalonic acid
↓
5-diphosphomevalonic acid
↓
isopentenyl-pyrophosphate
↓
3, 3-dimethylallyl-pyrophosphate
↓
geranyl-pyrophosphate→geranic acid
↓
farnesyl-pyrophosphate→farnesoic acid
↓
squalene
↓
lanosterol
↓
cholesterol

FIG. 44. Biosynthesis of cholesterol
(according to Popják *et al.*, 1960).

β-SITOSTEROL

The use of plant sterols, which constitute the main source of vegetable (or phyto) sterols for man and most animals as competitors for the intestinal absorption transfer-mechanism of cholesterol, has received a good deal of interest in the last decade. The substance which has been most studied is β-sitosterol which differs chemically from cholesterol only in the presence of an ethyl group at C_{24}. There is evidence that a reduction of 10–15% in the level of plasma cholesterol may be expected if suspensions of sitosterol up to 5 g. are taken before each meal (Page, 1958). This has been observed both in animal experiments and in man. In rats a decrease in the cholesterol content of the liver was also observed (Best and Duncan, 1956).

Feeding of *cholestenone* experimentally will reduce the plasma level of cholesterol, but since this leads to the accumulation of cholestanol in the plasma and other tissues, and since there is evidence that cholestanol will, like cholesterol, induce atherosclerosis, it would be expected that cholestenone would not be of value in the prevention and treatment of atherosclerosis (Tomkins *et al.*, 1957). Moreover, it has been shown that cholestenone can produce toxic effects, including marked inhibition of adrenal cortical secretion (Sternberg *et al.*, 1958).

NICOTINIC ACID

There is good evidence that large doses of nicotinic acid will reduce the serum cholesterol both in animals and in man. Clinically the administration of 3–6 g. of the drug per day in hypercholesteraemic patients will frequently bring about a marked reduction in cholesterol levels, though the lowering is less striking in subjects with normal levels. Flushing and pruritis occur at first, but subside within the first week of therapy in nearly all cases; occasionally other side effects are seen, e.g. urticaria, but so far no serious toxic reactions have developed. A variety of explanations have been advanced to account for this effect (Schade and Saltman, 1959) but there is good evidence that nicotinic acid interferes with the biosynthesis of cholesterol in the liver. Schön (1958) has actually shown that in rats the *in vivo* formation of total hepatic cholesterol is depressed in proportion to the amount of nicotinic acid fed in the diet. This author, as well as Schade and Saltman (1959), has suggested that the limiting factor is the amount of coenzyme A in the liver, for which detoxicating systems responsible for detoxication of nicotinic acid and lipid synthesizing systems compete. This is supported by the finding of Schön that both α-phenylbutyric acid and diphenylbutyric acid, which require coenzyme A for detoxication, also block cholesterol synthesis.

p-AMINOSALICYCLIC ACID

The administration of this drug in doses of 12 g. per day causes a decrease of about 30% in the serum cholesterol, even though PAS tends to produce decrease in thyroid activity. The mechanism of this action is unknown. Tygstrup *et al.* (1959) point out that a combination of blood-cholesterol lowering and a moderate anti-thyroid effect may be particularly desirable in coronary heart disease.

VITAMIN A

The oral administration of 100,000 units vitamin A acetate per day for 4–6 months significantly reduced the elevated total cholesterol levels in atherosclerotic patients. The greatest reductions were seen in patients with the highest initial levels. No effect was observed in subjects with normal cholesterol levels and no clinical history of coronary artery disease (Kinley and Krause, 1959). The mechanism of this action of vitamin A is unknown.

PARITOL (sulphated alginic acid)

This is a sulphated polymannurodide which was made following investigations with heparin. The clearing action of heparin on alimentary lipaemia and the associated degradation of large lipoprotein molecules have been known for some time and are now attributed to the activation or possibly release of a tissue lipolytic enzyme, the so-called 'lipoprotein-lipase' (Korn, 1958). It was then found that heparin could diminish hypercholesterolaemia in animals and decrease the development of atherosclerosis in rabbits fed cholesterol. This led to its use in various types of blood lipid abnormalities, but no striking effects were obtained.

In a search for more potent antilipaemic agents, sulphated derivatives of seaweed (alginic acid) polysaccharides with a mannuronic acid repeat unit gave very interesting results, being much more active than heparin in the prevention and treatment of hyperlipaemia in animals. This substance was also able to arrest the progress of aortic athero-sclerosis in rabbits. It is suggested that Paritol (which is a purified preparation of sulphated polymannuronides) produces its effect both by activating the lipoprotein lipase and by stimulating the reticulo-endothelial system, whereas heparin acts only by the former mechanism (Constantinides and Saunders, 1958).

These experimental results led to the clinical trial of Paritol in patients with hypercholesterolaemia which have given very interesting results. The drug was given either intravenously or intramuscularly to subjects, some of whom were survivors of myocardial infarction. Very striking reductions in the cholesterol blood levels were produced rapidly in nearly all cases (Constantinides *et al.*, 1960). The authors make the point that in the most responsive cases, the dramatic action of the drug on hyperlipaemia was comparable to the effect of insulin on hyper-glycaemia. The type of result obtained is illustrated in Fig. 45. It is well known that sulphated polysaccharides can produce an anticoagulant action and a variety of side effects, including alopecia, but the minimum effective dosage of Paritol (2·5 mg./kg.) showed no such side effects. It must be emphasized that these clinical experiments were of quite short duration—a few weeks at the most, and more prolonged investigations are obviously desirable.

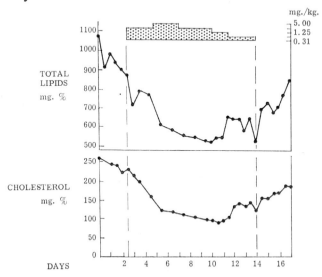

FIG. 45. Effect of Paritol on blood lipid and cholesterol levels (Constantinides *et al.*, 1960).

FARNESOIC ACID AND ITS ANALOGUES

It has been found that these substances inhibit the utilization of intermediates of cholesterol synthesis *in vitro*. This was first shown with farnesoic acid by Wright and Cleland (1957). More recently, Popják *et al.* (1960) have shown that some analogues of farnesoic acid are much more potent. The most active is 3, 7, 11-trimethyldodecanoate, but marked effects were also observed with three other related substances. It will be very interesting to see what effects are produced by these substances *in vivo*.

OESTROGENS AND TRIPARANOL

The blood lipid pattern in animals and man can be altered by the administration of oestrogens, and abnormal lipid values in subjects with atherosclerosis or in cholesterol fed animals can be lowered by such treatment (see Drill *et al.*, 1959). Eder (1959) investigated the effect of oestrogen administration to male subjects who were survivors of myocardial infarction and found, within 6 weeks, an appreciable decrease in the serum cholesterol (from 268 to 222 mg.% average). According to Oliver and Boyd (1959) a maximum effect on the blood cholesterol is obtained with 200 μg. of ethinyl oestradiol per day, and increasing the dose beyond this is no more effective while producing more side effects. These investigators also state that although oestrogens produced a depression of hypercholesterolaemia in 50 men investigated during a period of $2\frac{1}{2}$ years, there was no significant improvement in morbidity or mortality from coronary disease when contrasted with a comparable control group. In any case, oestrogens are not very suitable for continued administration since they frequently bring about gynecomastia and depression or loss of libido, as well as other side effects.

Various attempts have been made to produce derivatives of oestrogen which would retain the action on blood lipids without having any typical oestrogenic effects. Thus Drill *et al.* (1959) prepared a number of steroids related to oestrogens which had a more selective effect on the blood lipids.

A recent development is the synthesis of a compound related to triphenylethylene. Various derivatives of this compound are known to have quite marked oestrogenic effects and chlorotrianisene has been used clinically as a long acting oestrogen. Triparanol (MER 29) is related to triphenylethylene (also to ethamoxytryphetol, an oestrogen antagonist) and its structure is shown below.

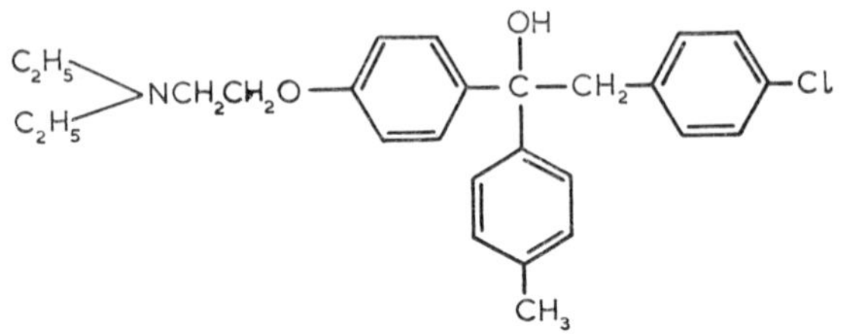

triparanol

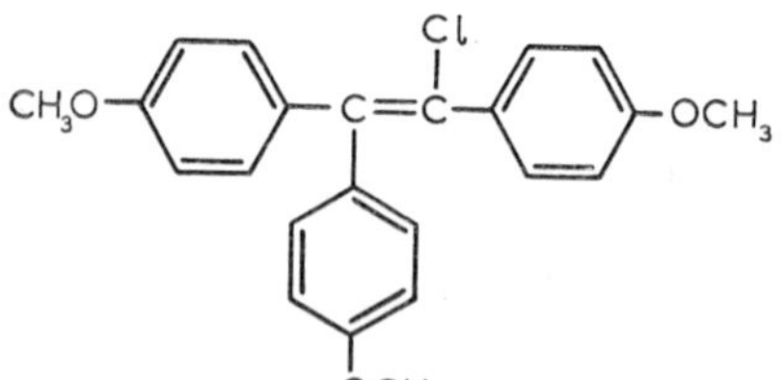

chlorotrianisene

Triparanol was synthesized by Palopoli and his co-workers (see Blohm and Mackenzie, 1959). It is a specific inhibitor of cholesterol biosynthesis, producing its effect at an advanced stage of the biosynthesis, i.e. after the formation of the steroid nucleus. Demesterol (24-dehydro-cholesterol) appears in large amounts suggesting that Triparanol blocks the synthesis of cholesterol from demesterol (Avigan *et al.*, 1960). Chronic administration of the drug to rats lowers the cholesterol level of plasma, erythrocytes, liver, skeletal muscle, lungs, adrenals and aorta, though not of the brain or of adipose tissue. Similar results were obtained in monkeys which received the drug orally over a period of 6 months (Blohm *et al.*, 1959). It has also been found that Triparanol decreases the production of cortisone and aldosterone in healthy subjects, and the excretion of adrenal cortical metabolites in patients with hyperadrenalism (Melby *et al.*, 1961).

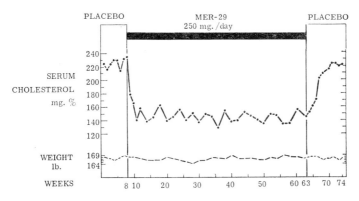

FIG. 46. Effect of Triparanol (MER-29) on serum cholesterol (Hollander *et al.*, 1960).

There have now been a number of clinical reports on the use of Triparanol and there is no doubt that it can lower the serum cholesterol in man, though it seems doubtful whether this can be fully maintained over long periods. This is for example reported by Carver *et al.* (1960; see also Annot., 1960). Another question which requires investigation is whether demesterol, which accumulates during Triparanol treatment, does not have atherosclerotic effects like cholesterol (assuming that cholesterol is in fact involved in the aetiology of vascular disease).

A particularly interesting study is that of Hollander *et al.* (1960) since they not only determined the effect of the drug over long periods (3–14 months), but also investigated the condition of the heart in these patients. They found that Triparanol depressed the cholesterol level and this was maintained during the period of therapy, after which it gradually returned to the former level and they gave a striking illustration of this effect which is shown in Fig. 46. Radioisotopic tracer studies moreover served to show that the drug decreased the total sterol and cholesterol content of the body by decreasing the formation of cholesterol. The clinical studies indicated that Triparanol reduced anginal attacks in 12 out of 28 subjects. This improvement occurred in subjects who had normal as well as high control serum cholesterol levels, but was associated in all subjects with a reduction of serum cholesterol. It is noteworthy, however, that out of the 43 subjects with evidence of coronary disease in this study, one developed a myocardial infarction after 4 months of therapy. The drug is usually well tolerated at a dose level of 250 mg. per day, which should not be exceeded. Occasionally, however, toxic effects occur and these may be serious. Skin reactions, including exfoliative dermatitis, have been observed, as well as loss of hair. Four cases of cataract are reported in patients who had previously had skin reactions and in whom treatment had nevertheless been continued. (Letter to the Medical Profession from the Merrell laboratories.) It is thus obvious that patients receiving the drug should be carefully watched for the appearance of toxic effects, and that Triparanol should not be given to subjects liable to any form of dermatitis.

THYROID HORMONES

It is well known that serum cholesterol levels are raised in hypothyroid subjects and that thyroid hormones can lower the serum cholesterol. The subject is reviewed by Kritchevsky (1960) who concludes that thyroid active compounds, which enhance cholesterol biosynthesis, exert their hypocholesterolaemic effect by stimulation of the processes of cholesterol degradation and excretion, which must thus be the predominant effect. The main degradation of cholesterol is to bile acids, 70–90% of the cholesterol synthesized daily being converted to bile acids. Cholesterol oxidation *in vivo* is controlled by a feed-back mechanism. The concentration of bile acids supplied to the liver via the portal circulation depresses the rate of bile acid synthesis by the liver, i.e. cholesterol degradation is affected by bile acid concentration.

Desiccated thyroid or thyroxine are unsuitable for administration to patients to reduce blood cholesterol since they would produce side effects, such as palpitation, nervousness, sweating, insomnia and loss of weight. There has thus been a search for synthetic thyroxine analogues which would have a potent hypocholesterolaemic action without any of these side effects. This is particularly important since death due to congestive heart failure can occur when patients with atherosclerosis are treated with normal doses of thyroid extract (Wallach *et al.*, 1958).

Boyd and Oliver (1960) investigated the effect of various thyroxine analogues on the serum cholesterol and on the heart rate of rats and found that some compounds had less effect on the heart in relation to their cholesterol lowering effect than others. Amongst the best compounds were tetra-iodo-D-thyronine, tri-iodo-D-thyronine, di-iodo-D-thyronine and tetra-iodothyroformic acid. Cuthbertson and his co-workers (1960) have done extensive work on the action of thyroxine

analogues on serum and liver cholesterol on experimental atherosclerosis in rats, in relation to their activity in causing enlargement of
the heart (as an index of metabolic activity) and have also found that
some compounds have a more specific effect on atherosclerosis and
cholesterol levels, e.g. di-iodo-D-thyronine and D-thyroxine.

A number of compounds have also been investigated clinically with
interesting results. Thus Corday *et al.* (1960) investigated the effect of
administration of tetraiodothyroformic acid in patients with marked
coronary atherosclerosis and hypercholesterolaemia. They were either
euthyroid, or hypometabolism had been previously induced by radio
iodine to relieve intolerable angina pectoris. A dose of 100 mg. per day
was well tolerated in all but one out of 26 patients and produced striking
reductions in the blood cholesterol in many cases (Fig. 47). 'Escape'
occurred occasionally after some months of treatment, but if the drug
was stopped for 2 weeks and then started again, the blood cholesterol
was again reduced.

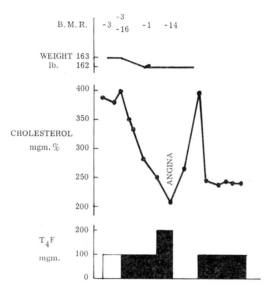

Fig. 47. Effect of placebo and tetra-iodothyroformic acid on the serum cholesterol concentration of a hyperthyroid patient with severe
coronary artery disease (Corday *et al.*, 1960).

The value of D-thyroxine in lowering the serum cholesterol in patients
with hypercholesterolaemia due to various conditions has also been
investigated. It can lower the blood cholesterol, in some cases without
producing any effect on the basic metabolic rate or on cardiac function
(Starr *et al.*, 1960). Triiodothyroacetic acid can also lower the blood
cholesterol, but the effect is not maintained and its administration has

led to the development of angina of effort (Oliver and Boyd, 1957). Lowering of the blood cholesterol has also been obtained with triiodothyropropionic acid (Bauer *et al.*, 1959).

AMINOPTERIN

This produced marked depression of the blood cholesterol and decrease of atheromatosis of the aorta, as compared with controls, in rabbits on an atherogenic diet (i.e. high cholesterol diet) but about one-fifth of the aminopterin treated rabbits died (Muschenheim *et al.*, 1960).

CONCLUSIONS

It has been suggested, and there is some evidence, that there is a causal relationship between atherosclerosis in man and a raised blood cholesterol (and other disturbances in blood lipids). This has led to the search for measures which would lower the blood cholesterol (and rectify the other disturbances in blood lipids). Blood cholesterol can be lowered by three main methods, namely (1) by decreasing the absorption from the intestine, (2) by decreasing the biosynthesis in the liver, and (3) by increasing the rate of metabolic breakdown. At present it would appear that the second method is the most hopeful.

A number of drugs have been found which will lower the blood cholesterol in man and decrease experimental atherogenesis in experimental animals. In some cases this can be brought about for long periods and with few or no side effects. There is as yet no evidence that any of these drugs are of value in the prevention or treatment of cardiovascular disease in man.

REFERENCES
*Denotes Review

ANNOTATION (1960). *Lancet*, **2**, 968

AVIGAN, J., STEINBERG, D., THOMPSON, M. J. and MOSETTIG, E. (1960). *Progr. cardiovascular Dis.* **2**, 525

BAUER, H. G., McGAVACK, T. H. and SWELL, L. (1959). *J. clin. Endocr.* **19**, 490

BEST, M. M. and DUNCAN, C. H. (1956). *Circulation*, **14**, 344

BLOHM, T. R., KARIYA, T. and LAUGHLIN, M. W. (1959). *Arch. Biochem.* **85**, 250

BLOHM, T. R. and MACKENZIE, R. D. (1959). *Arch. Biochem.* **85**, 245

*BOYD, G. S. and OLIVER, M. F. (1958). 'Cholesterol', p. 182. New York: Academic Press

BOYD, G. S. and OLIVER, M. F. (1960). *J. Endocr.* **21**, 25

CARVER, M. J., FREEMAN, J. G. and SMITH, J. A. (1960). *Ann. intern. Med.* **53**, 462

CONSTANTINIDES, P., JOHNSON, C., FAHRINI, B. M., NAKASHIMA, R. and MacINTOSH, H. W. (1960). *Brit. med. J.* **1**, 535

CONSTANTINIDES, P. and SAUNDERS, P. (1958). *Arch. Path. (Chicago)*, **65**, 499

*COOK, R. P. (1958). 'Cholesterol.' New York: Academic Press

CORDAY, E., JAFFE, H. and IRVING, D. W. (1960). *Arch. intern. Med.* **106**, 809

CUTHBERTSON, W. F. J., ELCOATE, P. V., IRELAND, D. M., MILLS, D. C. B. and SHEARLEY, P. (1960). *J. Endocr.* **21**, 45 and 69

DRILL, V. A., COOK, D. L. and EDGREN, R. A. (1959). In 'Hormones and Atherosclerosis', p. 247. Ed. Pincus, G. New York: Academic Press

EDER, H. E. (1959). In 'Hormones and Atherosclerosis', p. 335. Ed. Pincus, G. New York: Academic Press

FIELD, H., SWELL, L., SCHOOLS, P. E. and TREADWELL, C. R. (1960). *Circulation,* **22,** 547

*FLOREY, H. (1960). *Brit. med. J.* **2,** 1329

HATCH, F. T., ABELL, L. L. and KENDALL, F. E. (1955). *Amer. J. Med.* **19,** 48

HOLLANDER, W., CHOBANIAN, A. V. and WILKINS, R. W. (1960). *J. Amer. med. Ass.* **174,** 5

KEYS, A., ANDERSON, J. T. and GRANDE, F. (1958). *Lancet,* **2,** 959

KINLEY, L. J. and KRAUSE, R. F. (1959). *Proc. Soc. exp. Biol. (N.Y.),* **102,** 353

KORN, E. D. (1958). In 'Chemistry of Lipids', ed. Page, I. M. Springfield, Ill.: Thomas

KRITCHEVSKY, D. (1960). *Metabolism,* **9,** 984

MALMROS, H. and WIGAND, G. (1957). *Lancet,* **2,** 1

MELBY, J. C., AYR, M. S. and DALE, S. L. (1961). *New Engl. J. Med.* **264,** 583

MUSCHENHEIM, C., ADVOCATE, S. and HOSKINS, D. W. (1960). *Circulat. Res.* **8,** 759

OLIVER, M. F. and BOYD, G. S. (1957). *Lancet,* **1,** 124

OLIVER, M. F. and BOYD, G. S. (1959). In 'Hormones and Atherosclerosis', p. 403. Ed. Pincus, G. New York: Academic Press

PAGE, I. H. (1958). 'Cholesterol', p. 427. New York: Academic Press

PARSONS, W. B. (1958). *Circulation,* **18,** 489

POPJÁK, G. and CORNFORTH, J. W. (1960). *Advanc. Enzymol.* **22,** 281

POPJÁK, G., CORNFORTH, R. H. and CLIFFORD, K. (1960). *Lancet,* **1,** 1270

RUTHSTEIN, D. D., INGENITO, E. and MARTINELLI, M. (1958). *Lancet,* **1,** 545

SCHADE, H. and SALTMAN, P. (1959). *Proc. Soc. exp. Biol. (N.Y.),* **102,** 265

SCHÖN, H. (1958). *Nature (Lond.),* **82,** 534

STARR, P., ROEN, P., FREIBRUN, J. L. and SCHEISSNER, L. A. (1960). *Arch. intern. Med.* **105,** 830

STERNBERG, P., FREDRICKSON, D. S. and AVIGAN, J. (1958). *Proc. Soc. exp. Biol. (N.Y.),* **97,** 784

TOMKINS, G. M., NICHOLS, C. W., CHAPMAN, D. D., HOTTA, S. and CHAIKOFF, I. L. (1957). *Science,* **125,** 936

TURPEINEN, O., ROINE, P., PEKKARINEN, M., KARVONEN, M. J., RAUTANEN, Y., RUNEBERG, J. and ALIVIRTA, P. (1960). *Lancet,* **1,** 196

TYGSTRUP, N., WINKLER, K. and WARBURG, E. (1959). *Lancet,* **1,** 503

WALLACH, E. E., LUBASH, G. D., COHEN, B. D. and RUBIN, A. L. (1958). *J. Amer. med. Ass.* **167,** 1921

WRIGHT, L. D. and CLELAND, M. (1957). *Proc. Soc. exp. Biol. (N.Y.),* **96,** 219

CHAPTER 10

HYPOTENSIVE DRUGS

In the last few years there have been three major developments in the treatment of hypertension: the introduction of non-quaternary ganglion blocking agents, of compounds blocking postganglionic sympathetic nerves and of diuretics, more especially those belonging to the benzo-thiadiazine group. In addition the discovery of the hypotensive action of α-methyldopa and of the amine oxidase inhibitors has introduced possibilities which still need to be assessed. In the following account work published subsequent to 1957 will be principally considered; for earlier work the reader is referred to the Symposium edited by Harington (1957). The clinical aspects of the subject have been reviewed recently by Pickering, Cranston and Pears (1961) and by Aviado (1961).

GANGLION BLOCKING DRUGS

Of the quaternary ammonium compounds, those most convenient clinically for the prolonged treatment of hypertension are pentolinium, chlorisondamine, pentacynium and trimethidinium. All have the disadvantage that they are poorly absorbed from the alimentary canal, their action is therefore variable and unpredictable and they are liable to cause constipation and occasionally, ileus. Poor absorption is likely with all quaternary compounds, and the search for ganglion blocking agents has therefore been extended to tertiary and secondary amines and has resulted in the introduction of mecamylamine and pempidine. The absorption of these substances is indeed much more complete and their action more consistent and predictable. Their disadvantages are largely confined to the paralysis of the parasympathetic system. All attempts to find a ganglion blocking agent which has an action predominently on sympathetic synapses leaving parasympathetic synapses little affected, have so far proved unsuccessful, and it seems likely that these synapses are so similar in their mechanism that drugs blocking one will also block the other. However, with the introduction of bretylium and guanethidine, hypotensive agents have become available which have a marked action on adrenergic nerves and little effect on other nervous tissue. They are therefore free from many of the unpleasant effects of ganglion blocking agents though, with greater experience, other disadvantages have been disclosed and it cannot be said that a thoroughly satisfactory hypotensive agent has yet been found.

GANGLION BLOCKING DRUGS—QUATERNARY AMMONIUM
COMPOUNDS

Pentolinium, chlorisondamine and the short acting compound *trimeta-phan* (Arfonad) were described in the last edition of this book (Robson and Keele, 1956); more recent members of this group have little clinical value but will be described briefly.

Pentacynium (Presidal)

This is an unsymmetrical bisonium compound. Its pharmacological properties have been described by Green (1956) and its action on normal subjects and in the treatment of hypertension by McKendrick and Jones (1958). The hypotensive action reaches a maximum in about

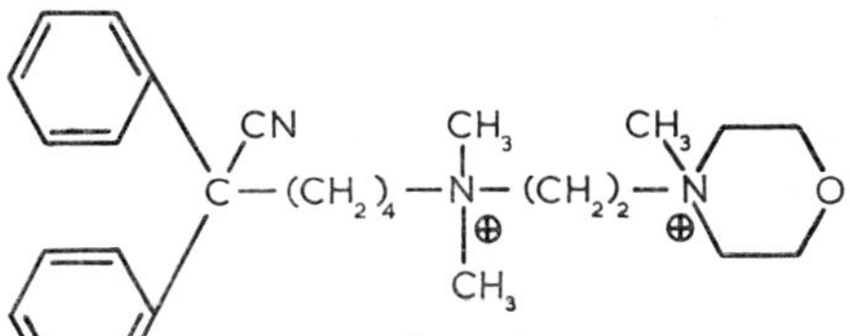

pentacynium

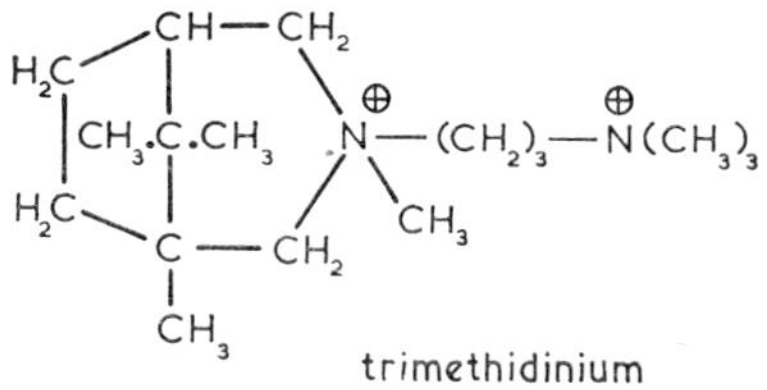

trimethidinium

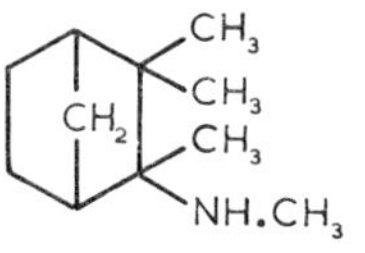

mecamylamine

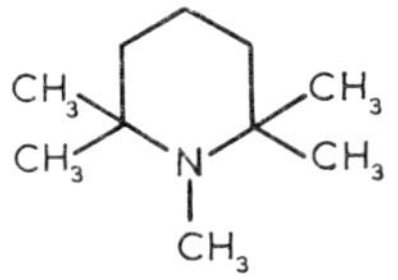

pempidine

an hour whether the drug is given by subcutaneous injection or by mouth. Its potency when given by injection is similar to that of chlorisondamine and mecamylamine, but given by mouth the dose needs to be increased 10 to 20 times to produce the same effect. The side effects observed with it are similar to those observed with other ganglion blocking agents.

Trimethidinium (Ostensin)

Trimethidinium (Ostensin), also an unsymmetrical bisonium compound with a long action, is similar to pentacynium in action. Treatment of hypertension with it has been described by Dunsmore *et al.* (1958).

Phenactropinium (Trophenium)

Phenactropinium (Trophenium), a quaternary derivative of homatropine, has a short action and has been used to produce hypotension during surgical operations. Clinically it appears to have no advantages over trimetaphan (Robertson and Armitage, 1959). It inhibits both pseudo- and true-cholinesterase and might therefore modify the action of muscle relaxants (Lehmann and Patston, 1958).

GANGLION BLOCKING DRUGS—NON-QUATERNARY
COMPOUNDS

Mecamylamine (formula p. 307)

Mecamylamine is a secondary amine, and is rapidly and completely absorbed from the intestinal tract. This is shown by the fact that after an oral dose none can be detected in the faeces and the action of a certain dose, whether given orally or parenterally, is the same. The plasma concentration is lower than would be expected from a uniform distribution throughout the body water and in experiments with rats the concentration in lung, kidney, spleen and heart was found to be considerably above that in the plasma. These results are explained by the penetration of mecamylamine into cells and its concentration there by fixation to intracellular protein (Milne *et al.*, 1957). This intracellular binding of mecamylamine may also explain its more gradual but sustained action compared with the quaternary compounds which do not penetrate cells to any extent. It also passes across the placenta into the foetus and into the cerebro-spinal fluid (Muggleton and Reading, 1959).

Mecamylamine is mainly eliminated by excretion in the urine but this is slow and incomplete. Only 37% of a single, injected dose given in man was recovered in the first 24 hours and appreciable amounts continued to be excreted in the next 24 hours. Excretion is depressed in renal failure and when the urine is rendered alkaline, whether this is done by the administration of sodium bicarbonate or by acetazolamide. The administration of ammonium chloride, resulting in an acid urine, increases excretion and the clearance may then exceed the glomerular filtration rate. Baer *et al.* (1956) explain this by tubular reabsorption when the urine is alkaline and secretion when it is acid. Milne *et al.* (1958) on the other hand suggest that this change in excretion with pH may reflect changes in ionization of the compound. If only the unionized form of the base were freely diffusible, diffusion into a more acid medium would be facilitated; thus an acid urine would increase excretion. The increased plasma concentration found by Payne and Rowe (1957) in cats after inhalation of 10% carbon dioxide may be similarly explained by the passage of intracellular amine into the more acid blood.

The action of mecamylamine at the neuromuscular junction and at the superior cervical ganglion has been investigated by Bennett *et al.* (1957). They found that mecamylamine potentiates the action of tubocurarine at the former site and modifies the action of depolarizing relaxants like suxamethonium, so that their action resembles that of tubocurarine, in that it can be antagonized by neostigimine. They also found that the response of the nictitating membrane to repeated stimulation of the preganglionic cervical sympathetic during partial blockade of the ganglion by hexamethonium, differed from the response when mecamylamine was used, and conclude that the action of mecamy-lamine at these sites is not produced by competition with acetylcholine but by modification of the cell on which the transmitter acts.

In *clinical use* the action of mecamylamine differs from that of the quaternary ammonium compounds in being slower of onset. Usually this is no disadvantage and the sustained action which it shows, together with the complete absorption from the gut, makes an even action more easily attainable, but when a rapid reduction in blood pressure is required a quaternary compound would be preferable. Of the usual concomitants of ganglionic blockade, constipation is the most troublesome and a number of cases of paralytic ileus have been reported. Tremor, mental confusion and delirium have been described by Harington and Kincaid-Smith (1958) in cases where large doses had been given to patients with impaired renal function. In these patients excretion was probably delayed. Mecamylamine is known to be con-centrated in the brain and the development of cerebral symptoms may be attributable to high concentrations in the brain.

Pempidine (formula p. 307)

Pempidine is a tertiary amine and was introduced by Corne and Edge (1958) and by Spinks *et al.* (1958). It is one of a number of poly-alkylpiperidines with ganglion blocking activity. The absorption, distribution and excretion of it has been described by Harington *et al.* (1958). Like mecamylamine its absorption from the gastrointestinal tract is complete but its excretion is more rapid and two-thirds of a single dose given either orally or by injection is excreted in the urine within 24 hours. Excretion is decreased when the urine is made alkaline by the administration of bicarbonate or acetazolamide but changes in reaction have less effect on excretion than they have with mecamylamine. It is not bound by plasma proteins and although concentrated in cells, the tissue/plasma ratios are lower than with mecamylamine. This may partly explain the more rapid excretion and also the more rapid onset of its action. Since elimination is nearly entirely by excretion through the kidney, it is very dependent on renal function. It is depressed in uraemia and also when, as a result of overdosage, there is severe hypotension.

In animal experiments pempidine has a weak neuromuscular blocking action and like mecamylamine potentiates the action of tubocurarine. On the superior cervical ganglion it has a similar, though weaker and more prolonged action than hexamethonium. Whether the prolonged effect is due to a difference in its mode of action or to slow release of drug bound in the ganglion cell has not been determined. Spinks *et al.* (1958) found that pempidine is roughly twice as potent as mecamylamine in blocking the superior cervical ganglion and pressor reflexes but only

11

half as potent in causing tremors and death from respiratory depression. This may be correlated with the lower concentrations of pempidine found in the brain.

Clinically, pempidine has been found effective in treating hypertensive patients. Harington *et al.* (1958) found that four oral doses daily between 7 a.m. and 10 p.m. were required to maintain a steady hypotensive action because of rapid excretion but this had the merit of allowing more rapid stabilization than can safely be done with the more slowly excreted mecamylamine. Moreover toxic effects passed off more quickly. These were all of the kind common with other ganglionic blocking drugs. Tolerance did not appear to develop with prolonged use.

DRUGS BLOCKING ADRENERGIC NERVES

Xylocholine

In 1952 Brown and Hey reported the properties of a series of choline ethers (see Hey and Willey, 1954). These included choline 2, 6-xylyl ether bromide (xylocholine, T.M. 10) which abolished the response of the cat nictitating membrane to postganglionic stimulation. The substance was found to have a powerful and long lasting local anaesthetic action and its action on sympathetic nerves was at first ascribed to this. More recently evidence has accumulated that this explanation

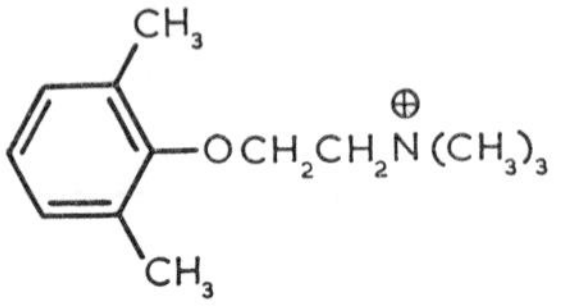

xylocholine

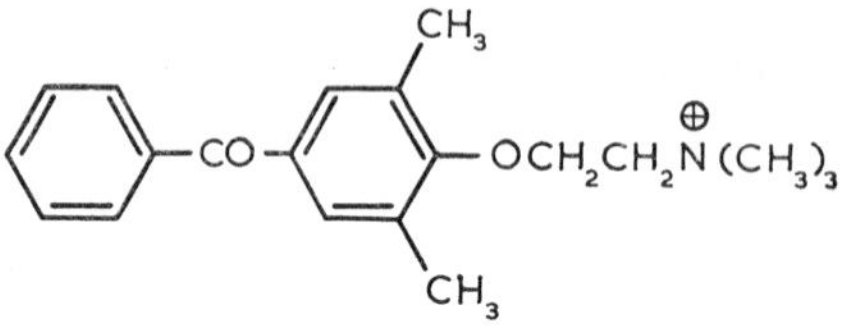

BW172C58

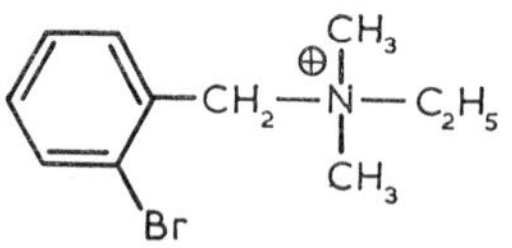

bretylium

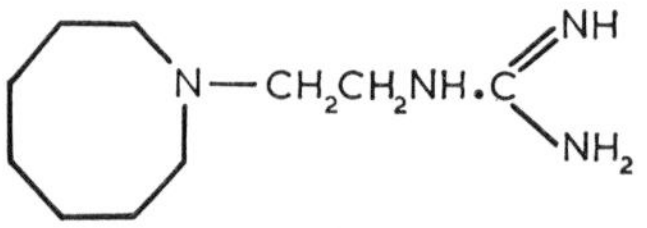

guanethidine

was incorrect (Bain, 1960) and that blockade of adrenergic nerves is brought about by depression of noradrenaline synthesis, most probably at the last step, the formation of noradrenaline from dopamine (see p. 98). Xylocholine has a variety of other actions. In addition to its local anaesthetic action it has muscarinic and nicotinic actions and is a weak antagonist of noradrenaline, acetylcholine and histamine. These actions limit its usefulness and McLean *et al.* (1960) have found that muscarinic activity can be reduced by methylation of the α- or β-carbon atoms in the chain. The α-compound has only a weak sympathetic blocking action but the β-compound is as potent in this respect as xylocholine.

The 4-benzoyl derivative of xylocholine (BW 172C58) also blocks adrenergic nerves and in animal experiments is 10 to 20 times as potent as xylocholine (Boura *et al.*, 1960a). Its action, which is similar to that of bretylium (*v. infra*) but more rapid in onset and shorter in duration, is however weak in man.

The discovery of substances with a specific action on adrenergic nerves provoked attempts to find a compound which might be effective in reducing vascular tone without having the other actions of xylocholine. Bretylium and guanethedine are two of the products of this search though their mode of action may be different.

Bretylium (formula p. 310)

The pharmacological properties of bretylium have been summarized by Green (1960). Like xylocholine it is a benzyl quaternary ammonium compound and is available as the *p*-toluene sulphonate (tosylate). It blocks postganglionic adrenergic nerves without depressing the sensitivity of the end organ to injected adrenaline or noradrenaline. Its action is thus different from that of substances like dibenyline and phentolamine, and unlike them can be reversed by noradrenaline infusion. The blocking action develops slowly, taking about 20 minutes to reach a maximum after the subcutaneous injection of 10 mg./kg. in a cat, and is accompanied by an accumulation of the drug in the nerve and a depression in the release of noradrenaline from its ending. These three changes disappear together during the subsequent hour. When large doses are given to animals with low sympathetic tone, a transient sympathomimetic action is to be seen which precedes block (Gaffney, 1961).

With repeated administration of bretylium additional changes are observed: increasing tolerance to bretylium, increasing sensitivity to injected adrenaline and noradrenaline and a gradual depletion of nerves and ganglia of their noradrenaline. These changes, occurring together, have a similarity to the results of nerve section. A further resemblance is in the decreased sensitivity to tyramine seen in both circumstances.

The development of tolerance to bretylium has been found to be a serious defect in the clinical use of the drug and is probably due to the increasing sensitivity of end organs to circulating and to locally liberated catechol amines.

The mode of action of bretylium in blocking adrenergic nerves by diminishing the release of noradrenaline at the endings is still not clear. Topical application of bretylium to nerves shows that conduction in non-adrenergic nerves can also be blocked but according to Boura *et al.* (1960b) they are in general less sensitive. The concentration in these nerves when the block develops is similar to that found in blocked adrenergic nerves and it therefore appears that the action may be similar to that of a local anaesthetic. The particular sensitivity of adrenergic nerves when the drug is given systemically is due to the very much higher concentration of the drug in them than in other nervous tissue (see also p. 112).

Intravenous injections in *man* in doses of 0·5 mg./kg. cause no change in the blood pressure of the supine subject but postural hypotension develops in about 10 minutes and persists up to 5 hours. The effect of bretylium on the blood flow through forearm and hand has been investigated by Blair *et al.* (1960) and by French and Matthews (1961), using venous occlusion plethysmography and the intra-arterial infusion of the drug. At first there was a small reduction in flow but after about ½ hour it increased to a level somewhat above that in the uninjected limb. When the infusion was made into an acutely nerve blocked forearm, the flow, at first very large compared with the control forearm because of the removal of constrictor tone, was reduced to a level similar to that on the control side, indicating a vasoconstrictor action of bretylium. However, a limb treated with bretylium alone failed to respond to a variety of procedures, such as the Valsava manoeuvre or general body heating and cooling, which normally change sympathetic tone reflexly. From these results Blair *et al.* conclude that the peripheral vascular actions of bretylium consist of a vasoconstrictor action and a longer lasting blocking action on sympathetic nerves.

Oral administration of bretylium has no effect on supine blood pressure but the blood pressure in the erect position usually falls in both normal and hypertensive subjects. The fall is however variable probably due to incomplete and irregular absorption. Dollery *et al.* (1960a) found that whereas about 75% of an intravenous dose can be recovered from the urine only 10 to 15% of an oral dose could be recovered. With impaired renal function the proportion recovered was less.

In the treatment of hypertensive patients sudden and unpredictable falls in blood pressure are not uncommon and are particularly undesirable in patients with occlusive vascular disease. A sudden fall in blood pressure is also likely to occur after exercise. The reason for this is not entirely clear but the following explanation has been suggested by Folkow (1960). During exercise, vasodilatation and the loss of blood volume caused by increased filtration from the vessels into the tissues of the exercised muscles calls for a considerable redistribution of vasomotor tone. In the absence of normal sympathetic innervation this is hampered and pooling of blood with a fall in cardiac output results.

Numerous side effects have been reported but these are less troublesome than those caused by ganglion blocking drugs as there is no interference with the parasympathetic system. Dollery *et al.* (1960a) concluded that two-thirds of their patients were not subjectively troubled to any important extent. Nausea and nasal stuffiness are not uncommon. Parotid tenderness and pain, accentuated by eating, has been frequently reported but has received so far no adequate explanation. Muscular weakness may be severe: it is sometimes associated with hypotension but not always. Campbell and Montuschi (1960) report a case in which there was electromyographic evidence of a lack of function of some of the muscle fibres in each motor unit. This, together with the similar change in the skeletal muscles of experimental animals treated with bretylium, reported by Vernikos-Danellis and Zaimis (1960), suggests that in some cases muscular weakness may be due to an action on skeletal muscles.

Bretylium is mainly excreted in the urine unchanged and so far no products of metabolism have been found (Duncombe and McCoubrey, 1960).

The low incidence of side effects made bretylium appear a valuable drug when it was first introduced but the variability of the response, leading to poor control or hypotensive attacks, the development of tolerance and the failure to bring about a satisfactory fall in blood pressure in a proportion of the patients has limited its use.

Guanethidine (formula p. 310)

This is a guanidine derivative and is structurally dissimilar from the foregoing compounds; and although its action resembles that of bretylium superficially, in that it diminishes sympathetic tone, the means by which this is brought about is probably quite different.

The immediate effect of an injection of 10 to 15 mg./kg. into an experimental animal is probably the release of catechol amines, for there is a rise in blood pressure and a contraction of the nictitating membrane, both effects being prevented by a previous injection of phentolamine. Moreover in the rabbit it causes a contraction of the non-gravid uterus (as does adrenaline) which is also abolished by phentolamine or by the previous treatment of the animal with reserpine. Following these changes there is a fall in blood pressure associated with a diminished response of the nictitating membrane to both pre- and post-ganglionic stimulation of the cervical sympathetic. Electrical recording from the post-ganglionic nerve during pre-ganglionic stimulation shows that, although conduction through the ganglion can be depressed, much larger doses are required than for inhibition of the nictitating membrane and the effect is much more transitory. The main site of action is thus distal to the ganglion but, although guanethidine has some local anaesthetic action, this appears to be too weak to explain the effects on the nictitating membrane.

Vascular reflexes, such as the pressor response to carotid occlusion and in man the cold pressor response and the reflex results of the Valsalva manoeuvre, are depressed. There is a reduction in cardiac output but no fall in peripheral resistance. In man too the fall in blood pressure is much less in the supine than in the erect position and is associated with a fall in cardiac output (Dollery *et al.*, 1961a) but little change in peripheral resistance. Page *et al.* (1961) point out that these findings would be explicable if the fall in cardiac output were mediated by diminished sympathetic tone in the veins and the pooling of blood in them. Guanethidine reduces the concentration of catechol amines in spleen, heart and arteries (see p. 112) and it has been suggested that the hypotensive effect, like that of reserpine, is brought about by depletion of noradrenaline stores, but Boura *et al.* (1961) point out that this is not an entirely satisfactory explanation. Guanethidine has no effect on the concentration of catechol amines in adrenal glands, nor does it affect their concentration or that of 5-hydroxytryptamine in the brain (Bein, 1960), into which it does not penetrate in any appreciable amount (Brodie and Kuntzman, 1960). Sensitivity to circulating noradrenaline, adrenaline and angiotensin is increased, but to tyramine and ephedrine it is diminished.

Dollery *et al.* (1960b) found that after an oral dose of guanethidine 36% was excreted in the urine in 72 hours and 20 to 25% in the faeces. In the same interval 72% of an injected dose can be recovered from the urine. Absorption from the intestine is thus incomplete but is appreciably better than the absorption of bretylium. Its action comes on more slowly than that of bretylium and continues for 3 to 4 days; this permits administration as a single daily dose when small doses only are needed.

Attacks of faintness and giddiness due to excessive fall in blood pressure have been most troublesome after exercise, as with bretylium (q.v.), or on first rising in the morning. A reduction in dose to overcome this may lead to poor control late in the day or while the patient is in bed.

The commonest side effect is looseness of the bowels but this rarely amounts to frank diarrhoea and when severe may be controlled by a small daily dose of pempidine or of codeine phosphate. Page *et al.* (1961) found that bradycardia was common and that it could be abolished by atropine. Parotid pain, nasal stuffiness and general weakness occur, as with bretylium, but possibly less frequently. A gain in weight due to fluid retention is not uncommon and Dollery *et al.* (1960b) report that 4 patients out of 80 developed the clinical picture of congestive heart failure without paroxysmal dyspnoea (Fig. 48). In some, fluid retention was accompanied by a rise in the blood pressure, which had previously been well controlled. Leishman *et al.* (1961) found that the administration of a benzothiadiazine diuretic caused a diuresis, a reduction in weight and a reduction in blood pressure, and recommend the regular weighing of patients on guanethidine to detect fluid retention and to distinguish failure of blood pressure control due to this cause from the development of true tolerance. Failure of ejaculation has been reported with both bretylium and guanethidine. The pressor action of guanethidine on injection makes this route of administration dangerous in hypertensive subjects and ganglion blocking drugs are preferable if a rapid fall in blood pressure is necessary.

One advantage of guanethidine over bretylium is that there is little evidence of the development of tolerance. Of 114 patients observed by Leishman *et al.* for more than 6 months, 71 were well controlled; only 8 had abandoned treatment.

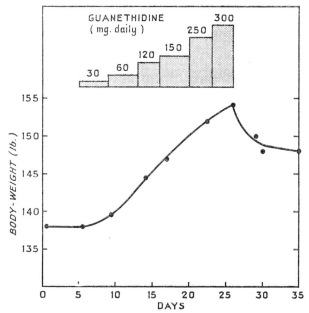

FIG. 48. Weight of a hypertensive patient who developed heart failure during treatment with guanethidine (Dollery *et al.*, 1960).

Reserpine

Reserpine which is also discussed on p. 48, has been much used in the treatment of hypertension. It causes a moderate fall in blood pressure which develops gradually: after an intravenous injection in an experimental animal the blood pressure may continue to fall for 1 to 3 hours. In acute experiments this is due to a fall in peripheral resistance but in man, Schuman (1954) has reported a reduction in cardiac output after prolonged treatment and Zaimis (1961) has described a toxic action on the myocardium in cats given 1 mg./kg. daily.

The cause of the fall in peripheral resistance has been ascribed to both a central and a peripheral action and has been linked with the loss from the tissues of catechol amines and of 5-hydroxytryptamine. This occurs both in the central nervous system, in peripheral nerves and in the adrenal medulla (p. 113). Recent work makes it probable that there is a fall in sympathetic tone after the administration of reserpine and that this is mainly due to the depletion of stores of catechol amines from adrenergic neurones and other peripheral sites. Muscholl and Vogt (1958) have shown that adrenergic neurones fail to excite the tissues they innervate when their store of amine is reduced to 10% or less. Moreover Iggo and Vogt (1960) found no reduction in the traffic in preganglionic sympathetic nerves in anaesthetized cats which had been treated for several days with reserpine in doses which cause severe amine depletion. They therefore concluded that there was little reduction in central sympathetic activity. If the results of these experiments are applicable to man it would appear that the central actions of reserpine contribute little to its hypotensive action. This subject is further discussed by Brodie and Kuntzman (1960).

The intravenous or intramuscular injection of reserpine in man causes a fall in blood pressure starting after about an hour and reaching a maximum in about 4 hours. With the oral administration of 1 mg. daily the blood pressure may continue to fall for 2 weeks or more and the hypotension may persist for up to 4 weeks after discontinuing medication. Tolerance does not develop.

Side effects with reserpine are common and the following have been reported: drowsiness, nasal congestion, nightmares, diarrhoea, oedema, flushing, Parkinsonism and depression. The latter may be severe and cases of suicide have been reported. As with other hypotensive agents, vascular reflexes are depressed and severe hypotension has been seen in patients on reserpine during anaesthesia and in late pregnancy (Editorial, 1961).

The value of reserpine in the treatment of hypertension is disputed. Its main value is probably in conjunction with other more potent hypotensive agents to enable the dose of these to be reduced and so to diminish side effects. When reserpine is used it is important to remember that all effects develop slowly and will be lost slowly when administration is discontinued, and that the depleted amines may not be restored for three weeks or more.

Other rauwolfia alkaloids, structurally similar to reserpine, are available and derivatives of reserpine have been prepared. Rescinnamine, deserpidine, syrosingopine and methoserpidine (10-methoxy-deserpidine) have been used in the treatment of hypertension. Side effects may be less with some of these substances but there is at present no convincing evidence that they have any advantage over reserpine.

SOME OTHER HYPOTENSIVE DRUGS

α-methyl dopa

The action of xylocholine in depressing the action of sympathetic nerves by inhibition of noradrenaline synthesis has been described above. Noradrenaline synthesis can also be depressed at an earlier stage by the use of inhibitors of dopa decarboxylase. This enzyme is responsible for the formation of dopamine, the immediate precursor of noradrenaline, from dopa. A number of inhibitors are known and are discussed on pages 18 and 128. One of these is α-methyl dopa and its administration was found to cause a fall in blood pressure. It depletes stores of noradrenaline and 5-HT both in the brain and peripherally (Goldberg *et al.*, 1960) but whether or not its hypotensive action is due to decarboxylase inhibition has not yet been established. Its use in the treatment of hypertension has been reported by Gillespie (1960) and by Oates *et al.* (1960) who found that with doses of 750 mg. to 4 G. daily postural hypotension, with little change in the recumbent blood pressure, developed in two days and was accompanied by sedation as in animal experiments. A depressive state occurred in three out of 40 subjects but this cleared up on discontinuing the drug. Excretion is rapid and doses need to be given 8 hourly. According to Gillespie only about 20% of an oral dose is absorbed. In a report on a recent trial on 15 hypertensive patients, Irvine *et al.* (1962) comment on the fact that both lying and standing blood pressure were equally reduced and that there was little postural hypotension. They found α-methyl dopa a valuable hypotensive, more especially for patients who do not respond adequately to rauwolfia alkaloids or diuretics. Though less potent than guanethidine, its side effects in their cases were of a minor nature and of short duration. The introduction of this substance is an interesting approach to the problem of devising a hypotensive drug, derived as it is from recent fundamental work on the synthesis and storage of catechol amines.

Diuretics

The newer diuretics are discussed in detail in chapter 7 (p. 235), where their formulae are given. In this section their action in relation to the treatment of hypertension will be described briefly.

Chlorothiazide and other benzothiadiazine diuretics will cause a fall in both systolic and diastolic pressure in some cases of hypertension; and Smirk *et al.* (1960) report that 15% of a group of 203 patients could be managed satisfactorily on chlorothiazide or hydrochlorothiazide alone. Used in conjunction with some more potent hypotensive drug, such as a ganglion blocking agent, they enable the blood pressure to be controlled in a larger proportion of cases and the doses of the hypotensive drug to be reduced.

The combination of chlorothiazide with a ganglion blocking agent is often very effective, but the cause of the potentiation is not entirely clear. Tapia *et al.* (1957) and Dustan *et al.* (1959) concluded that it is caused by sodium depletion and a reduction of blood volume. This has been supported by Dollery *et al.* (1959) who measured in hypertensive patients the fall in blood pressure caused by an intravenous injection of pentolinium both before and after they had been put on chlorothiazide. They found that only those patients whose blood volume was reduced during treatment with chlorothiazide became more sensitive to pentolinium, and that this sensitivity was lost when the blood volume was restored to its original value by an infusion of dextran. Hollander *et al.* (1960) however state that the blood pressure does not reach its initial level on replacing fluid and electrolytes and believe that there must be some other mechanism as well. Varnauskas *et al.* (1961) find that the fall in peripheral resistance on exercise is much smaller in hypertensive subjects than in normals and that after chlorothiazide the response of hypertensives is more nearly normal. They therefore suggest that chlorothiazide acts directly on the peripheral resistance. This view gains some support from the report of Rubin *et al.* (1961) of a newly synthesized benzothiadiazine with hypotensive but without diuretic properties. Evidence is needed however that the hypotensive action of this substance is similar to that of the diuretics. With mecamylamine, and probably also with pempidine, still another action has been suggested by Harington and Kincaid-Smith (1958). The excretion of the non-quaternary compounds is depressed, as explained above, by a rise in the pH of the urine; and chlorothiazide, probably because of its action as a carbonic anhydrase inhibitor, renders the urine more alkaline during the first few days of its administration, and the excretion of mecamylamine falls temporarily. This effect of diuretics on the excretion and distribution of ganglion blocking agents has been further investigated by Dollery, Emslie-Smith and Muggleton (1961b).

Chlorothiazide and related drugs are useful alone for treating mild cases of hypertension, or in conjunction with other drugs to obtain an adequate and well maintained effect with less severe side effects. The principal danger in the use of these diuretics is the production of potassium depletion. This can be guarded against by giving potassium chloride by mouth.

Amine oxidase inhibitors (see p. 57)

Postural hypotension is sometimes seen as an unwanted effect in the treatment of psychiatric patients with some amine oxidase inhibitors (see p. 75) and iproniazid has been used successfully in the treatment of hypertension. However, with other less toxic hypotensive substances available its use is probably not justified. Gillespie (1960) has found that pheniprazine has a consistent and powerful hypotensive action. This is unexpected from its action on the cardiovascular system of dogs (p. 66) which is more in accord with its amphetamine-like structure; but the effects of acute and chronic administration may well be different. The hypotension is accompanied by an elevation of mood and an increase in appetite, which by increasing activity and weight may be undesirable, and cases of retrobulbar neuritis and toxic hepatitis have been reported. Phenelzine, serine-*N*-isopropylhydrazine and tranylcypromine also cause postural hypotension in man. With the exception of tranylcypromine, all the substances mentioned are hydrazine derivatives and it may well be that their hypotensive action does not result from amine oxidase inhibition but is an independent action. Sjoerdsma (1960) suggests two possible mechanisms. Amine oxidase inhibitors, when given in high doses, depress conduction through the superior cervical ganglion (Gertner, 1961) and might therefore depress sympathetic tone. They also depress inactivation of dopamine, which is probably mainly brought about by amine oxidase, and the accumulation of this weakly pressor catechol amine might lead to the blocking of noradrenaline receptors.

The use of amine oxidase inhibitors in the treatment of hypertension is still in the experimental stage and further clinical assessment is needed before an opinion on its value can be expressed.

Mebutamate (2-methyl-2-*sec*-butyl-1,3-propanediol dicarbamate)

This compound differs from meprobromate by the substitution of a secondary butyl group for the propyl group in the latter compound; it was investigated because of the weak hypotensive action of meprobromate. Berger *et al.* (1961) report that it lowers the blood pressure of normal laboratory animals and of animals rendered chronically hypertensive by constriction of a renal artery and by the implantation of desoxycorticosterone acetate. From a variety of experiments they conclude that it acts on the brain stem vasomotor centres and that it does not alter cardiac output or have any important action on the autonomic nervous system. It caused a fall in both systolic and diastolic pressure in six hypertensive patients to whom it was administered orally, but further clinical assessment has not yet been reported.

CONCLUSION

A number of new compounds able to lower the blood pressure in hypertension have been discovered in the last few years. Some act in ways that are so far incompletely elucidated, but which are evidently quite different from those of established hypotensive drugs and thus present, not only a new field for the development of more effective and more convenient substances for the treatment of a common disease, but are already setting interesting problems in the mechanism of the actions of the sympathetic system and the maintenance of the blood pressure.

REFERENCES
* Denotes review

*Aviado, D. M. (1961). *Am. J. Med. Sci.* **241**, 650
Baer, J. E., Paulson, S. F., Russo, H. F. and Beyer, K. H. (1956). *Amer. J. Physiol.* **186**, 180

BAIN, W. B. (1960) in Adrenergic Mechanisms. Ed. Vane, J. R. London: Churchill
BEIN, H. (1960) in Adrenergic Mechanisms. Ed. Vane, J. R. London: Churchill
BENNETT, G., TYLER, C. and ZAIMIS, E. (1957). *Lancet,* **2,** 218
BERGER, F. M., DOUGLAS, J. F., KLETZKIN, M., LUDWIG, B. J. and MARGOLIN, S. (1961). *J. Pharmacol. exp. Ther.* **134,** 356
BLAIR, D. A., GLOVER, W. E., KIDD, B. S. L. and RODDIE, I. C. (1960). *Brit. J. Pharmacol.* **15,** 466
BRODIE, B. B. and KUNTZMAN, R. (1960). *Ann. N.Y. Acad. Sci.* **88,** 939
BOURA, A. L. A., COKER, G. G., COPP, F. C., DUNCOMBE, W. G., ELPHICK, A. R., GREEN, A. F. and MCCOUBREY, A. (1960a). *Nature (Lond.),* **185,** 925
BOURA, A. L. A., COPP, F. C., DUNCOMBE, W. G., GREEN, A. F. and MCCOUBREY, A. (1960b). *Brit. J. Pharmacol.* **15,** 265
BOURA, A. L. A., COPP, F. C., GREEN, A. F., HODSON, H. F., RUFFELL, G. K., SIM, M. P., WALTON, E. and GRIVSKY, E. M. (1961). *Nature (Lond.),* **191,** 1312
CAMPBELL, E. D. R. and MONTUSCHI, E. (1960). *Lancet,* **2,** 789
CORNE, S. J. and EDGE, N. D. (1958). *Brit. J. Pharmacol.* **13,** 339
DOLLERY, C. T., HARINGTON, M. and KAUFMANN, G. (1959). *Lancet,* **1,** 1215
DOLLERY, C. T., EMSLIE-SMITH, D. and MCMICHAEL, J. (1960a). *Lancet,* **1,** 296
DOLLERY, C. T., EMSLIE-SMITH, D. and MILNE, M. D. (1960b). *Lancet,* **2,** 381
DOLLERY, C. T., EMSLIE-SMITH, D. and SHILLINGFORD, J. P. (1961a). *Lancet,* **2,** 331
DOLLERY, C. T., EMSLIE-SMITH, D. and MUGGLETON, D. F. (1961b). *Brit. J. Pharmacol,* **17,** 488
DUNCOMBE, W. G. and MCCOUBREY, A. (1960). *Brit. J. Pharmacol.* **15,** 260
DUNSMORE, R. A., DUNSMORE, L. D., GOLDMAN, A., ELIAS, M. and WARNER, R. S. (1958). *Am. J. med. Sc.* **236,** 483
DUSTAN, H. P., CUMMING, G. R., CORCORAN, A. C. and PAGE, I. H. (1959). *Circulation,* **19,** 360
EDITORIAL: *Brit. med. J.* 1961. **1,** 1022
FRENCH, E. B. and MATTHEWS, M. B. (1961). *Clin. Sci.* **21,** 151
FOLKOW, B. U. G. (1960) in Adrenergic Mechanisms. Ed. Vane, J. R. London: Churchill
GAFFNEY, T. E. (1961). *Circulation Res.* **9,** 83
GERTNER, S. B. (1961). *J. Pharmacol.* **131,** 223
GILLESPIE, L. (1960). *Ann. N.Y. Acad. Sc.* **88,** 1011
GOLDBERG, L. I., DA COSTA, F. M. and OZAKI, M. (1960). *Nature (Lond.),* **188,** 502
GREEN, A. F. (1956). In Hypotensive Drugs. Ed. Harington, M. London: Pergamon
GREEN, A. F. (1960). In Adrenergic Mechanisms. Ed. Vane, J. R. London: Churchill
*HARINGTON, M. (1957). Hypotensive Drugs. London: Pergamon
HARINGTON, M. and KINCAID-SMITH, P. (1958). *Lancet,* **1,** 403
HARINGTON, M., KINCAID-SMITH, P. and MILNE, M. D. (1958). *Lancet,* **2,** 6
HEY, P. and WILLEY, G. L. (1954). *Brit. J. Pharmacol.* **9,** 471
HOLLANDER, W., CHOBANIAN, A. V. and WILKINS, R. W. (1960). *Ann. N.Y. Acad. Sci.* **88,** 975
IGGO, A. and VOGT, M. (1960). *J. Physiol.* **150,** 114
IRVINE, R. O. H., O'BRIEN, K. P. and NORTH, J. D. K. (1962). *Lancet,* **1,** 300
LEHMANN, H. and PATSTON, V. J. (1958). *Brit. med. J.* **1,** 708.
LEISHMAN, A. W. D., MATTHEWS, H. L. and SMITH, A. J. (1961). *Lancet,* **2,** 4
MCKENDRICK, C. S. and JONES, P. O. (1958). *Lancet,* **1,** 340.
MCLEAN, R. A., GEUS, R. J., MOHRBACHER, R. J., MATTIS, P. A. and ULLYOT, G. E. (1960). *J. Pharmacol. exp. Ther.* **129,** 11
MCLEAN, R. A., GEUS, R. J., PASTERNACK, J., MATTIS, P. A. and ULLYOT, G. E. (1960). *J. Pharmacol. exp. Ther.* **129,** 17
MILNE, M. D., ROWE, G. G., SOMERS, K., MUEHRCKE, R. L. and CRAWFORD, M. A. (1957). *Clin. Sci.* **16,** 599
MILNE, M. D., SCRIBNER, B. H. and CRAWFORD, M. A. (1958). *Amer. J. Med.* **24,** 709
MUGGLETON, D. F. and READING, H. W. (1959). *Brit. J. Pharmacol.* **14,** 202

MUSCHOLL, E. and VOGT, M. (1958). *J. Physiol.* **141,** 132

OATES, J. A., GILLESPIE, L., UDENFRIEND, S. and SJOERDSMA, A. (1960). *Science,* **131,** 1890

PAGE, I. H., HURLEY, R. E. and DUSTAN, H. P. (1961). *J. Amer. med. Ass.* **175,** 543

PAYNE, J. P. and ROWE, G. G. (1957). *Brit. J. Pharmacol.* **12,** 457

*PICKERING, G. W., CRANSTON, W. I. and PEARS, M. A. (1961). The treatment of hypertension. Springfield: Thomas

ROBERTSON, J. D. and ARMITAGE, P. (1959). *Anaesthesia.* **14,** 53

ROBSON, J. M. and KEELE, C. A. (1956). Recent advances in Pharmacology, 2nd edition. London: Churchill

RUBIN, A. A., ROTH, F. E., WINBURY, M. M. (1961). *Nature (Lond.),* **192,** 176

SCHUMAN, H. (1954). *Klin. Wschr.* **32,** 220

SJOERDSMA, A. (1960). *Ann. N.Y. Acad. Sci.* **88**

SMIRK, F. H., MCQUEEN, E. G. and MORRISON, R. B. I. (1960). *Brit. med. J.* **1,** 515

SPINKS, A., YOUNG, E. H. P., FARRINGTON, J. A. and DUNLOP, D. (1958). *Brit. J. Pharmacol.* **13,** 501

TAPIA, F. A., DUSTAN, H. P., SCHNECKLOTH, R. A., CORCORAN, A. C. and PAGE, I. H. (1957). *Lancet,* **2,** 831

VARNAUSKAS, E., CRAMÉR, G., MALMCRONA, R. and WERKÖ, L. (1961). *Clin. Sci.* **20,** 407

VERNIKOS-DANELLIS, J. and ZAIMIS, E. (1960). *Lancet,* **2,** 787

ZAIMIS, E. (1961). *Nature (Lond.),* **192,** 521

CHAPTER 11
BACTERIAL CHEMOTHERAPY

In this chapter it is intended to review briefly some recent progress on substances used in bacterial chemotherapy, and this will include newer antibiotics and long acting sulphonamides. Though new antibiotics continue to be discovered, it is possible that this will not keep up with the development of resistant strains of organisms. The natural resistance of the subject also plays an important part in the combating of infections and it may well be that, with the increasing development of resistant bacteria, more emphasis will be laid on this aspect. A discussion of bacterial endotoxin, particularly its relation to non-specific increase in resistance to bacterial infection, will therefore be included in this chapter, and reference will also be made to results obtained in tuberculosis with surface active agents, since these are believed to enhance resistance to infection.

LONG ACTING SULPHONAMIDES

Following the discovery of the sulphonamides, many new derivatives were rapidly introduced, some of which possessed advantages which led to their continued clinical use, e.g. sulphadimidine, sulphadiazine, sodium sulphacetamide and the slowly absorbed sulphonamides used in intestinal conditions.

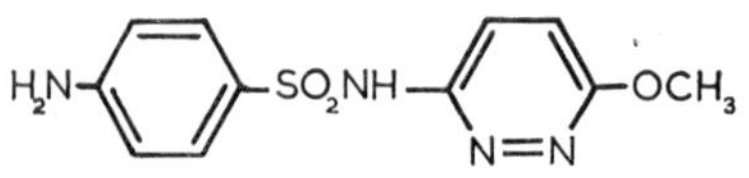

sulphamethoxypyridazine
(Midicel, Lederkyn, Kynex)

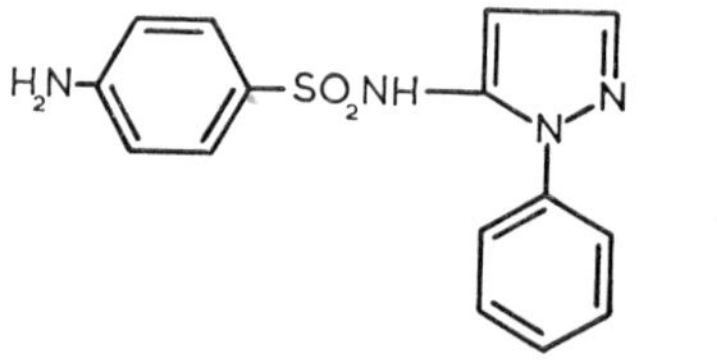

sulphaphenazole (Orisul)

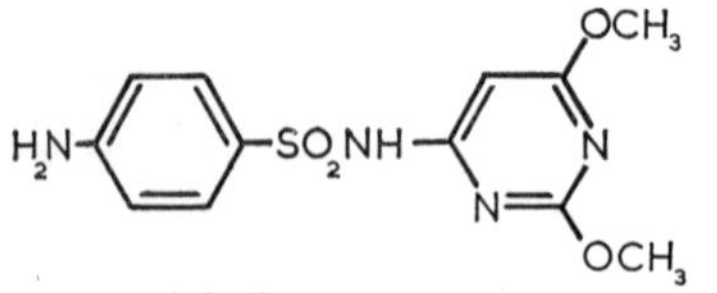

sulphadimethoxine (Madribon)

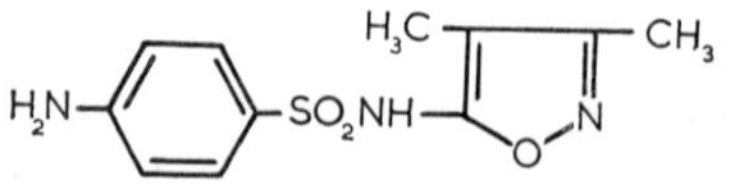

sulphafurazole (Gantrisin)

More recently, sulphonamides have been made which have a much more prolonged effect than the conventional ones (Editorial, 1959). Many findings are published in vol. 82 (1959) of the Annals of the New York Academy of Sciences. The formulae of the more important ones are shown above.

There are many factors which determine the value of a sulphonamide, e.g. intrinsic chemotherapeutic activity, blood and tissue concentrations, toxicity, etc. This is well illustrated by the careful experiments of Neipp *et al.* (1958) in which sulphaphenazole, sulphamethoxypyridazine and several other sulphonamides are compared. The results suggest that sulphaphenazole should have valuable therapeutic properties. Gold-hammer (1958) has made the interesting observation that the concentration of sulphaphenazole in various organs is appreciably higher than that in the serum, a finding which does not apply to sulphonamides like sulphadimidine. This may contribute to the long duration of action of sulphaphenazole and perhaps of other long acting sulphonamides.

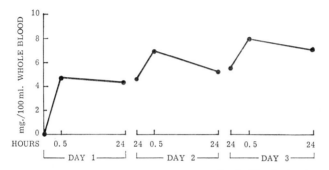

Fig. 49. Sulphamethoxypyridazine concentration in blood after 1 g. orally followed by 0·5 g. per 24 hours. (Finland *et al.*, 1957.)

The new sulphonamides have a chemotherapeutic activity which is equivalent to that of the most active conventional ones. Their prolonged effect is well illustrated by the work of Finland *et al.* (1957) on sulpha-methoxypyridazine. Fig. 49 shows the average blood levels obtained by the administration of an initial dose of 1·0 G. followed by 0·5 G. every 24 hours, and illustrates important clinical points, namely (1) the blood level gradually rises and may take a week to reach a maximum. This is also shown by the findings of Bogert and Gavin (1959) who also obtained evidence that this cumulation was more likely to occur in older subjects. (2) Following the first dose the blood level rises more slowly than with a conventional sulphonamide, so that in really acute infections a rapidly absorbed drug would be better, at least to start treatment. (3) There is marked individual variation in the blood level reached, as there is with other sulphonamides, but this needs more careful handling with the new drugs, since toxic effects are more likely with a long acting substance. (4) Little of the drug is acetylated. The compound is excreted quite slowly and urinary levels range around 20 mg. %. Great caution should therefore be used in patients with impaired renal function. It has also been found that the drug does not penetrate well into the cerebrospinal fluid and is thus unsatisfactory for the treatment of meningitis. Thus Rentchnick (1958) had to give 4 G. per day of sulphaphenazole to obtain a reasonable concentration in the cerebrospinal fluid. The properties described above suggest that the blood level of the new sulphonamides is more difficult to control than that of more rapidly eliminated drugs and toxic effects might be expected to be more common; this is in fact supported by the preliminary findings of Jackson and Grieble (1957) and Lindsay *et al.* (1958). On the other hand, Essellier *et al.* (1958) also investigated the fate of sulphaphenazole in man and treated many patients with this drug, and only rarely encountered side effects.

Newbould and Kilpatrick (1960) have found that some long acting sulphonamides are more extensively bound to plasma proteins than the older sulphonamides, such as sulphadimidine. Since the protein bound drug is chemotherapeutically inactive, this means that higher total plasma concentrations are needed with the newer drugs, thus increasing their liability to produce toxic effects.

It would be expected that long acting sulphonamides might be particularly suitable for prophylactic purposes when high blood levels are not required. Weekly doses of sulphadimethoxine (30 mg./kg.) were given by Lattimer *et al.* (1960) in the prevention of streptococcal infections in rheumatic patients, and appeared to be effective though 2 out of 28 patients developed symptoms for which the drug had to be stopped.

ETHAMBUTOL

This was synthesized in the Lederle Laboratories and the active substance is the dextro isomer of 2, 2'-(ethylenediimino)-di-1-butanol dihydrochloride (see formula below); the laevo isomer is inactive and the meso isomer is only one-sixteenth as active as the dextro form. The three isomers are equally toxic to mice. Ethambutol is a white crystalline substance, heat stable and highly soluble in water.

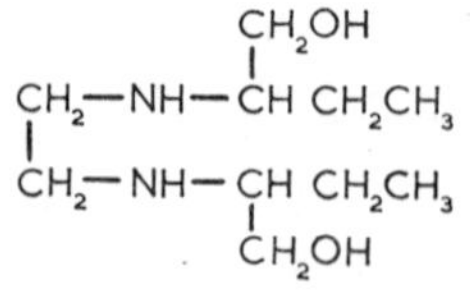

$$CH_2-NH-CH \overset{\displaystyle CH_2OH}{|} CH_2CH_3$$
$$CH_2-NH-CH \underset{\displaystyle CH_2OH}{|} CH_2CH_3$$

ethambutol

In vitro 1–4 μg./ml. of the racemate inhibits the growth of *M. tuberculosis* (various strains including H37Rv) and the inhibitory concentration has not increased appreciably through 8 consecutive passages in the presence of graded concentrations of the new compound.

This is active only against organisms of the genus Mycobacterium and inactive *in vivo* and *in vitro* against other bacteria, viruses and fungi.

In vivo tests in mice showed that ethambutol is appreciably less active than isoniazid but it is also a good deal less toxic so that the therapeutic ratio of the compound when given orally is of the same order as that of isoniazid. The new drug is fully active against strains of *M. tuberculosis* which are resistant to isoniazid and to streptomycin.

Karlson (1961) tested the effectiveness of ethambutol in experimental tuberculosis in guinea-pigs and found that the drug was highly active when given by subcutaneous injection, though less potent, on a weight for weight basis, than streptomycin and isoniazid. Schmidt found in established experimental tuberculosis in monkeys that the therapeutic effect of ethambutol comes on rather slowly, resembling streptomycin in this respect. With a dose of 100 mg./kg. this is followed by marked regression which is, however, not as satisfactory as is obtained with isoniazid. There is evidence that resistance to ethambutol can occur *in vivo* after relatively short exposures to the drug, and ethambutol should certainly not be used alone in the treatment of tuberculosis.

The metabolism of ethambutol has been investigated in a number of species including the monkey and the data given here are taken from a paper by Thomas *et al.* (1961) as well as from unpublished data made available by the Lederle Laboratories and a paper presented by Schmidt and his co-workers at the VA Conference on Pulmonary Diseases in January 1962. The drug is rapidly absorbed from the intestine and a maximum blood level is reached in about two hours; clearance is more or less complete within eight hours in mice and 100 hours in dogs. In the monkey there is still a small amount of drug in the serum twenty-four hours after a single oral dose of 100 mg./kg.

The LD 50 of ethambutol in mice is 8·9 G./kg. when given orally and 1·8 G./kg. when given subcutaneously. Subacute and chronic toxicity studies in rats and dogs show that the drug is well tolerated. At high dose levels (over 100 mg./kg./day) toxic effects on various organs, including the bone marrow, the liver and the central nervous system, have been observed. In monkeys, Schmidt found no toxic effects with doses up to 200 mg./kg. given daily for some six months. Higher doses produced toxic effects on the central nervous system and death. Schmidt also found that when the peak serum level of the drug did not exceed 5 µg./ml., there was no cumulation, but that this did occur with doses producing higher levels. It would be wise to take this into consideration during clinical trials of the drug.

Clinical data are still very scanty. Schmidt states that a number of patients treated with the racemate developed visual disturbances and peripheral neuritis. According to Litchfield (personal communication), ethambutol (i.e. the dextro isomer) has been given to patients resistant to the main anti-tuberculous agents in doses of 25 mg./kg. orally for 2–3 months. Favourable clinical responses and sputum conversion have been seen; no toxic effects were observed.

THE PENICILLINS (Fig. 50)

Up till quite recently, three preparations of penicillin were mainly used for therapeutic administration, namely (1) benzylpenicillin for intramuscular administration in acute infections—this produces a high blood level for several hours and has thus to be administered about 4 times a day, (2) procaine penicillin, also for intramuscular administration, with

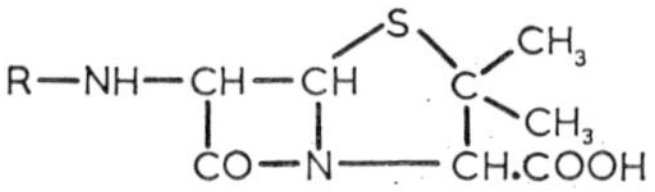

R = H	6-aminopenicillanic acid
R = CO.CH$_2$C$_6$H$_5$	benzyl penicillin
R = CO.CH$_2$OC$_6$H$_5$	phenoxymethyl penicillin
R = CO.CHOC$_6$H$_5$ CH$_3$	potassium salt is phenethicillin (Broxil, phenoxyethyl penicillin)

R = CO.CHOC$_6$H$_5$
    CH$_2$
    CH$_3$
	propicillin
	(Ultrapen; Brocillin)
	phenoxypropyl penicillin

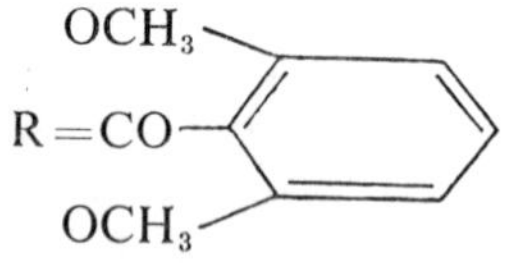 R = CO— (OCH$_3$ / OCH$_3$ ring)	methicillin sodium monohydrate is Celbenin (BRL 1241)
R = COCHC$_6$H$_5$ NH$_2$	ampicillin (Penbritin; BRL 1341)

Fig. 50. Formulae of penicillins

a more prolonged action than benzylpenicillin, but with correspondingly lower blood concentrations and thus not the preparation of choice in really severe infections, and (3) phenoxymethylpenicillin (Penicillin V) for oral administration, effective, though not as reliable as intramuscular benzylpenicillin. Benzathine penicillin, also given in the B.P. (1958) has a comparatively low solubility and has a very prolonged effect when given intramuscularly, though the injection is liable to be rather painful.

The general method of producing new penicillins has been a micro-biological one, i.e. to put various chemical substances into the culture medium, leaving it to the mould to incorporate the chemical grouping into the penicillin molecule. Substances like phenoxymethylpenicillin and allylmercaptopenicillin (Penicillin 'O') were so produced. Penicillin was synthesized by Du Vigneaud *et al.* (1946) and more recently the total synthesis of phenoxymethylpenicillin has been achieved (Sheehan and Henery-Logan, 1957) but this is at present essentially of theoretical interest.

In 1959 Batchelor *et al.* of Beecham Laboratories obtained 6-aminopenicillanic acid from a culture of penicillium chrysogenum. This substance possesses a low antibacterial activity, but its rate of destruction by penicillinase is much slower than that of benzylpenicillin. (The preparation and properties of 6-aminopenicillanic acid are des-cribed in a number of papers in *Proc. roy. Soc.* 1961, pp. 478–531.) The newly isolated substance has proved the starting point for the chemical production of new penicillins and important advances have already been made. The main ones have been the production of a form of penicillin (methicillin), effective against staphylococci which are resistant to the conventional form of penicillin (e.g. benzylpenicillin), and of another penicillin (ampicillin) effective against many gram negative organisms. In addition, new forms of penicillin have been produced which are claimed to be more suitable for oral administration than phenoxymethylpenicillin viz. phenethicillin, propicillin and phenoxy-benzylpenicillin. Unpublished data are also available about a form of penicillin (Prostaphlin) effective against benzyl penicillin resistant staphylococci, and reasonably well absorbed when given orally.

Gourevitch *et al.* (1960) describe the activity of a large number of new synthetic penicillins.

METHICILLIN ('Celbenin', BRL 1241)

This compound is sodium 6(2:6-dimethoxybenzamido) penicillinate monohydrate (see Fig. 50). It is a white crystalline solid extremely soluble in water giving a clear neutral solution. Such a solution loses about 50% of its activity in 5 days at room temperature, but only 20% in a refrigerator at 5°C. The substance is unstable in acid solutions.

Antibacterial activity

Cultures of *staphylococcus pyogenes* are sensitive to methicillin in concentrations of 1–4 µg. per ml., regardless of their resistance to benzyl penicillin, phenoxymethylpenicillin and other antibiotics (e.g. chloramphenicol, novobiocin, streptomycin, erythromycin, oleandomycin, tetracycline) (Rolinson *et al.*, 1960; Knox, 1960). This includes a wide range of penicillin-resistant, coagulase-positive staphylococci recently isolated in hospitals, some of which were resistant to concentrations of benzylpenicillin as high as 1,000 μg. per ml. Methicillin is bactericidal at concentrations only slightly higher than the minimum inhibitory concentration; its activity is not diminished in the presence of serum and is relatively unaffected by the inoculum size.

Methicillin is not affected by staphylococcal penicillinase which completely inactivates high concentrations of benzylpenicillin, but the new compound is inactivated by *Bacillus cereus* penicillinase, though at a much slower rate than benzylpenicillin; it is a powerful inducer of staphylococcal penicillinase. Cultures of *staphylococcus pyogenes* become tolerant to methicillin very slowly *in vitro*, and a few methicillin resistant staphylococci have already been encountered *in vivo* (Annotation, 1961).

Methicillin is an active agent against other organisms as is shown in Table 19, including β-haemolytic streptococci, streptococcus viridans and diplococcus pneumoniae; the table also shows that different penicillins show quite large differences in the range of their antibacterial activity. It is noteworthy that, weight for weight, methicillin is about 30–100 times less active than benzylpenicillin against staphylococcus pyogenes and other important pathogenic organisms.

Table 19

Antibacterial activity of different penicillins in vitro (*in mg./ml.*)

(The data above the line are from Knox (1960) and those below from Rolinson *et al.* (1960)

Staphylococcus	Benzyl	Ph.M.	Phenethicillin	Methicillin
Pyogenes (Oxford)	0·02	0·01	0·01	1·0
,, (resistant strain)	125	62	>250	2·0
Strep. pyogenes (Group A)	0·005	0·01	0·01	0·2
Strep. viridans	0·01	0·01	0·02	0·1
N. Meningiditis	0·2	0·2	0·2	6
Proteus vulgaris	15	>250	>250	>250
Ps. Pyocyanea	>250	>250	>250	>250
Salm. typhi	7·5	62	>250	>250
E. Coli	15	125	>250	>250
Dip. pneumoniae				0·05–0·5
Shigella shigae				250
Neis. catarrhalis				0·25
Strept. faecalis				50
Sarcina lutea				0·025
Corynebacterium hofmanni				0·6

The effectiveness of methicillin against infections in mice with a penicillin resistant staphylococcus has been demonstrated by Thompson *et al.* (1960), who have also demonstrated its value in an experimental pneumococcal infection.

Fate in the body

As methicillin is unstable in acid solutions and poorly absorbed when taken orally, it has to be given by injection, usually intramuscular. When so given in man, the blood concentration rises rapidly to reach a maximum at about 30 minutes and then falls to low values in 3–4 hours. In rabbits and dogs too, blood levels following intramuscular injection are similar to those following injection of benzylpenicillin. This is illustrated in Fig. 51. About 75% of the drug is excreted in the urine, mainly or entirely in unchanged form and both by tubular secretion and glomerular filtration (Acred *et al.*, 1961). The data suggest that 1 G. of methicillin should be injected at least every 4 hours in order to maintain chemotherapeutic levels in the blood. When given slowly by deep intramuscular injection, methicillin is no more painful than benzyl penicillin, though its use in combination with a local anaesthetic is advocated by Douthwaite *et al.* (1961). These investigators have also found that combination with probenecid (given orally) produces higher blood levels which are better maintained. Methicillin does not combine with serum protein to the same extent as benzyl penicillin, but there is usually, though not invariably, cross-sensitivity between the two drugs (Douthwaite *et al.*, 1961). The new penicillin, like the benzyl compound, does not penetrate well into the cerebro-spinal fluid. It is excreted in the bile in very high concentrations (Stewart, 1960; Acred *et al.*, 1961).

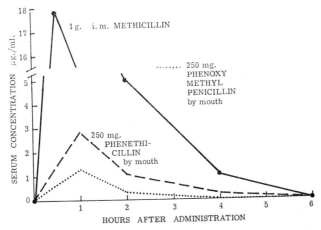

FIG. 51. Serum concentration following the administration of various penicillins (Knudson and Rolinson, 1959, 1960).

Toxicity

Brown and Acred (1960) have shown that the new compound has a very low toxicity when given to a variety of animals. No toxic symptoms were seen with doses of 2·5 G./kg. intravenously or 4·0 G./kg. subcutaneously. Repeated daily doses of 500 mg./kg. in rats for 12 weeks and twice daily doses of 250 mg./kg. in dogs for 4 weeks showed no evidence of toxicity. Daily application of a 1% solution to the rabbit eye caused no irritation. Given to anaesthetized cats at a dose of 500 mg./kg. there was no effect on the blood pressure or respiration. Some other aspects of the pharmacology of methicillin are described by Acred *et al.* (1961).*

Clinical Use

There are now a number of clinical reports which show the value of methicillin in infections with penicillin resistant staphylococci and also with streptococcal infections (Douthwaite *et al.*, 1960; 1961). In critically ill patients 2 grams should be given every four hours initially (Allan *et al.*, 1962). Apart from pain at the site of injection, there were no toxic effects, but superinfection was encountered and in one case this led to a fatal broncho-pneumonia. Two children showed superficial infections with *Candida albicans* which responded to therapy with nystatin (Stewart *et al.*, 1960). There is evidence that methicillin does not show cross-sensitivity with benzylpenicillin (Luton, 1961).

The importance of penicillin resistance in hospital practice is emphasized by a study by Thompson *et al.* (1960) who showed that of all the *staphylococci pyogenes* isolated in the Middlesex Hospital over a period of about 9 months, only 18% were sensitive to benzylpenicillin, whereas all were sensitive to methicillin. In this connection, the observations of Elek and Fleming (1960) are very interesting, since they showed that they could largely eliminate the growth of staphylococci in the nose of new born infants in a maternity unit by spraying methicillin into the air. Barber (1960) emphasizes that we know little about the development of resistance to methicillin and that the drug should thus be reserved for penicillin-resistant infections and not used indiscriminately. It is as yet too early to know to what extent methicillin is going to replace a number of other antibiotics (described in this chapter) which are used in the treatment of infections with penicillin resistant staphylococci, though it seems likely that in many of these cases methicillin will be the next drug of choice. Resistance of staphylococci to penicillin is a complex subject and it has indeed been suggested that there may be three types of penicillin resistance, due to either an inherent capacity to tolerate penicillin or to an ability to destroy it, either by means of penicillinase (giving penicilloic acid as the product) or by means of an amidase, giving 6-aminopenicillanic acid and a side chain as products (see Knox, 1961).

* Depression of the bone marrow has been reported (McElfresh, A. E. and Huang, N. N., 1962, *New Eng. J. Med.* **266**, 246).

Prostaphlin (Penicillin P-12)*

This has been prepared by the Bristol Laboratories and is 5-methyl-3-phenyl-4-isoxazolyl penicillin. It is soluble in water and a concentrated aqueous solution is stable for 24 hours at room temperature. The information given here is based on abstracts of a conference held in New York (see Branch *et al.*, 1962), on Editorial (1961), and on the data of Leduc and Fontaine (1962).

Prostaphlin is considerably more active than methicillin against a variety of benzylpenicillin resistant *staphylococcus aureus*, and is markedly resistant to the action of both *staphylococcus aureus* and *bacillus cereus* penicillinases. It is more active than methicillin against *diplococcus pneumoniae* and *streptococcus pyogenes*. Against experimental infections in mice, prostaphlin was found to be active when given orally.

Generally speaking the drug is also well absorbed when given orally in man, though occasionally adequate blood levels are not obtained by this route. The new penicillin diffuses well into most body fluids, though the level in the cerebro-spinal fluid is low. Clinical trials are at an early stage, but the results suggest that oral administration (in doses of the order of 1 G. every six hours) is effective in the treatment of infections with benzylpenicillin resistant staphylococci. Patients have complained of the bitter taste of the tablets. The drug has also been given by intramuscular injection.

AMPICILLIN (Penbritin)

Ampicillin ('Penbritin', BRL 1341) has also been prepared from 6-aminopenicillanic acid. It is of special interest because it is active against a wide range of gram negative as well as gram positive organisms, and is stable in acid solution and well absorbed when given orally. The compound is 6(D(-)α-aminophenylacetamido) penicillanic acid (formula, p. 326). The free acid is only sparingly soluble in water and at neutral pH the solubility is only about 10% at room temperature.

Antibacterial activity

Ampicillin has an activity similar to benzylpenicillin against sensitive staphylococci, haemolytic streptococci and pneumococci. It is, in addition, remarkably effective against many gram negative organisms, the activity being similar to that of tetracyclines and chloramphenicol. All species and strains of salmonella tested were inhibited by concentrations usually not above 1·25 µg./ml. Various strains of shigella and of *E. coli* are affected by concentrations up to 5 µg./ml. as are some strains of Proteus and *H. influenzae*. Other proteus, *Klebsiella aerogenes* and *Ps. pyocyanea* are much more resistant. Ampicillin is destroyed by penicillinase produced by staphylococci or by gram negative organisms

---

*Data about this, and two related compounds, are given by Barber, M. and Waterworth, P. M. (1962), *Brit. med. J.* (1), 1159.

and resistance of such organisms is thus due to penicillinase production. The drug is highly bactericidal. Resistance to it develops stepwise in the typical penicillin manner (Rolinson and Stevens, 1961).

The effects of the drug on experimental infections in mice were tested by Brown and Acred (1961). Not only in infections with gram positive (staph. aureus and strept. pyogenes) but also with gram negative (salmonella typhi-murium and Klebsiella pneumoniae) organisms, ampicillin compared favourably with tetracycline and chloramphenicol.

Fate in the body

This has been studied in man by Knudson *et al.* (1961). The drug is well absorbed when given orally, though rather more slowly than benzyl-penicillin and it is also more slowly excreted (Fig. 52). With single oral doses of 500–1000 mg. the maximum serum concentration is reached in about 2 hours and varies from around 4–7 µg./ml. Appreciable amounts (0·1–0·9 µg./ml.) are still present 6 hours after giving the drug. About 30% of the drug is excreted in the urine in that period, the urinary concentration varying between 250 and 2500 µg./ml. (Brown and Acred,

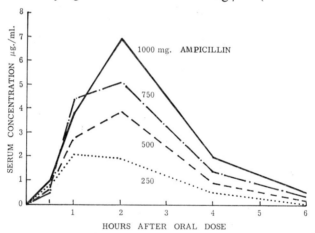

FIG. 52. Serum level of ampicillin following the oral administration of various doses (Knudson *et al.*, 1961).

1961). With repeated doses 30–50% of the drug is excreted in the urine. Only minute amounts penetrate into the cerebro-spinal fluid and only a trace can be detected in the faeces, though there is a marked suppressive effect on the faecal bacterial flora, even to the extent of producing sterile cultures aerobically (Stewart *et al.*, 1961).

Similar results are obtained in dogs. The maximum serum concentration with ampicillin is higher than with the same dose of either phenoxymethyl penicillin or phenethicillin, though again the absorption is rather slower. Large amounts of the drug are excreted in the urine, both by glomerular filtration and tubular secretion, and also in the bile. Preliminary investigations in mice, rats, dogs and cats show that ampicillin has a low toxicity (Brown and Acred, 1961).

Clinical results

Only preliminary results are available, but these are encouraging, the main trial being in kidney infections. Among 28 patients, three showed transient rashes and 3 infants passed some loose stools. The value of the new drug in a variety of intestinal infections, particularly in typhoid fever, remains to be established. The dose suggested is 250 mg. 6 hourly but more may be needed with relatively insensitive organisms.

p-Aminobenzylpenicillin (Penicillin T) was prepared chemically from *p*-nitrobenzylpenicillin, a biosynthetic type of penicillin (Tosoni *et al.*, 1958). According to Stewart *et al.* (1961) the aminobenzyl compound has the same order of activity against gram negative rods as ampicillin, though it is acid labile and has therefore to be given by injection. Like ampicillin, it is destroyed by penicillinase and is therefore ineffective against resistant strains of *staphylococcus aureus*.

PHENOXYMETHYLPENICILLIN AND PHENETHICILLIN

Phenoxymethylpenicillin has now been used for a number of years for oral administration and has proved very satisfactory in the treatment of various infections. Its absorption is reasonably reliable and good blood levels are maintained provided it is given several times a day.

More recently, Knudson and Rolinson (1959) have described the properties of *phenethicillin* ('Broxil', the potassium salt of 6(α-phenoxy-propionamido) penicillanic acid (see p. 326 for formula) made chemically from 6-aminopenicillanic acid. The new compound is as stable as phenoxymethylpenicillin in acid solutions and is better absorbed than the latter compound when given orally. The difference between the two is illustrated in Fig. 51; it is noteworthy that with phenoxymethylpeni-cillin, only 40% of the dose appeared in the urine within 6 hours, whereas the corresponding figure for phenethicillin was 60%.

These results have given rise to a good deal of controversy concerning their significance in practice. McCarthy and Finland (1960) have con-firmed the good absorption of phenethicillin, but state that these higher serum levels produce appreciably less antibacterial activity against haemolytic streptococci and pneumococci and are no more active against *staphylococcus aureus* than those produced by the oral adminis-tration of phenoxymethylpenicillin. They also state that with intra-muscular administration of benzylpenicillin, a high blood level is maintained for an appreciably longer time than is obtained with the oral administration of phenethicillin (or phenoxymethylpenicillin). Similar results have been obtained by Griffith (1960).

Another related compound, *propicillin* (phenoxypropylpenicillin), marketed under the trade names 'Ultrapen' and 'Brocillin', is said to produce blood levels somewhat higher than are attained with phenecillin, when given orally, and to be particularly suitable for the treatment of streptococcal infections (Williamson *et al.*, 1961). Another orally administered drug of this series is *phenoxybenzylpenicillin* (phenbenicillin), marketed under the name of Penspec (Rollo *et al.*, 1962; Carter and Brumfitt, 1962). At present there is no clear evidence that propicillin or phenoxybenzylpenicillin possess advantages over phenoxymethylpenicillin.

What is becoming quite obvious is that when a particular form of penicillin is to be used in the treatment of an infection, the sensitivity of the organism responsible for the infection against the form of penicillin used will have to be determined; it will not necessarily be possible to rely on a figure obtained for the sensitivity of the organism against benzylpenicillin. This will become even more important as new forms of penicillin are synthesized and made available for clinical use. A good example of this is the finding of Garrod (1960) that against *H. influenzae*, benzylpenicillin is much more active than either phenoxymethylpenicillin or phenethicillin.

Cephalosporin N (synnematin B) is a substance with the penicillin nucleus and a side-chain derived from D-α-aminoadipic acid i.e. (D-α-amino-4-carboxybutyl) penicillin. This substance has less than 1 % of the activity of benzylpenicillin against the Oxford strain of *staphylococcus aureus*, but is considerably more active against certain strains of *Salmonella typhi*. It has a low toxicity and shows no cross sensitivity with penicillin (Abraham, 1957; Abraham and Newton, 1961).

Work is also actively proceeding on derivatives of 7-aminocephalosporanic acid, such as cephalosporin C which, like cephalosporin N has a D-α-amino-adipoyl side-chain (Jago and Heatley, 1961).

DEMETHYLCHLORTETRACYCLINE ('Ledermycin')

The tetracyclines have the broadest spectrum of all the antibiotics, ranging from the rickettsias and some viruses through all the pyogenic cocci to the majority of gram negative bacilli.

The properties of three of them, i.e. chlortetracycline, oxytetracycline and tetracycline, are described by Robson and Keele (1956). Demethylchlortetracycline was discovered by McCormick *et al.* (1957) and its properties are reviewed by Finland and Garrod (1960). It is produced by a mutant of the original strain of *Streptomyces aureofaciens* from which chlortetracycline was originally obtained and its chemical structure is shown in Fig. 53.

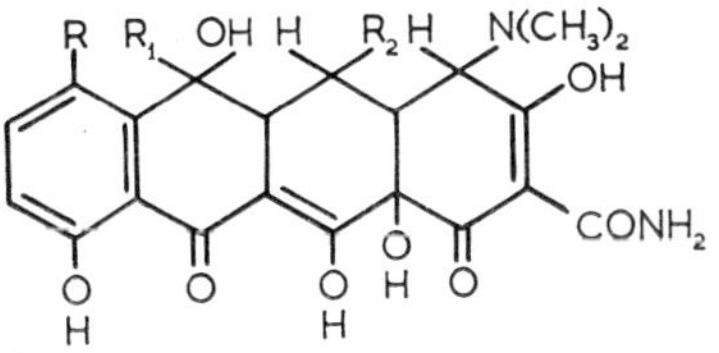

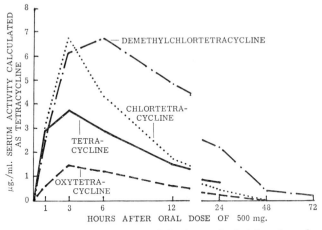

FIG. 53.

Demethylchlortetracycline is very stable and differs from its congeners in that it is more slowly eliminated from the body as is illustrated in Fig. 54, so that a single oral dose will produce a chemotherapeutic level in the blood for about twice as long as the other compounds. It is well absorbed from the intestine, though appreciable concentrations of unabsorbed substance are found in the faeces. In a small number of subjects (about 5%) the absorption of tetracycline is poor. Demethyl-chlortetracycline penetrates poorly into the cerebrospinal fluid.

The new compound is about twice as active as tetracycline against many bacteria and can be shown to be more active in experimental staphylococcal infections (Kuck and Redin, 1960).

It will take more time to make a final assessment of the new compound, but it would appear that two doses per day would be

FIG. 54. Serum concentrations following oral administration of various tetracyclines (Finland and Garrod, 1960).

sufficient to maintain a chemotherapeutic level and that smaller doses are necessary than of the other tetracyclines. In large doses, demethyl-chlortctracycline frequently produces gastro-intestinal disturbances. Very occasionally it produces an exaggerated sunburn reaction which may be quite severe with high fever, and which is not encountered with the other tetracyclines.

The properties of *erythromycin* are described by Robson and Keele (1956). It is the best known of a group of antibiotics produced by streptomyces, that consist of large lactone rings (called macrolides) linked glycosidically to novel diethylamino sugars and, in some cases, sugars without an amino group. Oleandomycin and spiramycin belong to the same group (see Abraham and Newton, 1960). The formula of erythromycin is shown below. Various esters of erythromycin have been made and it has been shown, in preliminary studies, that *propionyl*

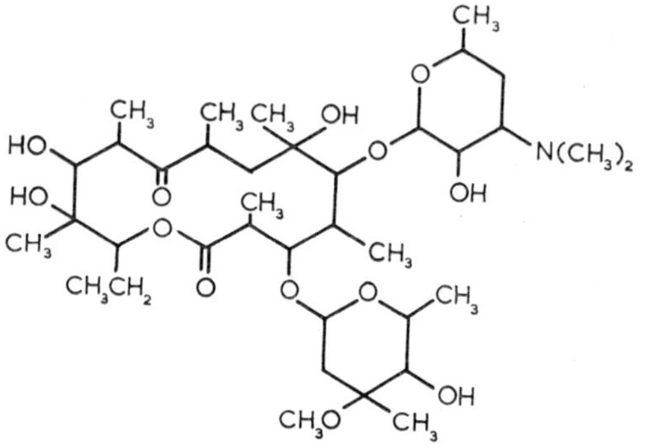

erythromycin

erythromycin produces a higher and more sustained level in the blood than erythromycin base (Griffith *et al.*, 1958).

Spiramycin and *oleandomycin* have properties similar to erythromycin; there is evidence that *triacetyloleandomycin* gives better antibiotic levels in the blood than does the parent compound (Hirsch *et al.*, 1959; Hinton and Wilson, 1959). Albright and Hall (1959) found that triacetyloleandomycin was consistently effective against infections with most gram positive organisms, but of little value in infections of the urinary tract with gram negative organisms. It has been found that prolonged treatment with triacetyloleandomycin, or with propionyl erythromycin, may produce liver damage, and it seems advisable to use the esters of these antibiotics for only short periods and employ the antibiotics themselves for more lengthy medication (Annotation, 1961).

Kanamycin ('Kannasyn') is derived from strains of *Streptomyces kanamyceticus* and is chemically related to neomycin. It consists of two amino-sugars glycosidically linked to deoxystreptamine (see p. 337).

The drug is only slightly absorbed from the gastro-intestinal tract and has to be given parenterally for systemic infections. It is absorbed rapidly from intramuscular sites and excreted in the urine by glomerular filtration. Some of it is excreted in the bile.

The antibacterial activity of kanamycin is identical with that of neomycin and there is complete cross-resistance between the two drugs. Kanamycin should be reserved for serious systemic infections caused

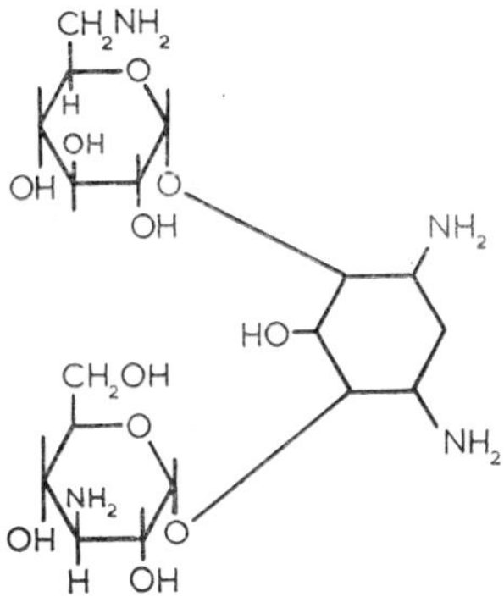

kanamycin

by staphylococci resistant to safer antibiotics and for urinary tract infections in which it is the only antibiotic to which the organism is sensitive (*Brit. med. J.*, 1960). It is given intramuscularly and there may be irritation at injection sites. Marmell and Prigot (1959–60) have used it successfully in the treatment of gonorrhoea.

The toxic effects are similar to those of neomycin, and in particular it can cause irreversible deafness. Damage to the kidneys also occurs, but this is usually reversible. Kanamycin should never be given to patients with poor renal function or with dehydration.

Vancomycin is produced by *Streptomyces orientalis*, and is an amphoteric substance with a molecular weight of 3200–3500 which appears to contain amino and phenolic groups and carbohydrate.

Its main action is against gram positive organisms, the chief indication being infection due to *staphylococcus aureus* resistant to other antibiotics. The drug must be given intravenously, preferably in an infusion in order to avoid thrombophlebitis (Dutton and Elmes, 1959), in order to produce any action other than on the intestine. After intravenous administration, vancomycin is rapidly excreted in high concentration in the urine and should, therefore, be given in several daily doses. It is not concentrated in the bile and is detectable in pleural, synovial and ascitic fluid, but does not diffuse into the cerebrospinal fluid. After oral administration, most of the drug is excreted in the faeces and only slight amounts can be detected in the blood or urine (Geraci *et al.*, 1956).

Vancomycin is toxic to the eighth nerve and is particularly dangerous in uraemic patients. Occasionally other toxic effects, e.g. chills, fever and rashes, may occur (Kirby *et al.*, 1960). Nephrotoxicity has also been observed.

Ristocetin is produced by an actinomycete, *Nocardia lurida* and has two components, ristocetin A and B, which have a similar range of activity. It is a substance similar to vancomycin and has also to be

given intravenously, well diluted. It has the same indications as vancomycin and produces similar toxic effects, though the incidence of skin
reactions is more frequent with ristocetin and in addition the drug has
been found to cause depression of the granulocytes in some patients
(Waisbren *et al.*, 1959–60). Thrombocytopenia occurs and is apparently
the result of a direct toxic effect of the drug on circulating platelets
(Gangarosa, 1959–60). In infants and small children, ristocetin has been
given intramuscularly, 1 mg. of hydrocortisone being added to each 100
mg. of the antibiotic to decrease the inflammatory response surrounding
the injection site (Koch *et al.*, 1956–60).

NOVOBIOCIN ('Albamycin', 'Cathomycin')

This is produced from cultures of *Streptomyces spheroides* or *Streptomyces niveus* and the history of its discovery is described by Finland and
Nichols (1957). The pure crystalline substance has the formula shown
below and has been prepared as the sodium or the calcium salt.
Novobiocin base is not absorbed and the calcium salt is more stable and
is therefore used when a liquid preparation, e.g. the syrup, is wanted for
pediatric use.

The sodium salt is rapidly absorbed when given orally, a peak level
in the blood being reached in 2–3 hours. The level remains high for some

novobiocin sodium

8 hours and there is still a small quantity left in the serum after 24 hours.
The antibiotic diffuses into pleural and aseitic fluid, but not appreciably
into the cerebrospinal fluid if the meninges are not inflamed. Novobiocin is concentrated in the liver and bile and excreted in the faeces,
with small quantities in the urine (Furesz, 1958). In dogs the urinary
excretion is very slow and it seems likely that the maintenance of high
concentrations in the blood is due to slow renal excretion and also
perhaps to binding to serum protein (Taylor *et al.*, 1956). Novobiocin
has also been administered intramuscularly and intravenously in
seriously ill patients and is well tolerated.

Novobiocin is effective against *Staphylococcus aureus*, including
strains resistant to many other antibiotics. Except for some strains of

Proteus vulgaris and coliform bacteria, it has little or no activity against most gram negative bacilli of the enteric group. Gram negative cocci are only moderately sensitive to the drug and its effect on enterococci is variable.

The main use of novobiocin is in staphylococcal infections in which other antibiotics have failed or proved unsuitable because of toxic effects. It has also been used in the treatment of Proteus infections, particularly those of the urinary tract that are resistant to other agents. Resistance to the drug does develop but no cross resistance with other antibiotics has so far been observed. There is no synergism between the action of novobiocin and tetracycline, indeed the administration of the two drugs resulted in a lower antibacterial activity in the serum against a tetracycline-resistant staphylococcus as compared with novobiocin alone (Hirsch and Finland, 1960).

Toxic effects are not uncommon and are essentially due to sensitization, including skin rashes often associated with eosinophilia and occasionally with haematuria, urticaria and fever. Transient leucopenia, possibly due to the drug, has been reported and hence the possibility of agranulocytosis should be borne in mind.

RIFOMYCIN

This was first isolated from the fermentation broth of a new streptomyces, *S. mediterranei* (Sensi *et al.*, 1959). It is a complex of substances (Sensi *et al.*, 1961), and the relation of the various components to one another is shown in Fig. 55.

Of these, Rifomycin B and SV have been studied fairly extensively. They are both highly active *in vitro* against various gram positive organisms, including *staphylococcus aureus, streptococcus pyogenes, D. pneumoniae*, and also against *M. tuberculosis* (Timbal, 1959–60). Against various gram positive organisms, Rifomycin SV appears to be appreciably

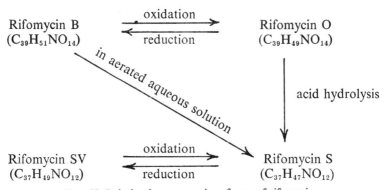

FIG. 55. Relation between various forms of rifomycin.

more active than Rifomycin B. Both show no cross resistance with other antibiotics in common use. Timbal (1959–60) has demonstrated the effectiveness of Rifomycin B against experimental infections in mice with *staphylococcus aureus, strep. haemolyticus* and *D. pneumoniae.* Its pharmacological properties have been studied by Maffii and Timbal (1959–60). It has a low toxicity in various animal species, e.g. the L.D.50 in mice, when given intravenously, is about 2·0 G./kg. It is not well absorbed when given orally, but after intramuscular injection, effective blood levels are maintained for several hours. The antibiotic does not cross the normal blood-brain barrier, but appears in high concentration in the bile. The treatment of patients with 2·0 G. daily of Rifomycin B given intramuscularly in 4 divided doses is described by Füresz and Scotti (1959–60). Good results were obtained in some cases and there were no side effects.

The value of Rifomycin SV in experimental infections in mice is described by Timbal and Brega (1961). It is more effective than Rifomycin B, particularly in infections with staphylococcus aureus. Encouraging results were also obtained in experimental tuberculosis in mice, though these were by no means as good as with isoniazid. When tested by the intracorneal method, Rifomycin SV is about 10 times less effective, weight for weight, than isoniazid (Robson and Sullivan, unpublished observations). The drug also produced striking effects in guinea pigs, though large doses (180 mg./kg.) had to be used (Monaldi *et al.*, 1961). These investigators also report on some very preliminary clinical results.

The pharmacological properties of Rifomycin SV have been studied by Maffii *et al.* (1961). Its acute toxicity is rather higher than that of Rifomycin B, as seen in experiments in mice, rats and dogs; for example the L.D.50 in mice (given i.v.) is 550 mg./kg. as compared with about 2·0 G. for Rifomycin B. There is some evidence of toxicity in chronic experiments in rats and dogs, in high daily doses, but this requires further investigation. The absorption and fate of the drug have been studied in dogs by Maffii *et al.* (1961). Following intramuscular administration to patients (500 mg.) therapeutic blood levels were detected up to 8 hours later. High concentrations of the drug are eliminated in the bile, but only small amounts appear in the urine. No drug was detected in the cerebro-spinal fluid. After oral administration, absorption was very irregular. There is some evidence that Rifomycin SV is apt to produce appreciable irritation when injected intramuscularly, even when combined with sodium ascorbate to prevent its conversion to the more irritant Rifomycin S (Maffii *et al.*, 1961).

At present it seems possible that Rifomycin may become of value in the treatment of resistant staphylococcal infections, of certain infections of the biliary tract, and possibly as an additional drug in tuberculosis.

PAROMOMYCIN (Humatin)

This was discovered by workers in the Parke-Davis Laboratories and is obtained from cultures of *streptomyces rimosus*. It is a white amorphous water soluble substance, and chemically is composed of glucosamine and a disaccharide joined to an inositol derivative (see formula below).

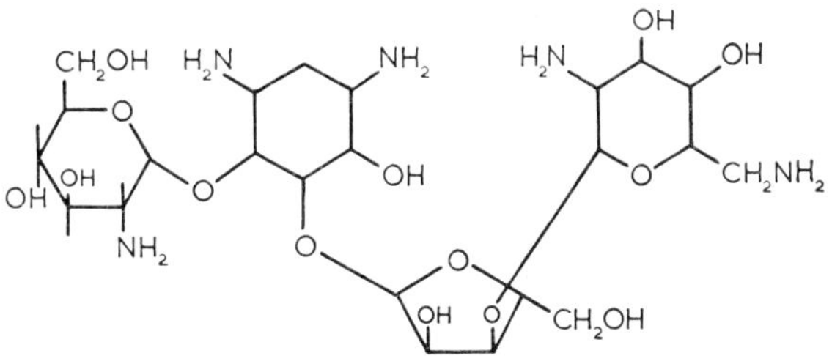

paromomycin

The activity *in vitro* of paromomycin is similar to that of neomycin and kanamycin and there is in fact cross resistance between these three antibiotics (Kunin *et al.*, 1958). The bacteria affected include staphylococci, Esch. Coli, and some strains of salmonella, shigella and proteus. In addition paromomycin is also effective against *Entamoeba histolytica*. Experimental infections in mice with these organisms yield to treatment with the drug, which is also active in dogs and rats. It has also shown some activity in experimental tuberculosis in mice and guinea pigs (Fisher *et al.*, 1959–60; Courtney *et al.*, 1959–60).

The acute *toxicity* of the drug is rather low, e.g. the L.D.50 in mice is 423 mg./kg. when given subcutaneously, but on subacute or chronic administration to various species of animals, there were toxic effects on the kidneys, so that paromomycin is not suitable for systemic administration. It is poorly absorbed when given orally and its use is therefore in infections of the intestine (Coffey *et al.*, 1959).

The main *clinical use* of paromomycin is in intestinal infections which have proved refractory to standard methods of treatment, particularly infections with salmonella and shigella and in amoebiasis. Sheikh (1960) found, however, that paromomycin was effective in acute amoebiasis but failed in most chronic cases. The drug is well tolerated when given orally but may cause nausea and looseness of stools. Overgrowth of *Candida albicans* may occur, which may occasionally result in oral thrush (Coles and Stewart, 1961). The drug has also been used as part of the treatment of hepatic coma to sterilize the intestine and prevent the formation of toxic nitrogenous substances by bacteria (Stormont *et al.*, 1958), the suggestion being that the drug (or neomycin) is less toxic than tetracyclines, which are absorbable. Doses up to 8 grams per day

12

have been given to adults but liability to toxic effects appears to increase with more than 2 grams per day. In children, Coles *et al.* (1960) gave 80 mg./kg. daily and obtained good results in salmonella and shigella infections.

ANTIFUNGAL ANTIBIOTICS

Griseofulvin was originally isolated by Raistrick and his colleagues (Oxford *et al.*, 1939) from *Penicillium griseofulvum,* and is in fact produced by several species of penicillium. Its chemical structure is shown below, and it has been synthesized by Brossi *et al.* (1960). It is a colourless, thermostable compound very slightly soluble in water and more soluble in alcohol (1 in 1000). It was first used to control pathogenic fungi in plants and its possible application in human and veterinary mycology was demonstrated by Gentles (1958) who studied its effect on ringworm infections in guinea pigs; when given orally the antibiotic is actually found in the hair (Gentles *et al.*, 1959).

After oral administration in man, griseofulvin is absorbed and reaches a maximum level in the serum after 4–8 hours with some still present at 24 hours (McNall, 1959–60) and much of the drug is excreted in the urine (Blank and Roth, 1959) mainly in the form of metabolites of which the chief one is 6-dimethylgriseofulvin (Barnes and Boothroyd, 1961). The inhibition of growth of *M. canis* by griseofulvin is partially reversed by various purines and purine derivatives, suggesting that its effect is at least partly due to inhibition of nucleic acid synthesis. When

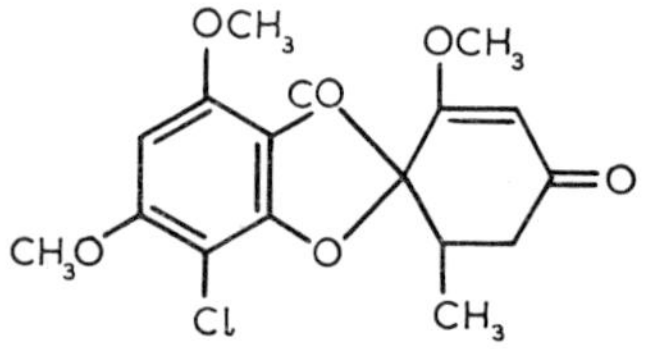

griseofulvin

the drug is injected intravenously at ten times the therapeutic dosage, arrest of mitosis is observed at metaphase. Toxic effects due to this have not been observed when the drug is used clinically (Symposium on Griseofulvin, 1960).

The main clinical use of the drug is in the treatment of ringworm of the scalp, though fungal infections of the skin have also been treated with success and it has indeed been described as a major advance in the therapy of superficial ringworm infections. Ringworm infections of the finger nails are cleared by prolonged treatment with griseofulvin, which is however not so successful when the toe nails are involved (Stevenson and Djavahiszwili, 1961). The dosage is 1–2 grams per day given orally. Beare and Mackenzie (1959) observed no serious toxic effect with doses of 0·25 G. three times daily given to children for periods of up to 10 weeks. Such effects as headache, urticaria and erythematous eruptions and diarrhoea have been reported, but on the whole the drug is remarkably non-toxic. The drug has also been shown to be effective against *Trichophyton verrucosum* in calves (Lauder and O'Sullivan, 1958).

Amphotericin B, as well as *Nystatin*, is produced by streptomyces. Both substances are amphoteric and consist of C_{40} structures linked to the same amino sugar, mycosamine. It is possible that they consist of large lactone rings (macrolides) similar to those found in erythromycin (Abraham and Newton, 1960).

Campbell and Hill (1959–60) have treated mice orally with a solubilized preparation of amphotericin B designed for infusion into human subjects and obtained good results in experimental histoplasmosis, coccidiodomycosis and cryptococcosis. Effective blood levels were demonstrated. Deep fungus diseases have been treated in human subjects, mainly with intravenous administration of the drug and the results appear to be encouraging, though side effects are by no means uncommon (Baum and Schwarz, 1959–60). Favourable results have also been reported in the treatment of American leishmaniasis (Furtado, 1959–60) and there is evidence that it can be of value in systemic moniliasis. There is a detailed discussion of Amphotericin B in New and Non-Official Drugs (1961).

A very new antifungal agent effective against systemic mycoses is at present known as *X 5079 C* and has been prepared in the laboratories of Hoffman La Roche. It is produced by a streptomyces and is a polypeptide containing sulphur. It has a low toxicity and is effective in experimental mycoses. Preliminary investigations show that it can cure a number of mycotic infections in man, when the drug is given subcutaneously every 6 hours at a daily dosage of about 4 mg./kg. for several weeks. No benefit was observed in Candida infections. During treatment there is a marked rise in sulphobromphthalein retention which falls promptly after cessation of administration. Microscopic observations of liver sections from patients showed the presence of periportal inflammation which disappeared after treatment was discontinued. (*See Amer. Rev. resp. Dis.*, 1961, **84**, pp. 504–547).

Nystatin inhibits the growth and cell division of species of candida and saccharomyces. It is not well absorbed when given orally. It has been used locally for infections of mucous membranes and also orally in patients with simple mycotic infections, mainly with *C. albicans*; rapid clearance of the infection was frequently observed and, apart from transient nausea, there were no toxic effects (Stewart, 1956). This result is rather at variance with the findings of Child (1956) on the failure of nystatin to clear *C. albicans* from the throat and sputum during therapy with tetracycline. Angioni and Gorecki (1960) however, found that orally administered nystatin could clear fungal infections (mostly due to candida) in cases of pulmonary tuberculosis.

The endotoxins produced by gram negative bacteria have been studied for many years and are known to produce a variety of reactions in animals and man. They are also known under the name 'pyrogen' and 'somatic antigen'. They are reviewed by Bennett and Cluff (1957) and by Westphal (1960). It is now known that these substances are produced in the wall of most, if not all, gram negative bacteria and constitute the heat stable filterable substance that is responsible for infectious fevers, i.e. the so-called *endotoxin* of gram negative bacteria. Recent studies by Stetson (1956) have shown that lysates of Group A haemolytic strepto-cocci possess similar toxic actions. The main actions produced by these substances are classified by Westphal as follows:

1. Acute reactions, essentially non-specific.
   Fever
   Activation of hormonal and enzymatic mechanisms (fibrinolysis, etc.)
   Alteration in white cell counts (leucopenia, leucocytosis, lym-phopenia, eosinopenia)
   Alteration in the titre of serum factors (complement, properdin)
   Alterations in the metabolic rate of numerous cellular systems (reticulo-endothelial system, etc.), leading to non-specific altera-tion in resistance to infections.

2. Less acute reactions, essentially specific.
   Formation of antibodies, leading to specific alterations in resistance to infections.

Among the interesting effects which have been obtained with these substances are haemorrhagic necrosis in normal and neoplastic tissues (the latter of which was in fact anticipated many years ago by the work of Coley on the treatment of sarcoma); extensive vasomotor disturbances (reviewed by Gilbert, 1960); and the production of the Schwartzman phenomenon. It is worth emphasizing that much work has been done in an attempt to separate hypothetical substances which may have these various effects, and particularly to remove the pyrogenic factor so as to leave a substance which will have valuable therapeutic effect without producing fever. One important aim in the chemical work has been to obtain a fraction suitable for increasing resistance to infection, and acting in a non-specific manner. Since Condie et al. (1955) and Johnson et al. (1959) have shown that concomitant administration of endotoxin with another antigen definitely enhances specific antibody formation, the non-specific and specific effects of endotoxin may be difficult to differentiate. This question is also discussed by Bloch (1960).

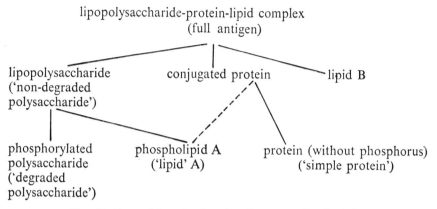

FIG. 56. Composition of endotoxins of gram negative bacteria.
(After Westphal, 1960.)

CHEMISTRY

The endotoxins extracted from various bacteria are complexes which contain a phosphorylated saccharide and protein component; in addition there is a lipoid component strongly bound to the complex, namely lipid A. Another lipid (lipid B) is weakly absorbed on to the complex; it is biologically inactive and not really part of the complex. The protein component is responsible for the antigenic activity of the complex (at least in the rabbit) but appears to play no part in its pharmacological activities.

In 1952, Westphal and his co-workers devised a method for the isolation of the lipopolysaccharide, i.e. a complex containing the polysaccharide bound to lipid A. The yield was 3–4% of the dry weight of the bacteria and the complexes have a molecular weight of 1 to 10 million in aqueous solution at a pH of 7·0. They contain 55–75% of phosphorylated saccharide and 20–45% of lipid A.

Analysis of *lipid A* shows that it contains about 20% of glucosamine, 7–8% of phosphoric esters, about 50% of higher fatty acids and a peptide chain in which serine is linked to dicarboxylic amino acids. Westphal (1960) suggests that lipid A plays an important part in the biological action of bacterial endotoxin and that the function of the specific polysaccharide and the protein is to disperse the complex and possibly to present it to the specific receptors in the appropriate steric positions.

The polysaccharides of gram negative bacteria contain 4–8% of phosphate esters and a variety of sugars, namely hexosamines, heptoses, hexoses, pentoses and desoxyhexoses. The sugar content of the bacterial polysaccharide plays an important part in determining the serological specificity of the endotoxins and reference should be made to the reviews by Westphal (1960) and of Staub (1960) for this very interesting aspect of the work.

DISTRIBUTION

When radioactive endotoxin is innoculated intravenously into rabbits or mice, the substance is at first partitioned between leucocytes and plasma and then becomes localized in the liver, spleen and lung. The toxin is cleared from the blood within two hours. Pretreatment of rabbits with thorium dioxide inhibits the uptake of the toxin by the reticuloendothelial cells and this is associated with an increase in the lethality of endoxin. Animals acquire tolerance to the action of endotoxin (particularly its pyrogenic action) and in such animals, 95% of the toxin disappears from the blood in 15 minutes and accumulates chiefly in the lung and liver (see Bennett and Cluff, 1957).

The plasma contains a heat labile substance which can rapidly inactivate endotoxic materials *in vitro*, so that they can no longer elicit their characteristic host responses. It has been suggested that a number of factors, i.e. the heat labile substance mentioned above, together with properdin, complement and specific antibody, participate in a series of reactions by which the host progressively modifies endotoxin so that it is rendered inactive (Skarnes *et al.*, 1958).

INFLUENCE ON NON-SPECIFIC RESISTANCE TO INFECTIONS

Rowley (1956) first showed that bacterial endotoxin has a marked and non-specific effect on the resistance of animals to bacterial infection. At first there is an increase in susceptibility, but this is followed by increased resistance so that animals so treated will survive infection with an inoculum many million times as large as is fatal in non-treated animals. Dubos and Schaedler (1956) have demonstrated a similar increase of resistance against staphylococci, Friedlander bacilli and also against bovine tubercle bacilli. An increase in resistance to infection has also been demonstrated following administration of acetone-extracted BCG cells (Boehme and Dubos, 1958).

It has been shown that injection of endotoxin in mice is followed by a considerable rise in the properdin level of the blood and there appears to be a close relationship between the level of serum properdin and non-specific resistance to infection, though this increased resistance may be the result of stimulation of other defense mechanisms, in addition to the properdin system, e.g. activation of the reticuloendothelial cells (Landy and Pillemer, 1956). A similar rise in the properdin level to 3–4

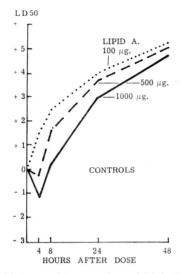

FIG. 57. Effect of lipid A on resistance to bacterial infection (Westphal, 1960).

times the normal has been observed in man following intravenous injection of endotoxin (Sanford and Landy, 1956).

Westphal (1960) and Howard *et al.* (1957) have shown that lipid A will also increase non-specific resistance though the doses required are appreciably larger than those of lipopolysaccharide. The results suggest that the preliminary decrease in resistance (negative phase) does not occur with lipid A as illustrated in Fig. 57. This finding may have practical implications.

SOME PHARMACOLOGICAL ACTIONS OF ENDOTOXIN

These have been extensively studied and can only be briefly discussed here.

Endotoxin is highly active. In the rabbit as small a dose as 0·001 μg./kg. will produce a febrile reaction. With larger doses this becomes more marked and there is the typical leucocytosis preceded by leuco-penia. The horse is also highly sensitive to the toxin. In man the minimum pyrogenic dose is about 0·02 μg. i.e. less per kg. of body weight than in the rabbit. Doses of 0·01–0·2 μg. in man produce febrile reactions not associated with leucopenia, thrombocytopenia or altera-tions in the differential count (Sanford and Landy, 1956).

There is good evidence that the pyrogenic effect is not produced by a direct action of endotoxin but through the liberation in the body of a thermolabile substance (endotoxin is thermostable) which then produces this action. Repeated administration of this endogenous pyrogen does not lead to tolerance such as occurs with continued administration of endotoxin. Moreover, the latent period for the production of fever is appreciably shorter with the endogenous pyrogen than it is with endotoxin. According to Westphal (1960), W. B. Wood and his colleagues of Baltimore have extracted and purified an endogenous pyrogen from the plasma of animals in which a rise in temperature had been produced by the injection of endotoxin.

That the production of endogenous pyrogen is essential for the production of fever has, however, not been established. In particular it has been shown that the intrathecal injection of very small amounts of endotoxin very rapidly produces fever and that no tolerance develops to this. Moreover, animals that are tolerant to endotoxin as a result of repeated intravenous injections show no decrease in their reactivity to intrathecal endotoxin. Bennett and Cluff (1957), who review these findings, conclude that the best explanation of the pyrogenic action of bacterial endotoxin would be a dual mechanism, involving a direct action of endotoxin and an indirect action of endogenous pyrogen. This might account for the biphasic fever curve that characterizes endotoxin fever.

Tatti (1960) has studied the effects of prolonged administration of endotoxin in patients suffering from tuberculosis. There were no toxic effects on the liver or on haemopoiesis, and no stimulation of the adreno-hypophyseal system was observed.

USE AS THERAPEUTIC AGENTS

These are reviewed by Bennett and Cluff (1957) while the use of fever as a mechanism of resistance is discussed by Bennett and Nicastri (1960). There is no doubt, according to these authors, that induced fever can be of value in some diseases and that the protective action of endotoxins can at least to some extent, be independent of their pyrogenic action. At the present state of our knowledge there is no justification for an extensive review here of the clinical use of endotoxins and the reader is referred to the reviews mentioned above.

These substances can produce a variety of side effects, but these are not common and proper control of dosage will largely avoid the more severe ones. The side effects include headache, malaise, nausea, muscle pain, lassitude, anorexia and a tendency to cardiovascular collapse; the general Schwartzman phenomenon with renal cortical necrosis, herpes labialis, hyperpyrexia, renal dysfunction, serum protein depletion and fatal bronchial asthma.

Recent clinical experiments with endotoxins include their use in tuberculosis and in venous thrombosis. Tatti (1960) treated a number of patients with pulmonary tuberculosis by intravenous injection of endotoxin (in conjunction with chemotherapy) for periods of up to 4 months. He concludes that such treatment can be of value in patients with subacute ulcero-caseous lesions which are tending to become chronic and no longer responding to chemotherapy. Stamms and Eichenberger (1958) have demonstrated that endotoxin increases the fibrinolytic activity of the blood and thus tends to lead to the disappearance of thrombi. They used endotoxin in the treatment of venous thrombosis, apparently with some success, and suggest that this treatment may be used in combination with anticoagulants.

MACROCYCLON

Since this drug is believed to exert its action by producing an increase in the resistance of the host, it is appropriately dealt with at this stage.

The work on this compound arose from a chance observation by Cornforth *et al.* (1951) that the commercial surface active agent 'Triton A20' produced a striking suppressive effect on the course of an acute tuberculous infection in mice. The commercial preparation is, however, rather toxic and produces lipaemia and liver damage. The results obtained with it led to the synthesis of a number of compounds which would have similar activity, but a sufficiently low toxicity to be suitable for clinical use, and the best of the compounds made was called macrocyclon, of which the formula is shown below. It has an average

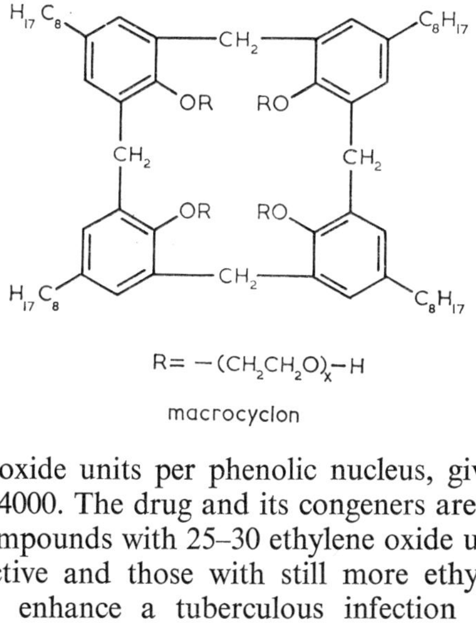

$$R = -(CH_2CH_2O)_x-H$$

macrocyclon

of $12\frac{1}{2}$ ethylene oxide units per phenolic nucleus, giving a molecular weight of about 4000. The drug and its congeners are extremely stable (Rees, 1958). Compounds with 25–30 ethylene oxide units per phenolic nucleus are inactive and those with still more ethylene oxide units (45–75) tend to enhance a tuberculous infection ('Protuberculous action'). A similar spectrum of activity, depending apparently on the physical properties of the compound, has also been found in another mycobacterial infection, namely rat leprosy.

Fate in the body

Macrocyclon is inactive when given orally, and has to be given by subcutaneous or intravenous injection. Studies with the compound labelled with 14C show that no radioactivity can be detected in the tissues following its administration *per os*. When given subcutaneously or intravenously in mice, the blood level drops rapidly in 2–3 days, during which time a small amount is excreted in the urine. The highest levels are found in the liver and relatively high concentrations are also found in monocytes (obtained from the peritoneal cavity), spleen and lungs. The level in these tissues falls slowly and macrocyclon can still be detected 8 weeks after a single injection. Approximately 50% of the dose given is excreted in the faeces in 4–6 weeks, presumably because of excretion in the bile (Rees, 1958).

Chemotherapeutic activity

Macrocyclon is inactive *in vitro* against *M. tuberculosis*, even at a concentration of 2%, and none of the 'protuberculous' compounds enhance growth of the bacilli *in vitro*. No tuberculostatic substance has been detected in the blood and tissue fluids of animals given large doses of the drug. It therefore seems unlikely that the drug produces a toxic effect on the organisms, and it probably acts by enhancing the effectiveness of the natural defences of the host or by making the organisms more susceptible to the natural defensive mechanisms. This is in agreement with the finding of Mackaness (1954) that tubercle bacilli grow slowly or not at all in monocytes derived from animals treated with the surface active agent, although the bacilli grow freely in monocytes from untreated animals.

Macrocyclon is effective in acute tuberculous infections in mice and in guinea pigs and in experimental rat leprosy. The activity in tuberculosis is of the order of streptomycin. The effect of the drug has been investigated in more detail by doing bacterial counts in infected mice. It has been found that treatment with macrocyclon will decrease multiplication of the bacilli in the lungs in an acute infection, but will have no effect in a chronic infection in which the bacilli do not appear to be multiplying (Hart and Rees, 1960). In a parallel investigation Niffenegger and Youmans (1960) found that the effect of macrocyclon is similar to that of previous immunization with B.C.G., suggesting that the drug may act by enhancing the power of acquired immunity.

Toxicity

The L.D.50 of macrocyclon in mice, rats and rabbits is low, i.e. 2·5 G./kg. Prolonged administration to mice only produced some vacuolation of the Kupffer cells of the liver and the reticulo-endothelial cells of the spleen and lymph nodes. Prolonged administration to monkeys also produces some vacuolation of the reticulo-endothelial cells, which disappeared after cessation of treatment, and also some rise in the blood cholesterol (Rees, 1958).

Clinical use

A pilot trial in patients with advanced pulmonary tuberculosis showed that even large doses of the drug produced no beneficial effect. This may be due to the fact that in such cases most of the bacilli are extra-cellular and therefore not exposed to the enhanced activity of the macrophages, if this is indeed the mechanism of action of macrocyclon. There is some evidence that the drug is active in human leprosy, in which disease the bacilli are intracellular.

Administration of the drug in man has so far produced no serious toxic effects. There was an increase in the serum cholesterol (also seen in monkeys) and pruritis with a maculopapular rash, which disappeared after cessation of treatment (Boyd *et al.*, 1959).

REFERENCES

* Denotes review

ABRAHAM, E. P. (1957). 'Biochemistry of some peptide and steroid antibiotics.' New York: John Wiley
ABRAHAM, E. P. and NEWTON, G. G. F. (1960). *Brit. med. Bull.* **16**, 3
ABRAHAM, E. P. and Newton, G. G. F. (1961). *Endeavour*, **20**, 92
ACRED, P., BROWN, D. M., TURNER, D. H. and WRIGHT, D. (1961). *Brit. J. Pharmacol.* **17**, 70
ALBRIGHT, J. G. and HALL, W. H. (1959). *Antibiot. Med.* **6**, 283
ALLEN, J. D., ROBERTS, C. E. and KIRBY, W. M. M. (1962). *New Engl. J. Med.* **266**, 111
ANGIONI, S. and GORECKI, Z. (1960). *Canad. med. Ass. J.* **82**, 1274
ANNOTATION (1961). *Brit. med. J.* **1**, 113
ANNOTATION (1961). *Brit. med. J.* **2**, 1415
BARBER, M. (1960). *Brit. med. J.* **2**, 939
BARNES, M. J. and BOOTHROYD, B. (1961). *Biochem. J.* **78**, 41
BATCHELOR, F. R., DOYLE, F. P., NAYLER, J. H. C. and ROLINSON, G. N. (1959). *Nature (Lond.)*, **183**, 257
BAUM, G. L. and SCHWARZ, J. (1959–60). *Antibiot. Ann.* p. 638
BEARE, M. and MACKENZIE, D. (1959). *Brit. med. J.* **2**, 1137
*BENNETT, I. L. and CLUFF, L. E. (1957). *Pharmacol. Rev.* **9**, 427.
BENNETT, I. L. and NICASTRI, A. (1960). *Bact. Rev.* **24**, 16
BLANK, M. and ROTH, R. J. (1959). *Arch. Derm. Syph.* **79**, 259
BLOCH, H. (1960). *Experientia*, **16**, 255
BOEHME, D. and DUBOS, R. J. (1958). *J. exp. Med.* **107**, 523
BOGERT, W. P. and GAVIN, J. J. (1959). *Ann. N.Y. Acad. Sci.* **82**, 18
BOYD, D. H. A., STEWART, S. M., SOMNER, A. R., CROFTON, J. W. and REES, R. J. W. (1959). *Tubercle*, **40**, 369
British Medical Journal (1960). **2**, 63
BROSSI, A., BAUMANN, M., GESECKE, M. and KYBUTZ, E. (1960). *Helv. chim. Acta*, **43**, 1444
BRANCH, A., RODGER, K. C., TONNING, H. O., LEE, R. W. and POWER, E. E. (1962). *Canad. me. Ass. J.* **86**, 97
BROWN, P. M. and ACRED, P. (1960). *Lancet*, **2**, 568
BROWN, D. M. and ACRED, P. (1961). *Brit. med. J.* **2**, 197
BRUMFITT, W., PERCIVAL, A. and CARTER, M. J. (1962). *Lancet*, **1**, 130
CAMPBELL, C. C. and Hill, G. B. (1959–60). *Antibiotics Annual*, p. 622
CARTER, M. J. and BRUMFITT, W. (1962). *Brit. med. J.* **1**, 80
CHILD, A. J. (1956). *Brit. med. J.* **1**, 660

COFFEY, G. L., ANDERSON, L. E., FISHER, M. W., GALBRAITH, M. L., HILLEGAS, A. B., KOHBERGER, D. L., THOMPSON, P. E., WESTON, K. S. and EHRLECH, J. (1959). *Antibiot. and Chemother.* **9,** 730.

COLES, H. M. T., MACNAMARA, B., MUTCH, L., HOLT, R. J. and STEWART, G. T. (1960). *Lancet,* **1,** 944

COLES, H. M. T. and STEWART, G. T. (1961). *Practitioner,* **186,** 379

CONDIE, R. M., ZAK, S. J. and GOOD, R. A. (1955). *Proc. Soc. exp. Biol. (N.Y.),* **90,** 355

CORNFORTH, J. W., HART, P. D., REES, R. J. W. and STOCK, J. A. (1951). *Nature (Lond.),* **168,** 150

COURTNEY, K. O., THOMPSON, P. E., HODGKINSON, R. and FITZSIMMONS, J. R. (1959–60). *Antibiotics Annual,* p. 304

DOUTHWAITE, A. H. and TRAFFORD, J. A. P. (1960). *Brit. med. J.* **2,** 687

DOUTHWAITE, A. H., TRAFFORD, J. A. P., McGILL, D. A. F. and EVANS, I. E. (1961). *Brit. med. J.* **2,** 6

DUBOS, R. J. and SCHAEDLER, R. W. (1956). *J. exp. Med.* **104,** 53

DUTTON, A. A. C. and ELMES, P. C. (1959). *Brit. med. J.* **1,** 1144

DU VIGNEAUD, V., CARPENTER, F. H., HOLLEY, R. S., LIVERMORE, W. H. and RACHELE, J. R. (1946). *Science,* **104,** 431

EDITORIAL (1959). *Brit. med. J.* **2,** 482

EDITORIAL (1961). *Canad. med. Ass. J.* **85,** 1355

ELEK, S. D. and FLEMING, P. C. (1960). *Lancet,* **2,** 569

ESSELLIER, A. F., HUNZIKER, H. and GOLDSAND, R. (1958). *Schweiz. med. Wschr.* **88,** 813

FINLAND, M. and GARROD, L. R. (1960). *Brit. med. J.* **2,** 959

FINLAND, M., JONES, W. F., ZIAL, M. and CHERRICK, G. R. (1957). *Amer. J. med. Sci.* **234,** 505

FINLAND, M. and NICHOLS, R. L. (1957). *Practitioner,* **179,** 84

FISHER, M. W., MANNING, M. C., GAGLIARDI, L. A., GAETZ, M. R. and ERLANDSON, A. L. (1959–60). *Antibiotics Annual,* p. 293

FÜRESZ, S. (1958). *Antibiot. and Chemother.* **8,** 446

FÜRESZ, S. and SCOTTI, R. (1959–60). *Antibiotics Annual,* p. 285

FÜRESZ, S. and SCOTTI, R. (1961). *Farmaco,* **16,** 262

FURTADO, T. A. (1959–60). *Antibiotics Annual,* p. 631

GANGAROSA, E. J. (1959–60). *Antibiotics Annual,* p. 536

GARROD, L. P. (1960). *Brit. med. J.* **1,** 527

GENTLES, J. C. (1958). *Nature (Lond.),* **182,** 476

GENTLES, J. C., BARNES, M. and FANTES, K. H. (1959). *Nature (Lond.),* **183,** 256

GERACI, J. E., HEILMAN, F. R., NICHOLS, D. R., WELMAN, W. E. and ROSS, G. T (1956). *Proc. Mayo Clin.* **31,** 564

GILBERT, R. P. (1960). *Physiol. Rev.* **40,** 245

GOLDHAMMER, H. (1958). *Dtsch. med. Wschr.* **2,** 1488

GOUREVITCH, A., HUNT, G. A. and LEIN, J. (1960). *Antibiot. and Chemother.* **10,** 121

GRIFFITH, R. S. (1960). *Antibiotic Medicine,* **7,** 129

GRIFFITH, R. S., STEVENS, V. C., WOLFE, R. N., BONIECE, W. S. and LEE, C. C. (1958). *Antibiotic Medicine,* **5,** 609

HARRELL, E. R. and BOCOBO, F. C. (1960). *Clin. Pharm. Ther.* **1,** 104

HART, P. D. and REES, R. J. W. (1960). *Brit. J. exp. Path.* **41,** 414

HINTON, N. A. and WILSON, D. L. (1959). *Antibiot. and Chemother.* **9,** 667

HIRSCH, H. A. and FINLAND, M. (1960). *New Engl. J. Med.* **262,** 209

HIRSCH, H. A., KUNIN, C. M. and FINLAND, M. (1959). *New Engl. J. Med.* **260,** 408

HOWARD, J. G., ROWLEY, D. and WARDLAW, A. C. (1957). *Nature (Lond.),* **179,** 314

JACKSON, G. G. and GRIEBLE, H. G. (1957). *Ann. N.Y. Acad. Sci.* **69,** 493

JAGO, M. and HEATLEY, N. C. (1961). *Brit. J. Pharmacol.* **16,** 170

JOHNSON, A. G., GAINES, S. and LANDY, M. (1959). *J. exp. Med.* **103,** 225

KARLSON, A. G. (1961). *Amer. Rev. resp. Dis.* **84,** 902

KIRBY, W. M. M., PERRY, D. M. and BAUER, A. W. (1960). *New Engl. J. Med.* **262,** 49

KNOX, R. (1960). *Brit. med. J.* **2,** 690
KNOX, R. (1961). *Guy's Hosp. Rep.* **110,** 134
KNUDSON, E. T. and ROLINSON, G. N. (1959). *Lancet,* **2,** 1105
KNUDSON, E. T. and ROLINSON, G. N. (1960). *Brit. med. J.* **2,** 700
KNUDSON, E. T., ROLINSON, G. N. and STEVENS, S. (1961). *Brit. med. J.* **2,** 198
KOCH, R., DRIES, C. P. and ASAY, L. D. (1959–60). *Antibiotics Annual,* p. 917
KUCK, N. A. and REDIN, G. S. (1960). *J. Pharmacol. exp. Ther.* **129,** 350
KUNIN, C. M., WILCOX, C., NAJARIAN, A. and FINLAND, M. (1958). *Proc. Soc. exp. Biol.* **99,** 312
LANDY, M. and PILLEMER, L. (1956). *J. exp. Med.* **104,** 383
LATTIMER, A., SIMON, A. J. and LEPPER, M. H. (1960). *Amer. J. med. Sci.* **239,** 548
LAUDER, I. M. and O'SULLIVAN, J. G. (1958). *Vet. Rec.* **70,** 949
LEDUC, A. and FONTAINE, J. (1962). *Canad. med. Ass. J.* **86,** 101
LINDSAY, D. G., PRLINA, I., BISCHOFF, A. J. and BECKER, S. W. (1958). *Arch. Derm. Syph. (Chicago),* **78,** 299
LOCKEY, E., EATON, B. R. and COMPSTON, N. (1962). *Brit. J. clin. Pract.* **16,** 13
LUTON, E. F. (1961). *J. Amer. med. Ass.* **177,** 152
MCCARTHY, C. G. and FINLAND, M. (1960). *New Engl. J. Med.* **263,** 315
MCCORMICK, J. R. D., SJOLANDER, N. O., HIRSCH, V., JENSEN, E. R. and DOERSCHUK, A. P. (1957). *J. Amer. chem. Soc.* **79,** 4561
MCNALL, E. G. (1959–60). *Antibiotics Annual,* p. 674
MACKANESS, G. B. (1954). *Amer. Rev. Tuberc.* **69,** 690
MAFFII, G., BIANCHI, G., SCHIATTI, P. and GALLO, G. G. (1961). *Farmaco,* **16,** 246
MAFFII, G., SCHIATTI, P., BIANCHI, G. and SERRALUNGA, M. G. (1961). *Farmaco,* **16,** 235
MAFFII, G. and TIMBAL, M. T. (1959–60). *Antibiotics Annual,* p. 277
MARMELL, M. and PRIGOT, A. (1959–60). *Antibiotics Annual,* p. 454
MONALDI, V., CURCI, G. and NITTI, V. (1961). *Arch. Tisiol. Mal. App. Resp.* **16,** 361
NEIPP, L., PADOWETZ, W., SACKMANN, W. and TRIFOD, J. (1958). *Schweiz. med. Wschr.* **88,** 835, 858
NEWBOULD, B. B. and KILPATRICK, R. (1960). *Lancet,* **1,** 887
NIFFENEGGER, J. and YOUMANS, G. P. (1960). *Brit. J. exp. Path.* **41,** 403
OXFORD, A. E., RAISTRICK, H. and SIMONART, P. (1939). *Biochem. J.* **33,** 240
REES, R. J. W. (1958). *Bull. Inst. Union. Tub.* **38,** 193
RENTCHNICK, P. (1958). *Schweiz. med. Wschr.* **88,** 362
ROBSON, J. M. and KEELE, C. A. (1956). 'Recent Advances in Pharmacology' 2nd ed. London: Churchill
ROLINSON, G. N. and STEVENS, S. (1961). *Brit. med. J.* **2,** 191
ROLINSON, G. N., STEVENS, S., BATCHELOR, F. R., WOOD, J. C. and CHAIN, E. B. (1960). *Lancet,* **2,** 564
ROLLO, I. M., SOMERS, G. F. and BURLEY, D. M. (1962). *Brit. med. J.* **1,** 76
ROWLEY, D. (1956). *Brit. J. exp. Path.* **37,** 223
SANFORD, J. P. and LANDY, M. (1956). *Clin. Res. Proc.* **4,** 134
SENSI, P., BALLOTTA, R., GRECO, A. M. and GALLO, G. G. (1961). *Farmaco,* **16,** 165
SENSI, P., MARGALITH, P. and TIMBAL, M. T. (1959). *Farmaco,* **14,** 196
SHEEHAN, J. C. and HENERY-LOGAN, K. R. (1957). *J. Amer. chem. Soc.* **79,** 1262
SHEIKH, A. E. (1960). *Antibiot. and Chemother.* **7,** 681
SKARNES, R. C., ROSEN, F. S., SHEAR, M. J. and LANDY, M. (1958). *J. exp. Med.* **108,** 685
STAMMS, H. and EICHENBERGER, E. (1958). *Geburts. u. Frauenheilk.* **18,** 451
STAUB, A. M. (1960). *Ann. Inst., Pasteur,* **98,** 814
STETSON, C. (1956). *J. exp. Med.* **104,** 921
STEVENSON, C. J. and DJAVAHISZWILI, N. (1961). *Lancet,* **1,** 373
STEWART, G. T. (1956). *Brit. med. J.* **1,** 658
STEWART, G. T. (1960). *Brit. med. J.* **2,** 694
STEWART, G. T., COLES, H. M. T., NIXON, H. H. and HOLT, R. J. (1961). *Brit. med. J.* **2,** 200
STEWART, G. T., NIXON, H. H. and COLES, H. M. T. (1960). *Brit. med. J.* **2,** 703

STORMONT, J. M., MACKIE, J. E. and DAVIDSON, C. S. (1958). *New Engl. J. Med.* **259**, 1145

SYMPOSIUM ON GRISEOFULVIN (1960). *Brit. med. J.* **1**, 1804

TATTI, V. (1960). *Schweiz. Z. Tuberk.* **17**, 1

TAYLOR, R. M., MILLER, W. L. and BROOK, M. J. V. (1956). *Antibiot. and Chemother.* **6**, 162

THOMAS, J. P., BAUGHN, C. D., WILKINSON, R. G. and SHEPHERD, R. G. (1961). *Amer. J. Resp. Dis.* **83**, 891

THOMPSON, R. E. M., HARDING, J. W. and SIMON, R. D. (1960). *Brit. med. J.* **2**, 708

THOMPSON, R. E. M., WHITBY, J. L. and HARDING, J. W. (1960). *Brit. med. J.* **2**, 706

TIMBAL, M. T. (1959–60). *Antibiotics Annual*, p. 271

TIMBAL, M. T. and BREGA, A. (1961). *Farmaco*, **16**, 191

TIMBAL, M. T., PALLANZA, R. and CARNITTI, G. (1961). *Farmaco*, **16**, 181

TOSONI, A. L., GLASS, T. G. and GOLDSMITH, L. (1958). *Biochem. J.* **69**, 476

WAISBREN, B. A., KLEINERMAN, L., SKEMP, J. and BRATCHER, G. (1959–60). *Antibiotics Annual*, p. 497

*WESTPHAL, O. (1960). *Ann. Inst. Pasteur*, **98**, 789

WILLIAMSON, G. M., MORRISON, J. K. and STEVENS, K. J. (1961). *Lancet*, **1**, 847

FUCIDIN

This is an antibiotic isolated from the fermentation broth of *Fusidium coccineum*. It is a steroid related in structure to helvolic acid. The sodium salt is very soluble in water.

In vitro it is highly effective against *staphylococcus pyogenes*, though the effect is mainly bacteriostatic (affecting both penicillin sensitive and penicillin resistant organisms) and is considerably decreased in the presence of serum. Resistant forms develop rather readily. A synergistic effect of Fucidin with penicillin and also with erythromycin has been demonstrated.

Following oral administration in man, the drug is well absorbed and with a dose of 500 mg. a maximum blood concentration of around 25 µg./ml. is observed after 1–2 hours, with appreciable amounts still present at 24 hours. The drug is slowly excreted and with repeated administration cumulation occurs and the blood concentration rises.

Fucidin has a low toxicity in animals. There are no published data on the effectiveness of the drug in experimental infections. Preliminary investigations in man show that it can be valuable in the treatment of various staphylococcal infections, given either alone or in combination with penicillin. The dosage has varied from 500–1,500 mg. per day given for periods up to three months. No serious toxic effects have so far been observed. (See *Lancet*, 1962, **1**, 928–937.)

CHAPTER 12

ANTIMALARIAL
AND ANTHELMINTIC DRUGS

ANTIMALARIALS

The past ten years have shown great changes in the campaign against malaria. From being a vast unsolved problem of the tropics, malaria has become an eradicable disease, and the methods by which eradication can be achieved are known. It has been banished from a number of islands, such as Ceylon, Cyprus and Mauritius; islands have the great advantage that reintroduction of the disease can be prevented if the control of immigrants is efficient. The disease has also disappeared from the U.S.A. and the U.S.S.R., and great strides have already been made in the even more difficult problem of eradication in India. In 1960 the W.H.O. announced an all-out campaign based upon the use of residual insecticides and chemotherapy which, used together, can interrupt transmission by reducing the numbers of mosquitos and parasites to such low levels that the life-cycle of the parasite has little chance of completion. During the 'attack phase' of the campaign the parasite and vector are reduced to low levels of incidence. Two years of consolidation follow, during which all people with fevers which are likely to be caused by malaria are treated with antimalarial drugs. Consolidation is followed by surveillance to ensure that parasites are not reintroduced by immigrants, and that any previously undetected foci of infection are immediately wiped out. After a successful eradication campaign, and under adequate conditions of surveillance, it does not matter if the *Anopheles* mosquito returns. There are no parasites for it to transmit. The effectiveness of good surveillance can be seen in the Southern States of the U.S.A. in which even the extensive movements of people to and from malarious areas during the Korean war did not give rise to more than a handful of cases of malaria. These were rapidly detected and treated, and no epidemics occurred. Such an attack on a widespread disease costs a great deal of money and calls for many teams of experienced workers. It also requires the co-operation of the people of the country and if this cannot be achieved by persuasion or compulsion, an expensive eradication programme may come to nothing.

INSECTICIDES

For the control of the malaria mosquito, potent residual insecticides such as Dicophane (DDT), Benzene hexachloride (Gammexane) and Dieldrin are now available. Many malaria-transmitting *Anopheles* mosquitos bite during the night while the people are indoors and, having taken a meal of blood, the female mosquitos rest for a while on the walls of the room. If the walls are sprayed regularly so that the mosquito picks up a lethal dose on contact, the vectors rapidly decline in numbers, because dead female mosquitos do not lay eggs.

The matter is not quite so simple in areas such as the forests of Venezuela, where some species of mosquito which act as malaria transmitters bite people out in the fields while they are at work. It is very difficult and expensive to spray large tracts of tropical forest. However, a measure of control can be brought about by locating and dealing with the main breeding places if these are not too widely distributed. The tactics of each campaign must depend upon the species and habits of the vector, the type of country, and the way of life of the human host.

Unfortunately, mosquitos can become resistant; strains which are no longer killed by the standard range of insecticides have been reported from several parts of the world.

LIFE-CYCLE

The life-cycle of the malaria parasite is illustrated in Fig. 58. The small 'ring-form' of the parasite grows and divides asexually in the erythrocyte to form a schizont. The infected cell bursts, and more erythrocytes are infected. A small number of parasites grow into male or female gametocytes, which when taken up by the mosquito develop into gametes; the female gamete is fertilized by the male and the motile zygote burrows into the wall of the mosquito's stomach. Here the oocyst develops, and the nucleus of the parasite divides into numerous sporozoites, which migrate to the salivary glands. When the mosquito feeds again, the sporozoites are injected into the new human host with the saliva of the insect and find their way to the parenchymal cells of the liver. Here they develop into large exoerythrocytic schizonts which, when mature, release parasites which infect the red cells of the blood, and the sexual cycle is complete.

Once out of the liver cells and into the blood, *P. falciparum* does not return, but the exoerythrocytic forms of *P. vivax* may infect other liver cells. *P. vivax* malaria may therefore persist in the liver for considerable periods and unless cured it will relapse.

CHEMOTHERAPY

If every person in a malarious area could be treated effectively so that no parasites remained in the blood or tissues, the disease would quickly die out even if the mosquitos remained. The life of a mosquito in the tropics is usually short and the parasite is not transmitted to the egg. A recent World Health Organization Technical Report (1961) states that

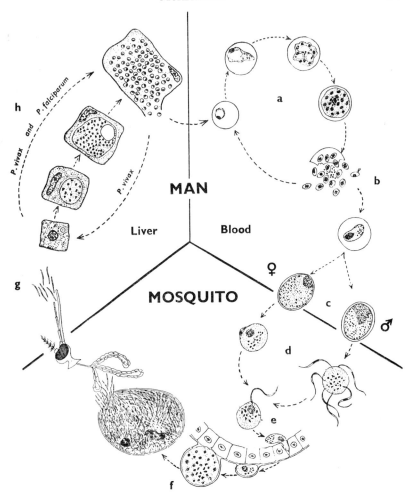

a. Erythrocytic cycle   e. Zygote
b. Segmenting schizont   f. Oocysts
c. Gametocytes   g. Sporozoites
d. Gametes   h. Exoerythrocytic stages

Fig. 58. The life-cycle of the malaria parasite.

'in ideal conditions of a stable, fully co-operative population, given the guarantee of a complete drug coverage of an epidemiologically delimited area, a well-organized mass administration of schizonticidal and sporonticidal drugs may eradicate malaria within a year, barring its reintroduction from the outside'.

In practice however, except under military discipline, such a campaign meets with difficulties. In intensely malarious areas, although most of the surviving population is infected, the people are sufficiently immune to be free from symptoms for most of the year; they are therefore not unduly concerned about taking drugs regularly for prolonged periods. Health education is essential, and it may be necessary to initiate a system of rewards for those who co-operate. The distribution of tablets requires close supervision, and cannot usually be entrusted to any but the members of a trained team of paid employees of the health organization. Depending upon the habits and traditions of the people, certain age-groups, religious or farming groups may be very difficult to treat and constitute a reservoir for future transmission. Small children, who are often the main source of the malarial gametocytes which infect the mosquitos, are usually difficult to treat, especially with bitter medicines. In remote areas where regular distribution of drugs is impossible, some success has been achieved by adding chloroquine or pyrimethamine to domestic salt.

A drug which acts upon the asexual parasites in the erythrocytes is called a *schizonticide*, and rapidly acting, efficient drugs of this kind are used for the treatment of malarial fever. Quinine and mepacrine have now been almost completely superseded by the less toxic 4-amino-quinoline derivatives chloroquine and amodiaquine. If taken regularly, a schizonticide will also suppress malaria by killing the asexual forms as soon as they reach the red cells, but it will not affect exoerythrocytic stages of *P. vivax* in the liver.

Exoerythrocytic parasites are killed by 8-aminoquinoline compounds; the most widely used is primaquine. They are also affected and are often killed by proguanil, chlorproguanil and pyrimethamine. Drugs which act in this way are called *tissue schizonticides* and are used for the radical cure of people who have left malarious areas, and for treating infections which develop after the attack phase of an eradication campaign. In addition, primaquine kills gametocytes. Proguanil, chlorproguanil and pyrimethamine also affect gametocytes, rendering them incapable of development in the mosquito. These drugs are therefore called *sporonticides*. They act too slowly on asexual erythrocytic forms to be of much value in the treatment of acute malaria in a patient who has no immunity to the infection, but all three drugs are effective prophylactics if taken regularly. No drug is yet known which has unquestionable activity against sporozoites. Such a drug would constitute a true causal prophylactic and prevent malarial infection from the outset.

Quinine and Mepacrine

These drugs are not now widely used. Quinine is given for the treatment of cerebral malaria, an acute, dangerous development of *P. falciparum* infection in which the central nervous system is involved.

For this purpose quinine is given intravenously. Large stocks of mepacrine were left over from the 1939–1945 war, and these are still being used in developing countries with limited money to spend on imports, but little is now manufactured. Mepacrine stains the skin, but is a valuable antimalarial drug and the incidence of serious side-effects such as skin affections and psychotic illness is very low.

4-aminoquinoline derivatives

Chloroquine and amodiaquine are of equal activity and are the most widely used and most efficient schizonticides. For the treatment of malarial fever in an indigenous patient who has some immunity to the infection, a single dose of chloroquine phosphate equivalent to 600

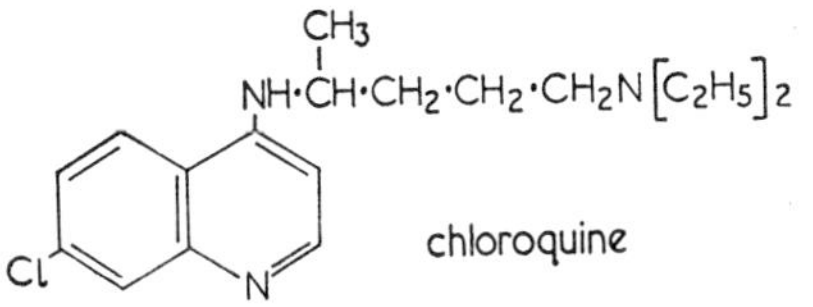

$$NH \cdot CH(CH_3) \cdot CH_2 \cdot CH_2 \cdot CH_2N[C_2H_5]_2$$

chloroquine

$$CH_2N[C_2H_5]_2$$

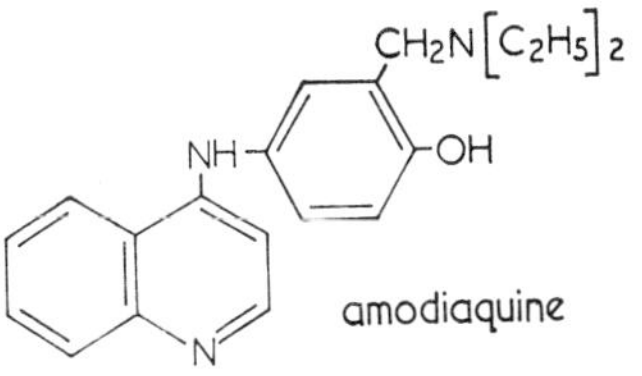

amodiaquine

mg. of base is usually sufficient to bring about a rapid clinical cure. Patients from non-malarious countries who have no acquired immunity are usually given a total dose of 1·5 g. over the course of 3 days. A similar regimen is followed for amodiaquine.

The drugs are also used to suppress malaria in doses of 300 mg. (base) given once weekly. They have no serious toxic side-effects at these dose-levels and their only disadvantage is their bitter taste. An attempt to overcome the flavour of chloroquine by giving it as the sparingly soluble hydroxynaphthoate or tannate met with little success because in these forms it was poorly absorbed from the intestine and its antimalarial action was low and irregular (Clyde, 1960a). Chloroquine is concentrated and stored in the liver, and although it has no action against exoerythrocytic malaria parasites, it is effective in amoebic hepatitis. It has also been used in very large doses (up to 1·0 g. daily) for the alleviation of rheumatoid arthritis and discoid lupus erythematosus and in these quantities may cause side-effects, especially ocular changes and alimentary disturbances. The ocular lesions are of two kinds. Corneal changes were found by Hobbs et al. (1961) in a third of the cases being treated for these two conditions. They caused no impairment of vision and cleared upon discontinuing the drug. Retinal changes occurred in only 3% cases but in these vision was permanently impaired. A drug with such diverse properties must have an interesting pharmacology, but very little is known of its mode of action.

Proguanil, Chlorproguanil and Pyrimethamine

These three drugs have very similar modes of action but differ in potency and degree of persistence in the body; proguanil needs to be given once a day as a prophylactic, whereas chlorproguanil and pyrimethamine are given once weekly. Pyrimethamine is the most persistent of the three (Smith and Ihrig, 1957) and in some parts of the world is effective when given at monthly intervals. Widely-spaced doses are not, however, recommended because they are liable to induce drug-resistance (see below).

As long ago as 1948, Hawking and Perry showed that proguanil was without activity against malaria parasites in tissue culture, but that serum from animals treated with the drug was highly active. It was therefore clear that proguanil must yield an active metabolite, and this was finally isolated in 1951 (Carrington, Crowther, Davey, Levi and

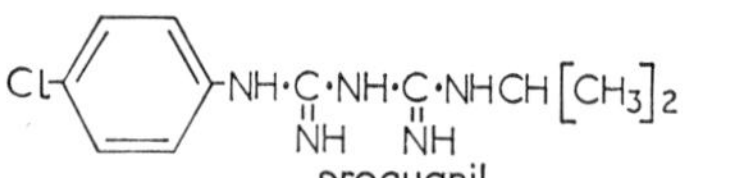

proguanil

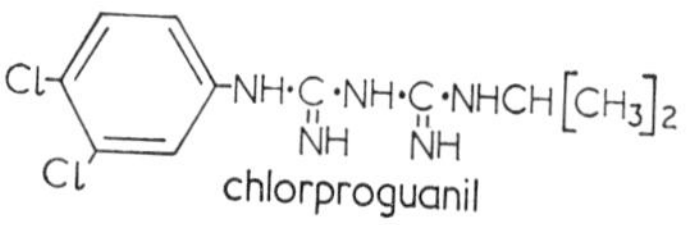

chlorproguanil

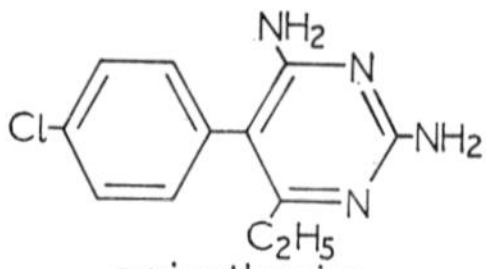

pyrimethamine

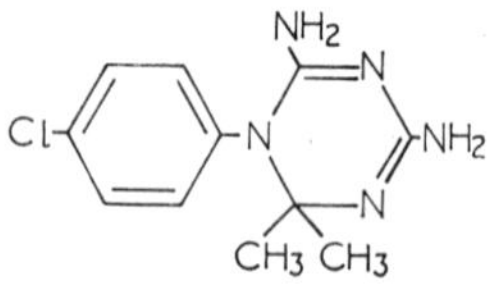

metabolite of proguanil

Rose, 1951; Crowther and Levi, 1953) and it was shown that the biguanide chain of proguanil forms a dihydrotriazine ring. In the meantime, Hitchings and his co-workers, in the course of an investigation of diaminopyrimidine derivatives designed as antimetabolites of possible value in the chemotherapy of cancer, noted that the powerful antagonism to folic and folinic acids exerted by these compounds to cultures of *Streptococcus faecalis*, was shown to a lesser degree by proguanil. The diaminopyrimidines were therefore tested as antimalarials and the most active, pyrimethamine, had 200 times the activity of proguanil against experimental infections of *P. gallinaceum* in chicks (Falco, Goodwin, Hitchings, Rollo and Russell, 1951). The high activity of pyrimethamine was soon confirmed in human malaria (Archibald, 1951) and the drug is now widely used for prophylaxis. The similarity in the structure of pyrimethamine and the proguanil metabolite is clear.

Pyrimethamine acts by depriving the malaria parasite of folinic acid at the points in its life history when this metabolite is most in demand —during division of the nucleus. It has no great activity on the growing parasite and its action in acute malaria may therefore be slow unless the schizonts are reaching maturity at the time the drug is administered. Schizonticides such as chloroquine and amodiaquine affect all stages of the asexual cycle and therefore act more rapidly.

The toxicity of pyrimethamine to the malaria parasite is high because the parasite relies upon the synthesis of folic acid from p-aminobenzoate; toxicity to the host is much lower because human cells make use of pre-formed folic and folinic acid absorbed from the gut.

Sulphonamides and sulphones are quite active antimalarials, because they compete with p-aminobenzoate, and in experimental malaria infections in chicks and mice (Rollo, 1955) they potentiate the action of pyrimethamine (Fig. 59). This is because they block different points

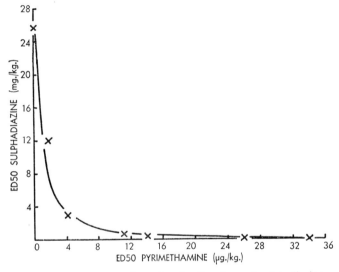

FIG. 59. Potentiating effect of pyrimethamine and sulphadiazine in chicks infected with *Plasmodium gallinaceum* (Rollo, 1955).

along the same metabolic pathway (Fig. 60) and their joint action is more powerful than could be expected from the sum of their separate effects (Goodwin and Rollo, 1955; Goodwin, 1956). This has been confirmed in human malaria in the Gambia by Hurly (1959). A single dose of 0·1 to 0·25 mg./kg. of pyrimethamine alone was sufficient to clear the blood of *P. falciparum* malaria parasites. A dose of 1 g. of sulphadiazine was without effect. When the two drugs were given together, one-tenth of the dose of pyrimethamine with one-quarter of the dose of sulphadiazine were fully effective against the asexual forms of *P. falciparum*, *P. malariae* and *P. ovale*. This combination of drugs is also effective against *Toxoplasma* infections (Eyles and Coleman, 1952, 1953; Ryan, Hart, Culligan, Gunkel, Jacobs and Cook, 1954) and against coccidiosis (Kendall and Joyner, 1956).

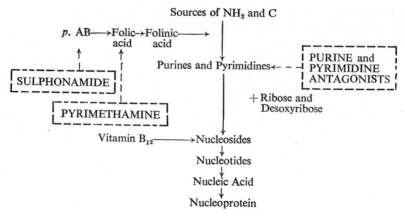

FIG. 60. The points of action of sulphonamides and pyrimethamine in metabolic processes of micro-organisms (Goodwin, 1956).

Chlorproguanil was shown by Robertson (1957) to be an effective prophylactic in experimental *P. falciparum* infections in East Africa. Its mode of action is similar to that of proguanil and pyrimethamine.

Primaquine

The first synthetic antimalarial, introduced in 1926, was the 8-aminoquinoline derivative, pamaquin (Schulemann, 1932). The activity of this drug against gametocytes, and its ability to cure *P. vivax* malaria have been known for many years, although the existence of the exoerythrocytic form of the parasite was only established in recent years (Shortt, Garnham, Covell and Shute, 1948). The relatively high toxicity of pamaquin to human erythrocytes, especially when given

together with mepacrine, has limited its usefulness. Research carried out since 1945 in Chicago on human volunteers by Alving and his associates showed that certain other 8-aminoquinoline derivatives had high activity against the tissue forms of *P. vivax*. The most active and least toxic of the compounds tested was primaquine, the primary amine corresponding to pamaquin. Other related derivatives, such as pentaquine, had less favourable margins of safety.

In 1950, large numbers of American servicemen were exposed to *P. vivax* malaria during the Korean war (Alving, Arnold and Robinson,

1952). Chloroquine was given once weekly to suppress malarial fever, and, in order to prevent the reintroduction of malaria to the United States, all were given treatment with primaquine, 15 mg. (base) daily for 15 days on the return voyage, to kill the tissue parasites. This measure was immensely successful (Archambeault, 1954) and about 250,000 troops were treated. The course of treatment is now widely used for the radical cure of *P. vivax* malaria.

'*Primaquine-sensitivity*'

The chief danger associated with the use of 8-aminoquinoline derivatives is intravascular haemolysis, which may be so severe as to be diagnosed as blackwater fever. Such haemolytic crises occur most frequently in dark-skinned peoples and certain other racial or ethnic groups, such as Sardinians and Sephardic Jews. The reactions are precipitated by daily doses of 30 mg. of primaquine and also by other synthetic drugs such as acetanilide, sulphonamides and sulphones. An extensive biochemical study of the phenomenon has been carried out by Alving and his collaborators in Chicago since 1950. It has been shown quite clearly that 'primaquine-sensitivity' occurs in persons with a genetically transmitted abnormality of their erythrocytes, the most characteristic and severe evidence of which is a deficiency of the enzyme, glucose 6-phosphate dehydrogenase (G-6-PD), (Carson, Schrier and Kellermeyer, 1959). Primaquine-sensitivity is also associated with 'favism', the severe haemolysis which occurs when some people eat partially cooked or uncooked broad-beans.

Beutler, Dern, Flanagan and Alving (1955) discovered that primaquine-sensitive cells show a diminished content of reduced glutathione, a substance which appears to protect erythrocytes against a variety of physical and chemical agents. Glutathione is maintained in the reduced state by the enzyme glutathione reductase, with the assistance of reduced triphosphopyridine nucleotide (TPNH) as a coenzyme. In mature erythrocytes, reduction of triphosphopyridine nucleotide (TPN) to TPNH requires the oxidation of glucose *via* the pentose-phosphate pathway; the first enzyme in this pathway is G-6-PD. It is therefore clear that a deficiency in the activity of G-6-PD will lead through the chain of interrelated biochemical reactions to an inability to maintain a protective level of reduced glutathione in the erythrocyte (Fig. 61).

The first stage in the metabolism of primaquine is the removal of a methyl group to form a 6-hydroxy compound with a powerful oxidizing capacity. Such a substance would be expected to affect erythrocytes deficient in reduced glutathione.

The details of the mechanism have not yet been fully explained, but it is certain that this is a fruitful investigation which may go far to explain conditions which have hitherto been very imperfectly understood.

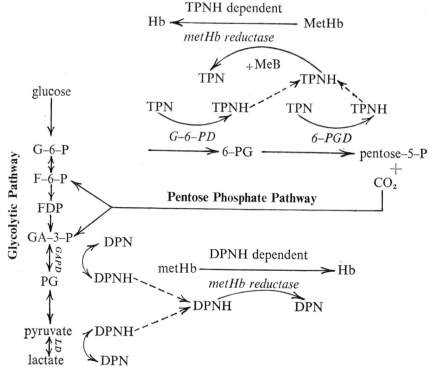

FIG. 61. Pathways of carbohydrate metabolism and specific enzymatic methaemoglobin reduction in the mature mammalian erythrocyte (Brewer, Tarlov and Alving, 1960).

Abbreviations: DPN, diphosphopyridine nucleotide; DPNH, reduced diphosphopyridine nucleotide; FDP, fructose diphosphate; F-6-P, fructose-6-phosphate; G-6-P, glucose-6-phosphate; G-6-PD, glucose-6-phosphate dehydrogenase; GAPD, glyceraldehyde phosphate dehydrogenase; GA-3-P, glyceraldehyde-3-phosphate; Hb, haemoglobin; MetHb, methaemoglobin; MeB, methylene blue; 6-PG, 6-phosphogluconate; PG, phosphoglycerate; Pentose-5-P, pentose-5-phosphate; LD, lactic dehydrogenase; TPN, triphosphopyridine nucleotide; TPNH, reduced triphosphopyridine nucleotide; 6-PGD, 6-phosphogluconic dehydrogenase; CO_2, carbon dioxide.

The pentose phosphate pathway functions as an alternative (TPNH-dependent) route for the reduction of methaemoglobin in the presence of electron carriers, such as methylene blue. The reduction of methaemoglobin in this pathway in primaquine-senstive erythrocytes is probably limited by the deficiency of G-6-PD activity, which characterizes this inborn error of metabolism.

For the sake of simplicity, many enzymes and many steps in both pathways have not been included in the figure.

Methaemoglobin is reduced to haemoglobin in the normal red cell by a specific reductase. This enzyme is dependent upon TPNH for its regeneration (Fig. 61), and it is therefore not surprising that primaquine-sensitive red cells have a diminished capacity for reducing methaemoglobin. This defect has been used in the design of a simple *in vitro* test for the identification of sensitive individuals (Brewer, Tarlov and Alving, 1960) which should prove of great value in forecasting the occurrence of haemolytic reactions when 8-aminoquinoline drugs are used in the mass treatment of populations.

Older red cells appear to be more susceptible to haemolysis than those that have recently left the bone marrow, and it was shown by Dern Beutler and Alving (1954) that if the treatment of a sensitive patient with large doses of primaquine was continued in spite of haemolysis, there was a brisk reticulocytosis. The lysed, older cells were soon replaced by less sensitive younger cells and the blood picture returned to normal (Fig. 62). The resistance of the younger cells was, however, less than that of normal erythrocytes, and excessive doses of primaquine caused a chronic haemolytic anaemia of great severity.

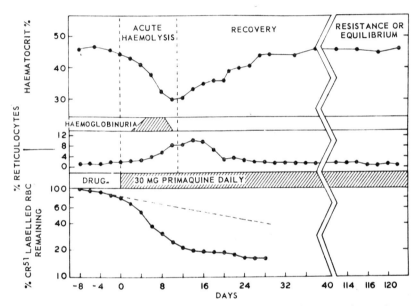

FIG. 62. Clinical course of primaquine haemolysis, shown by composite results from three sensitive males with major expression of the genetic defect (Alving *et al.*, 1960). The haemolysis is self-limited even though the standard challenge dose of 30 mg. daily is continued, because it stimulates erythropoiesis by the bone marrow. Reticolucytes and younger erythrocytes are relatively more resistant to haemolysis by the oxidized degradation products of primaquine than are the older cells. If the daily dose of primaquine is excessively great, chronic haemolytic anaemia results, unless the medication is terminated.

4-Aminoquinoline-Primaquine Combinations

With the increased speed of transport, it is now no longer practicable to rely upon a return voyage from the tropics which lasts for 15 days. Alving and his team have therefore recently tried doses of primaquine at more widely spaced intervals throughout the time of exposure to *P. vivax* infection. They found that 60 mg. of primaquine, given once weekly together with 300 mg. chloroquine to kill erythrocytic parasites, protected a high percentage of volunteers experimentally infected with *P. vivax*. Moreover, such a dose-regime of primaquine had a negligible haemolytic effect upon the red cells of primaquine-sensitive individuals (Alving, Johnson, Tarlov, Brewer, Kellermeyer and Carson, 1960). Similar studies have also been conducted with primaquine and amodiaquine (Courtney, Hodgkinson, Ramsey and Haggerty, 1960). It is likely that the association of an 8-amino- and a 4-aminoquinoline compound will afford a suppressive-curative effect against all forms of malaria.

Such drug associations are not new. Sinton used quinine and pamaquin in India many years ago. Proprietary preparations such as 'Rhodopraequine' and 'Premaline' have been used for many years in the former French colonies and have proved their value. The 8-aminoquinoline ingredients of such preparations, pamaquin and 'rhodoquine' (6-methoxy-8- (diethylamino-*n*-propylamino) quinoline) are, however, considerably more toxic to man than primaquine, and the new combinations introduced by American workers are likely to have a greater margin of safety. Even with primaquine, the effective dose is too close to the toxic dose to be completely reassuring, and Alving *et al.* (1960) recommend that in populations over which full supervision cannot be assured the weekly dose should be 45 mg. instead of 60 mg. It is possible that other curative drugs may be found with a more favourable chemotherapeutic index.

Other Combinations of Drugs

Apart from mixtures of 4-amino- and 8-aminoquinolines, there is an increasing tendency to give antimalarial drugs in combination, in order to obtain the benefit of their different types of activity against the various stages of the malaria parasite.

Pyrimethamine or chlorproguanil is given together with chloroquine to exert a three-fold action—on the asexual blood parasites, the tissue forms in the liver and the gametocytes. Such combinations are frequently given to people during malaria eradication campaigns, and to those in areas in which campaigns have been carried out. Facilities are not always available for complete investigation and treatment, and people with fever must be presumed to be infected with the malaria parasite. A dose of a schizonticide plus a sporonticide will help to ensure that such people will not act as foci from which the spread of malaria may begin again. Trials with pyrimethamine and primaquine are also in progress.

Drug Resistance

Strains of the malaria parasite are sometimes found which are resistant to proguanil or pyrimethamine. They may arise because of inadequate treatment, or because prophylactic doses are given too infrequently. Parasites are therefore exposed to ineffective concentrations of drug in the blood; resistant variants are selected and may be transmitted by the mosquito. In other instances resistant strains have been encountered very soon after the use of the drugs in a new area; resistance, or a remarkable facility for its rapid development, must be presumed to have existed in the original parasite population. An excellent review of drug-resistance in the malaria parasite has been made by Bishop (1959).

Pyrimethamine- and proguanil-resistant strains are sensitive to 4-aminoquinolines and are therefore less likely to be encountered when these two types of drugs are used in combination. Very little is known of the ability of drug-resistant strains to survive in the field, and evidence presented by Clyde and Shute (1959) and Clyde (1960b) suggests that pyrimethamine resistance may be localized, variable and short-lived.

Resistance to chloroquine has, until recently, been encountered only very rarely in human malaria, and the instances reported have not been well-substantiated. The 4-aminoquinolines were regarded as completely free from the danger of losing their efficacy. However, recent events in South America have shown that this is not necessarily so. Malarial infections in Venezuela, Colombia and Brazil have been found which do not respond to very large doses of chloroquine (Moore and Lanier, 1961). True resistance has been proved by transmission of such strains to volunteers (Young and Moore, 1961). At present the areas from which these strains have come are limited, and are being fully investigated by W.H.O. observers. It is of the utmost importance that foci of this nature should not be allowed to spread.

Malaria is an eradicable disease. The chief difficulties in removing it from the face of the earth are difficulties of communication, population control and finance. Every area is different and must be treated differently. If waste of money and effort is to be avoided, and if the development of resistance to chemical substances by mosquitos and parasites is to be prevented, intelligent, full-scale attacks with adequate surveillance will have to be organized. In connection with another tropical disease Morris (1960) wrote . . . 'Meanwhile, the generations of a trypanosome are measured in hours, not years; epidemic diseases are no more respecters of time than of international frontiers. If the return of possibly disastrous epidemics is to be avoided, the solution must lie in the action of a body, such as the World Health Organization, with the vision and status to put forward a realistic programme of eradication on international lines.' This is equally true of malaria.

ANTHELMINTICS

In spite of the hindrances afforded by political boundaries and shortage of money in the developing countries of the tropics, considerable progress has been made in the fight to loosen the grip of the diseases which have sapped the health of the indigenous populations for centuries. The major killing diseases are in many areas on the wane; West Africa is no longer the 'white man's grave' and epidemics of malaria, trypanosomiasis, plague and smallpox have not of recent years caused the depopulation of large tracts of country. Helminthic infections, which are relatively unimportant in the presence of the greater scourges, are now being recognized as the cause of much chronic ill-health and inefficiency. Helminths in the tissues may cause severe damage; in the alimentary tract they use up nutrients which can ill be spared from the diet of the host—a diet which is often deficient in calories, proteins and vitamins. The extent of this diversion of foodstuff from the vertebrate to the invertebrate kingdom can be gauged from the calculations made by Stoll (1947), who estimated the total weight of roundworms in the Chinese bowel in that year to be equal to the weight of an army of 200,000 men. The annual output of eggs by these worms, largely composed of protein and a direct loss to the host, was about 8,000 tons. More than half the population of the world carries worm infections of one kind or another and many people harbour several species at the same time. Domestic animals also carry large burdens of parasitic worms which make further inroads upon human food supplies.

Efficient sanitation drastically reduces the opportunities of parasitic worms to complete their life-cycles; if sewage can be kept out of food and water supplies, most parasitic helminths find it impossible to get from one host to another. Unfortunately, rural areas in all parts of the world (including Britain) are unable to bear the expense of water-borne sanitation and sewage works. Much can be done, however, by education, by less expensive methods of sewage disposal and by the protection of drinking and washing water. Measures may be taken against mollusc and insect vectors and, if the worm burden of the population can be reduced by treatment with safe and efficient drugs at the same time, there is a possibility of great improvement in the health of human and animal populations.

The parasitic helminths of man include:

Nematodes   Threadworms (*Enterobius*), roundworms (*Ascaris*), hookworms (*Necator* and *Ancylostoma*), whipworms (*Trichuris*), *Strongyloides*, and filarial worms (*Wuchereria, Loa, Onchocerca*).

Trematodes   *Schistosoma* and other flukes.

Cestodes   Tapeworms (*Taenia, Diphyllobothrium, Hymenolepis*).

Very few of the helminths of man will infect laboratory animals and, in the search for new drugs, species are used which are natural parasites of small rodents, and which are related zoologically and in their habitat to the corresponding human parasites. These methods (Standen, 1962) have led to the introduction of a number of useful anthelmintics and it is to be expected that the rate of development of new drugs of this kind will increase.

DRUGS EFFECTIVE AGAINST NEMATODES

Piperazine
   The pharmacological history of piperazine as an anthelmintic is an interesting one. Piperazine urate is a soluble substance and in the days when it was thought that the symptoms of gout and rheumatism were caused by the presence of uric acid crystals in the tissues, piperazine

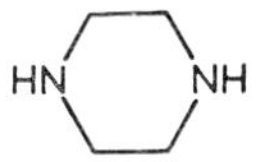

piperazine

was introduced for the treatment of these conditions. The uric acid theory fell into disrepute and the drug was deleted from official British pharmaceutical publications, although it continued to be used fairly extensively in other parts of Europe. In 1949, a thesis submitted to the University of Paris by Fayard described the anthelmintic action of piperazine hydrate against roundworms (*Ascaris lumbricoides*). However, it is made quite clear in the text of the thesis that the original observation of the effectiveness of piperazine against roundworms was made by a Rouen pharmacist, M. Boismare, who recommended Fayard to try the drug and provided him with a preparation of piperazine hydrate flavoured with apple syrup for the purpose. Monsieur Boismare should have the credit for an observation that has revolutionized the treatment of roundworm and threadworm infections during recent years.
   Many reports on a variety of salts of piperazine have now been published and confirm that the drug is effective, has a wide margin of safety, and causes few side-effects.
   For the mass-treatment of populations in the tropics it is difficult to administer more than a single dose of a drug. Goodwin and Standen (1954; 1958) showed that a single dose of a piperazine salt equivalent to 4 g. of the hexahydrate was sufficient to render the stools free from roundworm eggs in more than 80% of African patients. Purgation neither increased nor diminished the effectiveness of the drug.
   The use of piperazine salts for the treatment of threadworms began in 1951 (Mouriquand, Roman and Coisnard, 1951), and in 1953 White and Standen showed that piperazine citrate was more effective than gentian violet in the treatment of threadworms in children. Under the

conditions of the out-patient clinic in Britain a single dose of piperazine, with or without the simultaneous administration of a purgative, was sufficient to remove evidence of threadworm infection from over 90% of children (White and Scopes, 1960). However, it is generally considered advisable to give several daily doses of piperazine in order to kill worms which develop from ova ingested at the time of the first dose.

Piperazine is absorbed from the intestine of man and is excreted in the urine (Rogers, 1958). It is not easy to understand how it reaches threadworms which inhabit the lower part of the bowel. It acts upon roundworms as a narcotic; the worms become flaccid and unable by their muscular movements to maintain their position in the small intestine (Fig. 63). They are swept onwards by the peristalsis of the gut

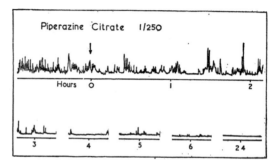

FIG. 63. Kymograph record of the effect of piperazine citrate on the movements of *Ascaris in vitro*. The movements gradually diminish and the worm becomes quiescent in about 6 hours (Goodwin, 1958).

and expelled. They recover some measure of activity if washed in Ringer solution to remove the piperazine. During narcosis, roundworms *in vitro* show no preliminary phase of stimulation (Goodwin, 1958). If stimulation occurs, roundworms may knot together and cause intestinal obstruction, may migrate into the bile duct or appendix or may cause perforation of the gut wall; this is a disadvantage of drugs such as oil of chenopodium, hexylresorcinol and tetrachloroethylene (Fig. 64). Norton and de Beer (1957) showed that piperazine blocks the response of *Ascaris* muscle to small concentrations of acetylcholine; the blocking effect with mammalian muscle is much weaker. Piperazine also reduces the production of succinate by *Ascaris*, and a study of the relationships between metabolism, muscular activity and the conditions at the myoneural junction might throw light on the mode of action of the drug and on the biochemistry of the worm (Bueding and Swartzwelder, 1957).

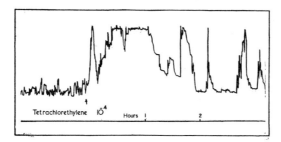

FIG. 64. The effect of tetrachloroethylene on the movements of *Ascaris in vitro*. The worm is stimulated to violent and incoordinated activity (Goodwin, 1958).

Piperazine has no effect upon larval stages of *Ascaris* during their migration through the tissues of the host, and has no useful anthelmintic action on whipworms or filarial worms.

Diethylcarbamazine

Diethylcarbamazine is a derivative of piperazine, but its use as an anthelmintic preceded that of the parent compound. It has an effect on roundworms but is less well tolerated and is more expensive than

$$CH_3-N\underset{\diagdown\diagup}{\diagup\diagdown}N-CON(C_2H_5)_2$$

diethylcarbamazine

piperazine. Its chief value is in the treatment of filarial infections and the drug was discovered as a result of laboratory trials on a filarial worm which lives in the thorax of the cotton rat (Hewitt, Kushner, Stewart, White, Wallace, and SubbaRow, 1947).

Adult filarial worms live in the lymphatics of man and cause elephantiasis (*Wuchereria*) or in the subcutaneous tissues and produce nodules or swellings (*Loa, Onchocerca*). The fertilized females liberate broods of small larval worms which swim in the blood stream or the subcutaneous tissue-spaces where they are within the reach of the insect vector when it comes to feed.

The action of diethylcarbamazine on adult *Wuchereria* and *Loa* worms is slow, and on *Onchocerca* it is not very great. The effect on the larvae (microfilariae) is more spectacular. The drug has no apparent effect upon the movements of the larvae in the host or *in vitro*. Their surfaces nevertheless become modified in such a way that they are immediately recognized by the defence mechanisms of the host as intruders and they are trapped and devoured by histiocytes in the capillaries of the lung and the liver (Hawking, Sewell and Thurston,

1948). This action of diethylcarbamazine, which is not understood, has been likened to the opsonization of bacteria.

Diethylcarbamazine is used in veterinary medicine to kill the lungworm *Dictyocaulus viviparus*, which causes 'husk' in cattle. The drug kills both the adult worms in the bronchial passages and the larvae in the lung tissue.

One of the problems associated with the killing of relatively large worms such as *Wuchereria* or *Onchocerca* in the tissues of the human host is the local or general reaction to the foreign protein liberated when the worms die. Helminth infections give rise to a greater or lesser degree of immunity in the host; complement fixation tests may be used in some instances to show that worm infection is present, and the skin frequently becomes sensitized to intradermal injection of proteins derived from one or more stages in the life history of the worm. The sudden death of the worms as a result of chemotherapy releases a massive dose of antigen, and severe allergic reactions sometimes ensue. The reactions may be alleviated by antihistamine drugs and corticosteroids, but great care must be taken in the treatment of *Onchocerca* infections which involve the eye.

Bephenium

Hookworms (*Ancylostoma* and *Necator*) live in the duodenum of man; they attach themselves to the mucous membrane and pump blood from the host through their bodies. Unwanted blood drips from the worms and if the number of parasites is large the blood loss to the host may be considerable. Roche, Perez-Gimenez, Layrisse and Di Prisco (1957) using ^{51}Cr-tagged red cells have calculated that the loss to a patient with a heavy infection of hookworms may amount to 250 ml. of blood daily. Similar figures have been reported from West Africa (Gilles, Watson-Williams and Worlledge, 1961) and from Malaya (Tasker, 1961), and there is little doubt that hookworm infection contributes to the severity of the iron-deficiency anaemia which is common in these countries. The diet is frequently deficient in available iron and it is not uncommon for patients with heavy hookworm infections to have haemoglobin values of 3 g. per cent. The anaemia may be relieved by giving iron, but if the hookworms are not expelled the loss of blood continues.

Tetrachloroethylene was introduced for the treatment of hookworm infections in 1924. In spite of the fact that it is a chlorinated hydrocarbon and therefore a potential liver poison, serious toxic effects have seldom been reported in the literature, although millions of doses have been given in the course of annual mass-treatments in many tropical countries. Abdominal discomfort is common after tetrachloroethylene and the frequent occurrence of dizziness indicates that the drug may be absorbed from the intestine. Many clinicians regard the drug with misgiving, especially for the treatment of patients who are severely ill and who, because of their nutritional state, are likely to have fatty livers.

Copp, Standen, Scarnell, Rawes and Burrows (1958) reported the activity of a new series of quaternary ammonium compounds against *Nippostrongylus* infections in rats. This nematode has a habitat and mode of existence which are related to those of the hookworm in man.

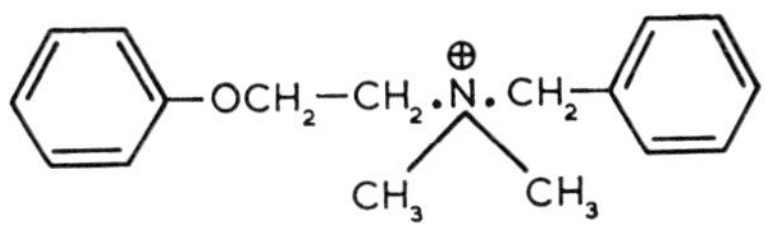

bephenium

It was subsequently shown that bephenium, one of the most active and least toxic compounds of the series, was also active against *Nematodirus* infections in sheep (Rawes and Scarnell, 1958), and against the dog hookworm *Ancylostoma caninum* (Burrows, 1958).

Bephenium hydroxynaphthoate was tested by Goodwin, Jayewardene and Standen (1958) against human *Necator* infections in Ceylon. Many reports have followed and show the drug to have low toxicity and a degree of activity against hookworms comparable with that of tetrachloroethylene. Bephenium is bitter and sometimes causes vomiting; the dose is large, 2·5 g. of the base being required as a single dose for the expulsion of *Necator*, and larger doses are sometimes needed (Gilles et al., 1961). *Ancylostoma*, the hookworm found in more temperate regions (North Africa, Pakistan and Japan) is more sensitive to the drug than *Necator*. Bephenium is effective against a wide variety of species of parasitic nematodes including *Ascaris* and *Trichostrongylus* and it has some activity against whipworms (*Trichuris*). It is also reported to expel *Heterophyes*, a trematode which passes one stage of its life-cycle in the small intestine of man (Nagaty and Khalil, 1961). Bephenium hydroxynaphthoate is poorly absorbed by the host and is therefore likely to act by contact with the cuticle of the hookworm. The chemical structure of the drug would suggest that it may act on the neuromuscular system of the worm, but little is known of the mechanism of action.

Dyes

It is inconvenient to use deeply coloured substances in human medicine, but the disadvantages of dyes are sometimes overshadowed by their usefulness in the treatment of otherwise intractable infections. Gentian violet was for many years the drug of choice in the treatment of threadworm infections. Welch, Peters, Bueding, Valk and Higaski (1947)

13

showed that a series of cyanine dyes had activity against filarial worms in the laboratory. Pyrvinium, given as the insoluble pamoate (embonate), was introduced in 1956 for the treatment of threadworms (Sawitz and Karpinski, 1956). It is red in colour, but has the advantage of being effective in a single small dose. Dithiazanine, a blue cyanine

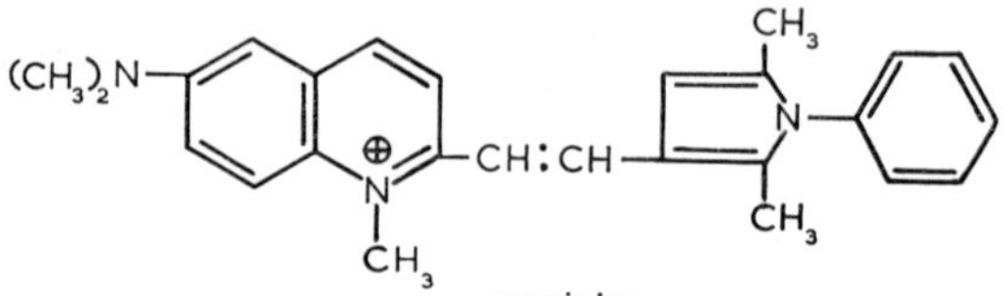

pyrvinium

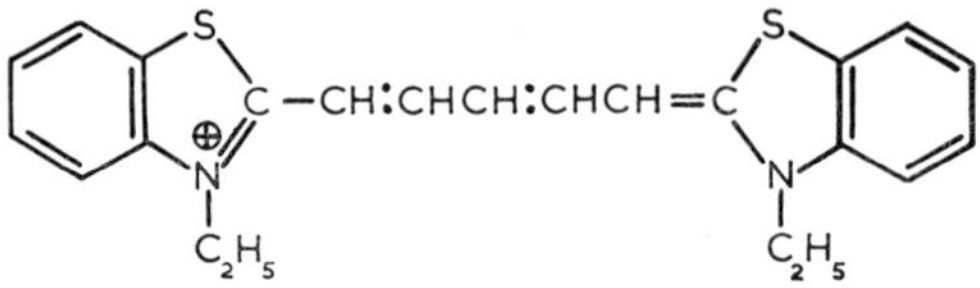

dithiazanine

dye, was introduced in 1957 (Swartzwelder, Frye, Muhleisen, Miller, Lampert, Chavarria, Abadie, Anthony and Sappenfield, 1957). It has the property of eliminating whipworm and *Strongyloides* infections in man; in addition, it has some effect against roundworms, hookworms and threadworms. It has the disadvantage of being very toxic when absorbed by an inflamed intestinal mucosa.

The cyanine dyes have been shown to have powerful inhibitory effects on the carbohydrate metabolism of helminths, but no generalizations can be made. In schistosomes they inhibit oxidative processes but do not affect the anaerobic glycolytic reactions on which the trematode depends; they are therefore ineffective in the treatment of schistosomiasis. In whipworms, both aerobic and anaerobic mechanisms are inhibited and the worms are killed (Bueding and Swartzwelder, 1957).

DRUGS EFFECTIVE AGAINST TREMATODES

The most important parasitic trematodes of man are the schistosomes. Schistosomiasis (Bilharziasis) is widespread in Africa, South America, China and Japan. The intermediate host of the helminth is a fresh-water snail, and the infection is contracted by bathing in, or drinking the water into which the infective forms of the parasite have emerged from the tissues of the snail. There are millions of cases of the disease in the Nile valley and the infection is a constant hazard in all irrigation schemes which are developed in the tropics to improve soil fertility and food production. The adult flukes live within the blood vessels of the gut or the bladder of man. Chronic illness and severe damage to tissues is caused by the passage of the eggs shed by the females through the

ANTIMONIALS

375

mucous membranes. Eggs which enter the portal system lodge in the liver and cause fibrosis. One of the species of schistosome which infect man (*Schistosoma mansoni*) can be readily transmitted to mice and the action of drugs can be tested against it. The chemotherapy of schistosomiasis leaves much to be desired.

Organic antimonials

Trivalent organic antimony compounds were among the earliest remedies to be discovered; they are still in use today. Sodium antimonyltartrate, if given intravenously for a sufficient number of injections, will kill the worms. The side-effects are often serious and coughing, vomiting, and pains in the abdomen and the joints frequently drive away the out-patient, and he fails to complete the course of treatment. Stibophen is less toxic than sodium antimonyltartrate and may be given intramuscularly. It is also less effective; long and repeated courses of treatment are necessary and cure is uncertain. Sodium antimonyl gluconate is less toxic than the tartrate, and a course of treatment may be completed in six days, but no antimonial is completely free from toxic effects upon the heart muscle. The electrocardiogram frequently shows inversion of the T-wave towards the end of a course of treatment. The most recent addition to the list of organic antimonials is sodium antimonyl dimercaptosuccinate. This may be given intramuscularly, but is more toxic than stibophen.

Schistosomes are dependent upon a high rate of carbohydrate metabolism and Bueding and Mansour (1957) have shown that trivalent antimony is a powerful inhibitor of schistosome phosphofructokinase, the enzyme which catalyses the phosphorylation of fructose-6-phosphate by adenosine triphosphate. Mammalian phosphofructokinase is much less sensitive to inhibition and it is probable that the chemotherapeutic action of antimony in schistosomiasis depends upon this difference in sensitivity of the host and parasite enzymes.

Lucanthone

Lucanthone was discovered in Germany (Kikuth, Gönnert and Mauss, 1946). It has an action against schistosomes when given to the patient by mouth. Lucanthone hydrochloride often causes abdominal discomfort, and sometimes affects the mental state of patients, making

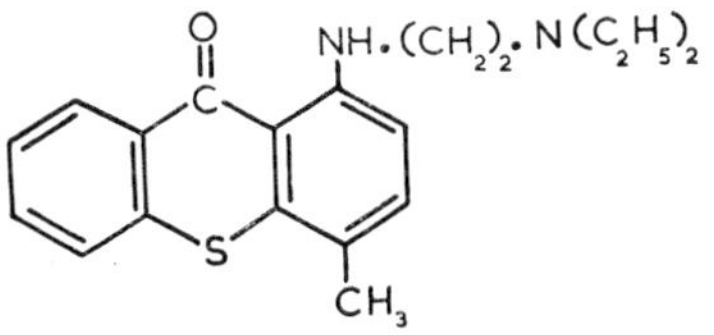

lucanthone

13*

them depressed and very anxious for the treatment to stop. Unless a sufficiently high concentration of drug can be maintained in the tissues for a sufficiently long time, the infection will relapse and the treatment will have been of little value. Many compounds have been made which are chemically related to lucanthone, but so far no significant improvement has been achieved. Recently a new approach has been made by combining lucanthone with a synthetic resin. The drug remains attached to the resin until it reaches the alkaline environment of the small intestine; it is then released slowly over a considerable period. In this way the concentration of the drug in the blood is maintained at a more steady level and the high peaks which follow successive doses of the soluble and rapidly-absorbed hydrochloride are avoided. A clinical trial of this preparation has been made in East Africa and it appears that the resinate is better tolerated than the hydrochloride and is equally effective (Davis, 1961). Further work on preparations of this kind is needed before their value can be assessed.

Phenoxyalkanes

The discovery of the high activity of phenoxyalkane derivatives against schistosome infections in mice was made simultaneously in two research laboratories in Britain (Raison and Standen, 1954; Collins, Davis and Hill, 1954). A large number of derivatives has been made and there are many which have low toxicity for the mouse. Activity is linked with chemical structure and reaches its maximum in a series of diaminodiphenoxy-alkanes with a central chain of 7 carbon atoms (Raison and Standen, 1955). Compounds of a related type prevent the uptake of glucose by schistosomes but have no direct action upon the enzymes involved in carbohydrate metabolism. The drugs may perhaps interfere

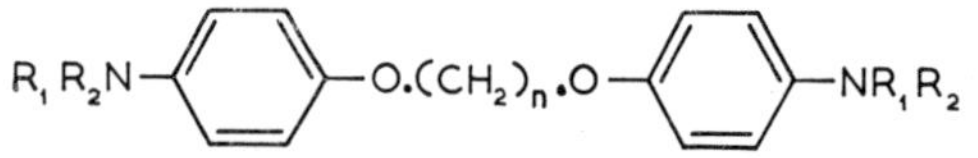

diaminodiphenoxyalkanes

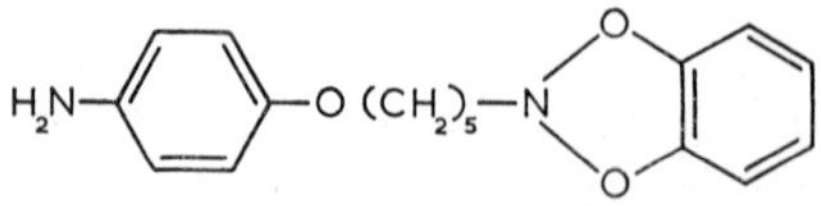

M and B 2948A

with the uptake or transport of exogenous glucose (Bueding and Swartzwelder, 1957). Unfortunately these compounds have a specific toxic effect on the pigment layer of the retina in cats, rabbits and monkeys. Tentative clinical trials with the least toxic members of the series have shown that visual disturbances also occur in man. Even the monophenoxy-compound, 'M & B 2948A' (*N*-(5-*p*-aminophenoxy-pentyl)phthalimide); which has low retinotoxicity and which was shown to have some effect in human schistosomiasis in Africa (Schneider and Sansarricq, 1959), when used in Hong Kong caused signs of visual disturbance in some patients, and its use was discontinued (Collins, Davis, Edge, Hill, Reading and Turnbull, 1959; Alves, Harper and Hill, 1961).

Apart from metabolic poisons such as sodium azide, very few substances have any specific effect on the retina and it is curious that this series of potential schistosomicides should be retinotoxic. Retino-toxic potency may be assayed in frogs (Goodwin, Richards and Udall, 1957). Frogs which have been given injections of the drug in a bright light are unable to resynthesize so much visual purple in the retina as untreated control frogs when they are subsequently placed in the dark. Large doses of the drugs in mice cause intravascular haemolysis, suppression of urine and symmetrical patches of alopecia. So far no member of this series has been widely used in human schistosomiasis.

DRUGS EFFECTIVE AGAINST CESTODES

Tapeworms are found in the small intestine of man. When cattle or pigs feed on land contaminated with human faeces they ingest the eggs of the worm. The eggs hatch in the gut and larvae migrate to the skeletal muscles where they encyst. If 'measly' pork or beef is insufficiently cooked, the parasites survive and the life-cycle is completed. Beef tapeworms (*Taenia saginata*) are very common in Africa and are not uncommon in Europe. The fish tapeworm (*Diphyllobothrium*) is common in Scandinavia where uncooked fish is eaten. The small tapeworm *Hymenolepis nana* is a common parasite of man in some countries; this species does not require an intermediate host. It infects laboratory rodents and may be used to test new drugs for anthelmintic activity.

Echinococcus is a tapeworm of the dog. The cystic stage occurs in the muscles of sheep and the infection is common in Australia. If the infective eggs in dog faeces are ingested by man, the cystic form develops, usually in the liver. This is a very dangerous disease and as yet there is no effective drug for its treatment. An attempt is being made in Australia to rid the dogs of their tapeworms to reduce the reservoir of infection.

Little advance has been made of recent years in the chemotherapy of tapeworm infections in man. Extract of male fern is still widely used, although many consider large doses of mepacrine to be more effective and to cause less side-reactions. Organic derivatives of tin were for a time considered to be promising as a result of tests on laboratory infections in chicken (Kerr and Walde, 1956), but these substances are now known to be too toxic for use in man.

Dichlorophen, introduced as a veterinary anthelmintic, is now being used for the treatment of tapeworm in man. After treatment with this drug, the worm is expelled in a partially digested state, and it is therefore not possible to find the head of the worm in the faeces and to

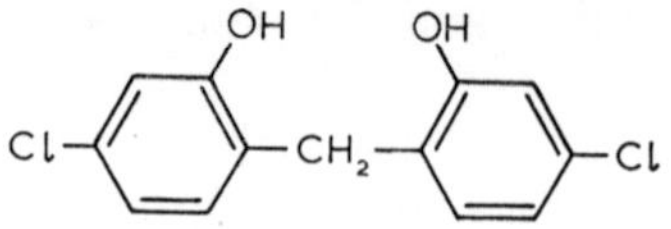

dichlorophen

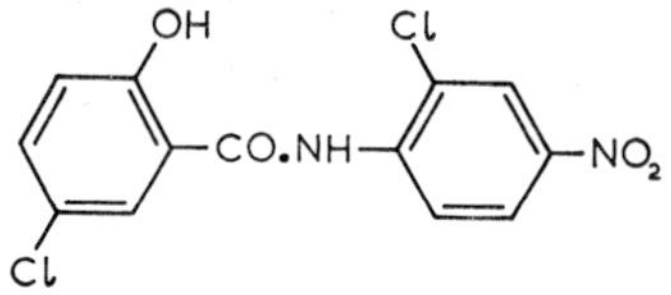

Yomesan

be sure that it will not grow again. It is necessary to re-examine the patient about eight weeks after treatment. Very few comparisons of the relative activities of drugs have as yet been carried out in which this factor has been taken into account.

A new compound related to dichlorophen, N-(2'-chloro-4'-nitro-phenyl)-5-chlorosalicylamide, or 'Yomesan', has recently been shown to have high activity against *Hymenolepsis* and other tapeworm infections in experimental animals (Gönnert and Schraufstätter, 1960) and preliminary trials in man are encouraging (Donckaster, Donoso, Atias, Faiguenbaum and Jarpa, 1960).

REFERENCES

ALVES, W., HARPER, J. and HILL, J. (1961). *Trans. roy. Soc. trop. Med. Hyg.* **55**, 40

ALVING, A. S., ARNOLD, J. and ROBINSON, D. H. (1952). *J. Amer. med. Ass.* **149**, 1558

ALVING, A. S., JOHNSON, C. F., TARLOV, A. R., BREWER, G. J., KELLERMEYER, R. W. and CARSON, P. E. (1960). *Bull. Wld. Hlth. Org.* **22**, 621

ARCHAMBEAULT, C. P. (1954). *J. Amer. med. Ass.* **154**, 1411

ARCHIBALD, H. M. (1951). *Brit. med. J.* **2**, 821

BEUTLER, E., DERN, R. J., FLANAGAN, C. L. and ALVING, A. S. (1955). *J. Lab. clin. Med.* **45**, 286

BISHOP, A. (1959). *Biol. Rev.* **34**, 445

BREWER, G. J., TARLOV, A. R. and ALVING, A. S. (1960). *Bull. Wld. Hlth. Org.* **22**, 633

BUEDING, E. and MANSOUR, J. M. (1957). *Brit. J. Pharmacol.* **12**, 159

BUEDING, E. and SWARTZWELDER, C. (1957). *Pharmacol. Rev.* **9**, 329

BURROWS, R. B. (1958). *J. Parasitol.* **44**, 607

CARRINGTON, H. C., CROWTHER, A. F., DAVEY, D. G., LEVI, A. A. and ROSE, F. L. (1951). *Nature (Lond.)*, **168**, 1080

CARSON, P. E., SCHRIER, S. L. and KELLERMEYER, R. W. (1959). *Nature (Lond.)*, **184,** 1292
CLYDE, D. F. (1960a). *E. Afr. med. J.* **37,** 543
CLYDE, D. F. (1960b). *Trans. roy. Soc. trop. Med. Hyg.* **54,** 87
CLYDE, D. F. and SHUTE, G. T. (1959). *Trans. roy. Soc. trop. Med. Hyg.* **53,** 170
COLLINS, R. F., DAVIS, M. and HILL, J. (1954). *Chem. & Ind.* 1072
COLLINS, R. F., DAVIS, M., EDGE, N. D., HILL, J., READING, H. W. and TURNBULL, E. R. (1959). *Brit. J. Pharmacol.* **14,** 467
COPP, F. C., STANDEN, O. D., SCARNELL, J., RAWES, D. A. and BURROWS, R. B. (1958). *Nature (Lond.)*, **181,** 183
COURTNEY, K. O., HODGKINSON, R., RAMSEY, R. and HAGGERTY, M. (1960). *Amer. J. trop. Med. Hyg.* **9,** 149
CROWTHER, A. F. and LEVI, A. A. (1953). *Brit. J. Pharmacol.* **8,** 93
DAVIS, A. (1961). *Lancet,* **1,** 201
DERN, R. J., BEUTLER, E. and ALVING, A. S. (1954). *J. Lab. clin. Med.* **44,** 171
DONCKASTER, R., DONOSO, F., ATIAS, A., FAIGUENBAUM, J. and JARPA, A. (1960). *Bol. chil. Parasit.* **16,** 4
EYLES, D. E. and COLEMAN, N. (1952). *Publ. Hlth. Rep. (Wash.)*, **67,** 249
EYLES, D. E. and COLEMAN, N. (1953). *Antibiot. and Chemother.* **3,** 483
FALCO, E. A., GOODWIN, L. G., HITCHINGS, G. H., ROLLO, I. M. and RUSSELL, P. B. (1951). *Brit. J. Pharmacol.* **6,** 185
FAYARD, C. (1949). Thesis for Doctor of Medicine, Paris
GILLES, H. M., WATSON-WILLIAMS, E. J. and WORLLEDGE, S. M. (1961). *Ann. trop. Med. Parasit.* **55,** 70
GÖNNERT, R. and SCHRAUFSTÄTTER, E. (1960). *Arzneimittel-Forsch.* **10,** 881
GOODWIN, L. G. (1958). *Brit. J. Pharmacol.* **13,** 197
GOODWIN, L. G., JAYEWARDENE, L. G. and STANDEN, O. D. (1958). *Brit. med. J.* **2,** 1572
GOODWIN, L. G., RICHARDS, W. H. G. and UDALL, V. (1957). *Brit. J. Pharmacol.* **12,** 468
GOODWIN, L. G. and STANDEN, O. D. (1954). *Brit. med. J.* **2,** 1332
GOODWIN, L. G. and STANDEN, O. D. (1958). *Brit. med. J.* **1,** 131
GOODWIN, L. G. (1956). *Proc. roy. Soc. Med.* **49,** 871
GOODWIN, L. G. and ROLLO, I. M. (1955). 'Biochemistry and Physiology of Protozoa', Vol. II. Ed. by Hutner, S. H. and Lwoff, A. New York: Academic Press
HAWKING, F. and PERRY, W. L. M. (1948). *Brit. J. Pharmacol.* **3,** 320
HAWKING, F., SEWELL, P. and THURSTON, J. P. (1948). *Lancet,* **2,** 730
HEWITT, R. I., KUSHNER, S., STEWART, H. W., WHITE, E., WALLACE, W. S. and SUBBAROW, Y. (1947). *J. Lab. clin. Med.* **32,** 1314
HOBBS, H. E., EADIE, S. P. and SOMERVILLE, F. (1961). *Brit. J. Ophthal.* **45,** 284
HURLY, M. G. D. (1959). *Trans. roy. Soc. trop. Med. Hyg.* **53,** 412
KENDALL, S. B. and JOYNER, L. P. (1956). *J. comp. Path.* **66,** 145
KERR, K. B. and WALDE, A. W. (1956). *Exp. Parasit.* **5,** 560
KIKUTH, W., GÖNNERT, R. and MAUSS, H. (1946). *Naturwissenschaften,* **33,** 253
MOORE, D. V. and LANIER, J. E. (1961). *Amer. J. trop. Med. Hyg.* **10,** 5
MORRIS, K. R. S. (1960). *Science,* **132,** 652
MOURIQUAND, G., ROMAN, E. and COISNARD, J. (1951). *J. Méd. Lyon,* **32,** 189
NAGATY, H. F. and KHALIL, H. M. (1961). *J. trop. Med. Hyg.* **64,** 263
NORTON, S. and DE BEER, E. J. (1957). *Amer. J. trop. Med. Hyg.* **6,** 898
RAISON, C. G. and STANDEN, O. D. (1954). *Trans. roy. Soc. trop. Med. Hyg.* **48,** 446
RAISON, C. G. and STANDEN, O. D. (1955). *Brit. J. Pharmacol.* **10,** 191
RAWES, D. A. and SCARNELL, J. (1958). *Vet. Rec.* **70,** 251
ROBERTSON, G. I. (1957). *Trans. roy. Soc. trop. Med. Hyg.* **51,** 457
ROCHE, M., PEREZ-GIMENEZ, M. E., LAYRISSE, M. and DI PRISCO, E. (1957). *J. clin. Invest.* **36,** 1183
ROGERS, E. W. (1958). *Brit. med. J.* **1,** 136–137
ROLLO, I. M. (1955). *Brit. J. Pharmacol.* **10,** 208

RYAN, R. W., HART, W. M., CULLIGAN, J. J., GUNKEL, R. D., JACOBS, L. and COOK, M. K. (1954). *Trans. Amer. Acad. Ophthal. Otolaryng.* **58,** 867

SAWITZ, W. G. and KARPINSKI, F. E. (Jr.). (1956). *Amer. J. trop. Med. Hyg.* **5,** 538

SCHNEIDER, J. and SANSARRICQ, H. (1959). *Méd. Trop.* **19,** 412–424

SCHULEMANN, W. (1932). *Proc. roy. Soc. Med.* **25,** 897

SHORTT, H. E., GARNHAM, P. C. C., COVELL, G. and SHUTE, P. G. (1948). *Brit. med. J.* **1,** 547

SMITH, C. C. and IHRIG, J. (1957). *Amer. J. trop. Med. Hyg.* **6,** 50

STANDEN, O. D. (1962). Chapter in 'Experimental Chemotherapy: An Advanced Treatise', Vol. I. Ed. Hawking, F. and Schnitzer, R. J. (In the press.) New York: Academic Press

STOLL, N. R. (1947). *J. Parasitol.* **33,** 1

SWARTZWELDER, J. C., FRYE, W. W., MUHLEISEN, J. P., MILLER, J. H., LAMPERT, R., CHAVARRIA, A. P., ABADIE, S. H., ANTHONY, S. O. and SAPPENFIELD, R. W. (1957). *J. Amer. med. Ass.* **165,** 2063

TASKER, P. W. G. (1961). *Trans. roy. Soc. trop. Med. Hyg.* **55,** 36

WELCH, A. D., PETERS, L., BUEDING, E., VALK, A. (Jr.) and HIGASKI, A. (1947). *Science,* **105,** 486

WHITE, R. H. R. and SCOPES, J. W. (1960). *Lancet,* **1,** 256

WHITE, R. H. R. and STANDEN, O. D. (1953). *Brit. med. J.* **2,** 1272

WORLD HEALTH ORGANIZATION. *Tech. Rep. Ser.* 1961, **226,** 40

YOUNG, M. D. and MOORE, D. V. (1961). *Amer. J. trop. Med. Hyg.* **10,** 317

CHAPTER 13

HYPNOTICS, ANTICONVULSANTS, ANALGESICS AND ANTI-TUSSIVES

HYPNOTICS AND ANTICONVULSANTS

In recent years there has been a steady production of new hypnotics and anticonvulsants. No attempt will be made here to review these systematically and the reader is referred to 'New and Non-official Drugs' for a practical assessment of the more important substances; here a few members of the group which appear to be of special interest will be described.

The substance glutarimide (Fig. 65) has proved to be a fruitful source of compounds having both stimulant and sedative actions on the central nervous system and several derivatives have become available for clinical use. The best known of these is glutethimide which was introduced as an hypnotic in 1954.

Glutethimide (α-phenyl-α-ethylglutarimide, Doriden) has an hypnotic action which comes on about half an hour after the oral administration of a suitable dose and has a duration of action of about 6 hours. In these respects it is comparable to a medium action barbiturate. Its metabolism has been studied by Hoffmann and Kebrle (1955). Inactivation is by de-ethylation to α-phenyl-glutarimide, which is not hypnotic, and is mainly excreted in the urine conjugated with glucuronic acid. No unchanged glutethimide is found in the urine.

Fastier (1958) has compared glutethimide with pentobarbitone in a trial on students. He found that 200 mg. had little more hypnotic effect than dummy tablets but that 700 mg. was equivalent to 150 mg. pentobarbitone and with these doses drowsiness next day was about the same. Nausea and skin rashes very occasionally occur with glutethimide and addiction has been described (Cohen, 1960). Cases of poisoning due to overdosage have been collected by McBay and Katsas (1957), Schreiner *et al.* (1958) and Winters and Grace (1961). The lethal dose in untreated cases is between 10 and 20 G. Severe hypotension and sudden variation in the depth of coma has been noted and the use of bemigride (see below) has been advocated by Rowell (1957) and by Schreiner *et al.* (1958), who also used external haemodialysis with satisfactory results.

The anticonvulsant properties of glutethimide were noted in the first laboratory reports but the *p*-amino-phenyl derivative (*amino-glutethimide*, Elipten) was found to be more potent in protecting mice against electro-shock and leptazol convulsions and to have no demonstrable hypnotic action in doses with a marked anticonvulsant action. In clinical

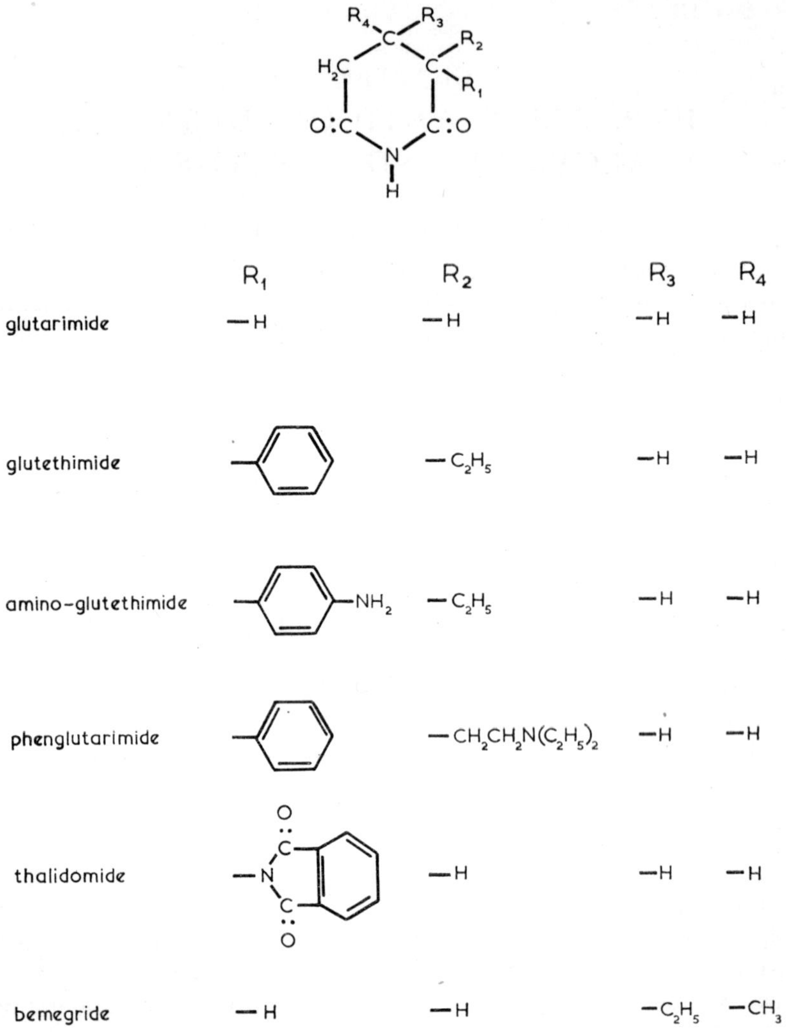

	R_1	R_2	R_3	R_4
glutarimide	—H	—H	—H	—H
glutethimide	(phenyl)	—C_2H_5	—H	—H
amino–glutethimide	(phenyl)—NH_2	—C_2H_5	—H	—H
phenglutarimide	(phenyl)	—$CH_2CH_2N(C_2H_5)_2$	—H	—H
thalidomide	(phthalimido)	—H	—H	—H
bemegride	—H	—H	—C_2H_5	—CH_3

FIG. 65. Derivatives of glutarimide.

use it has been somewhat disappointing (Fabisch, 1959) though it may find a place, given with other anticonvulsants, in the treatment of some resistant cases of grand mal (Carter, 1960; La Veck, 1960).

The substitution of a diethylaminoethyl group for the ethyl group of glutethiamide gave a compound with strong atropine-like properties and this has been introduced as phenglutarimide for the treatment of Parkinsonism.

Phenglutarimide (Aturbane) has been investigated by Bein and Tripod (1958). In animal experiments it was found to antagonize the muscarinic actions of acetylcholine on plain muscle and on salivary and gastric secretion. It has a potency of one-third to one-tenth that of atropine, has little ganglion blocking or antihistamine actions and is not sedative or anticonvulsant. In man similar effects on salivary and gastric secretion and on gastro-intestinal movements have been reported by Peremans (1958) and by Wyant and Haley (1959).

The assessment of drugs in the treatment of Parkinsonism is notoriously difficult but good results in the relief of the rigidity and excessive salivation have been reported, and Hughes, Keevil and Gibbs (1958) concluded from a small trial that in these respects phenglutarimide is as good or better than other drugs. The main undesired effects were nausea, vomiting, dryness of mouth, euphoria and mental confusion.

Thalidomide (α-phthalimidoglutarimide, Distaval) has been introduced as a mild hypnotic. Its pharmacological properties have been described by Somers (1960). It has no anticonvulsant action. Oral toxicity cannot be determined in animals as deaths do not occur even with very large doses; in man doses 20 to 40 times the normal hypnotic dose, taken with suicidal intention, cause only sleep and a severe headache. The mildness of the effects of over-dosage is probably due to poor absorption. After therapeutic doses about 40% is excreted in the urine, mainly as unidentified metabolites. Some cases of peripheral neuritis, with both sensory and motor symptoms, have occurred, usually in patients over 40 years of age who have been taking 100 mg. or more daily for several months. The cause of this is not known but the condition appears to clear up rapidly if the drug is discontinued as soon as symptoms develop.

Lasagna (1960) compared the effect of 100 mg., 200 mg. and a dummy capsule on sleep and found only the larger dose to be significantly different from the dummy in hypnotic action. The main value of thalidomide appears to be as a sedative and hypnotic in patients who do not tolerate barbiturates well or who are suspected of suicidal intentions. The drug has recently been withdrawn as there have been reports of congenital abnormalities, many involving the limbs, in the children of mothers who had taken it during early pregnancy (Annotation, 1962).

In considering glutarimide derivatives reference must be made to *bemigride* (β-ethyl-β-methyl-glutarimide, Megimide) a central nervous stimulant used since 1954 in the treatment of barbiturate poisoning. At first it was thought to be a specific antagonist of barbiturates. It is now known to act as an analeptic in other forms of narcotic poisoning and there is other evidence that its antagonism of barbiturates is non-competitive and closely resembles that of leptazol. This is reviewed by Hahn (1960). Like leptazol, bemigride stimulates respiration by a central action, not through the chemoreceptors, and like it has central pressor, hypoglycaemic and hypothermic actions. The relative merits of bemigride and other analeptics in the treatment of narcotic poisoning is not yet established. Overdosage causes increased reflexes, muscular twitching and convulsions. To the depressant glutarimides it thus has a similar relationship as the convulsant barbiturates (Domino *et al.*, 1955; Jolly and Domino, 1956) have to hypnotic barbiturates.

OTHER HYPNOTICS

Methaqualone (Melsedin). The hypnotic action of methaqualone was discovered accidentally during the investigation of quinazolone derivatives for antimalarial action (Fig. 66). Parsons and Thomson (1961) found that 150 mg. of it was equivalent to 200 mg. cyclobarbitone on patient assessment in a double blind trial. It also has an antitussive action, roughly equivalent to codeine, and anticonvulsant properties. The latter have been investigated for a number of related compounds by Bianchi and David (1960).

Acetylenic carbinols and their derivatives. In the search for non-barbiturate hypnotics pharmaceutical manufacturers have turned to unsaturated carbinols of which methylpentynol (Fig. 66) is an example (P'an *et al.*, 1953). *Ethchlorvynol* (Placidyl) is such a compound and differs from methylpentynol in that the methyl group of the latter is

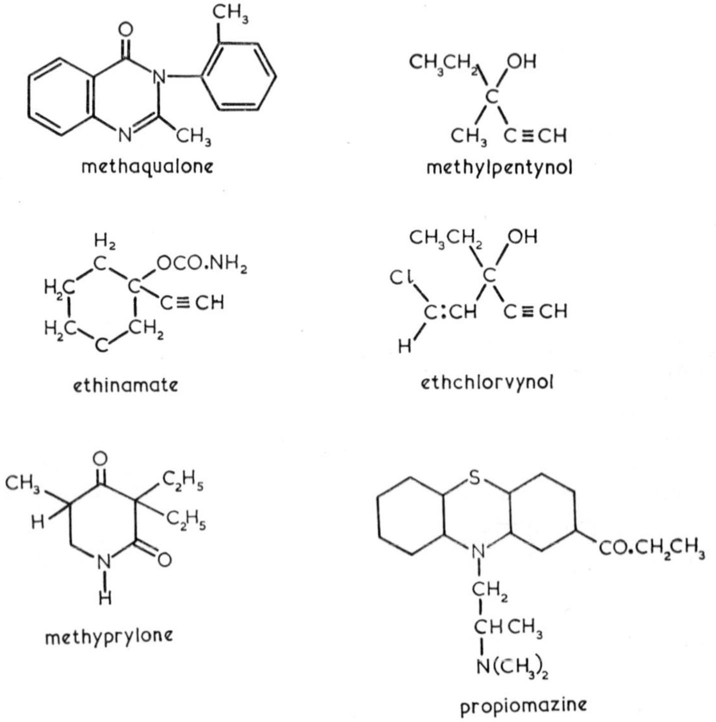

FIG. 66. Hypnotics.

replaced by a chlorvinyl group. Its potency and duration of action is very similar to *ethinamate* (Valmidate), a carbamic acid ester of an unsaturated carbinol. Gruber *et al.* (1954), in hospital patients, found a dose of 500 mg. of this substance to be roughly equivalent to 100 mg. quinalbarbitone but to have a slightly shorter action. Both substances appear to be of value in the treatment of mild cases of simple insomnia and both have anticonvulsant properties when tested on animals (Langecker *et al.*, 1953).

Other recently introduced non-barbiturate hypnotics are *acetylurea* (Levanil) a non-toxic sedative, and *methyprylone* (Noludar), a piperi-dinedione (Fig. 66), comparable in potency and duration of action to quinalbarbitone. Structurally it has similarities to the barbiturates.

The hypnotic action of promethazine is sometimes a desirable, some-times an undesirable feature of the action of this antihistamine. *Propiomazine* (Fig. 66) (Indorm) is the 2-propionyl derivative of prome-thazine and has a more marked hypnotic action but much weaker atropine-like and antihistamine actions. It has been introduced as an hypnotic and has a duration of action of about 5 hours. Dobkin (1960) found that in common with promethazine and certain other phenothia-zines, it prolongs considerably the action of intravenous thiopentone. Like chlorpromazine (see p. 43), which is the 2-chloro derivative of promethazine, it has an anti-emetic action.

OTHER ANTICONVULSANTS

The treatment of epilepsy is still far from satisfactory and a number of new anticonvulsants have been introduced. Some of these are related to compounds already known. *Methsuximide* (Celontin) and *ethosuximide* (Zarontin) are succinimides and related to phensuximide (Milontin). Methsuximide has caused fatal bone marrow aplasia and renal damage but ethosuximide appears to be much less toxic and to be a valuable drug in the treatment of petit mal.

Ethotoin (3-ethyl-5-phenyhydantoin, Peganone) is a recently introduced hydantoin. It has mainly been used on patients resistant to other treatment. Good results in grand mal, petit mal and psychomotor

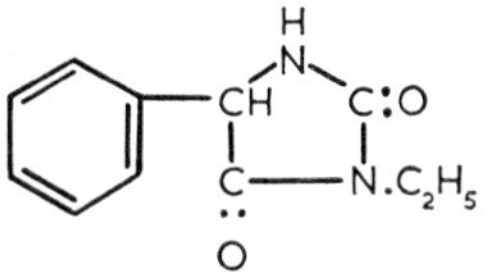

ethotoin 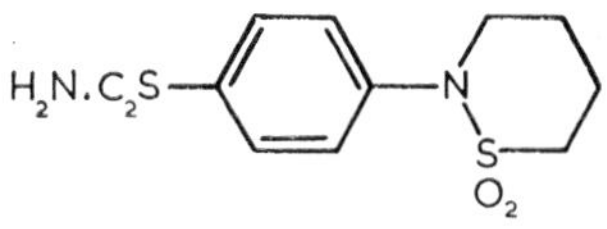   Ospolot

attacks have been reported (for references see Zimmerman and Burge-meister, 1958) without evidence of liver, renal or bone marrow damage and only very rarely of gum hyperplasia.

Ospolot. An entirely new group of compounds with actions on the central nervous system are the *N*-aryl-sultam derivatives. Members of this series have been found to have stimulating, sedative, anticonvulsant and antipyretic actions (Friebel and Sommers, 1960) and are structurally unrelated to other drugs used for their central actions. Ospolot (tetrahydro-2-*p*-sulphamoyl phenyl-1, 2 thiazine 1, 1-dioxide) antagonizes electroshock and leptazol convulsions in mice and has little hypnotic action. In clinical use it has been found to be especially useful in temporal lobe epilepsy. It is less effective than hydantoins in grand mal, and petit mal showed little improvement with it. Apart from paraesthesia, common during the first two weeks of treatment, side effects are said to be rare and of a minor nature (Engelmeier, 1960).

NEWER ANALGESICS

The search for potent analgesics, capable of taking the place of morphine or pethidine, has led to the introduction of several new compounds. These will be discussed in two categories: (i) drugs structurally related to morphine and (ii) drugs related to pethidine or methadone (Fig. 67).

(i) In the first catgeory only two drugs merit description, oxymorphone and phenazocine.

Oxymorphone (hydroxydihydromorphinone, Numorphan) is the 14–OH derivative of dihydromorphinone (Dilaudid) and resembles it closely in properties. Its potency, weight for weight, is 8 to 10 times that of morphine (Eddy *et al.*, 1957) and it is as effective as morphine in controlling intense pain, but not more so. Like morphine it causes sedation, euphoria, respiratory depression, nausea and vomiting, but it has little antitussive action. Respiratory depression of the foetus is probably sufficiently great to contra-indicate its use in labour, but it is valuable for pre- and post-operative medication and as an analgesic in neoplastic disease. Addiction and tolerance develop as with morphine.

Phenazocine (Narphen) is a benzomorphan derivative with a potency similar to that of oxymorphone. Clinical experience with it is at present limited, but it appears to have a similar range of usefulness. Respiratory depression has been noted with medicinal doses but opinion is divided as to the importance of this when phenazocine is used as an adjuvant to anaesthesia. There is some evidence that central depressant effects are potentiated by other central depressant drugs and this should be taken into account in considering the dose to be prescribed. Sandove *et al.* (1960) report favourably on its use in labour.

(ii) *Anileridine* (Leritine) is very similar to pethidine in its properties and has the same uses and limitations but is about 2½ times as potent.

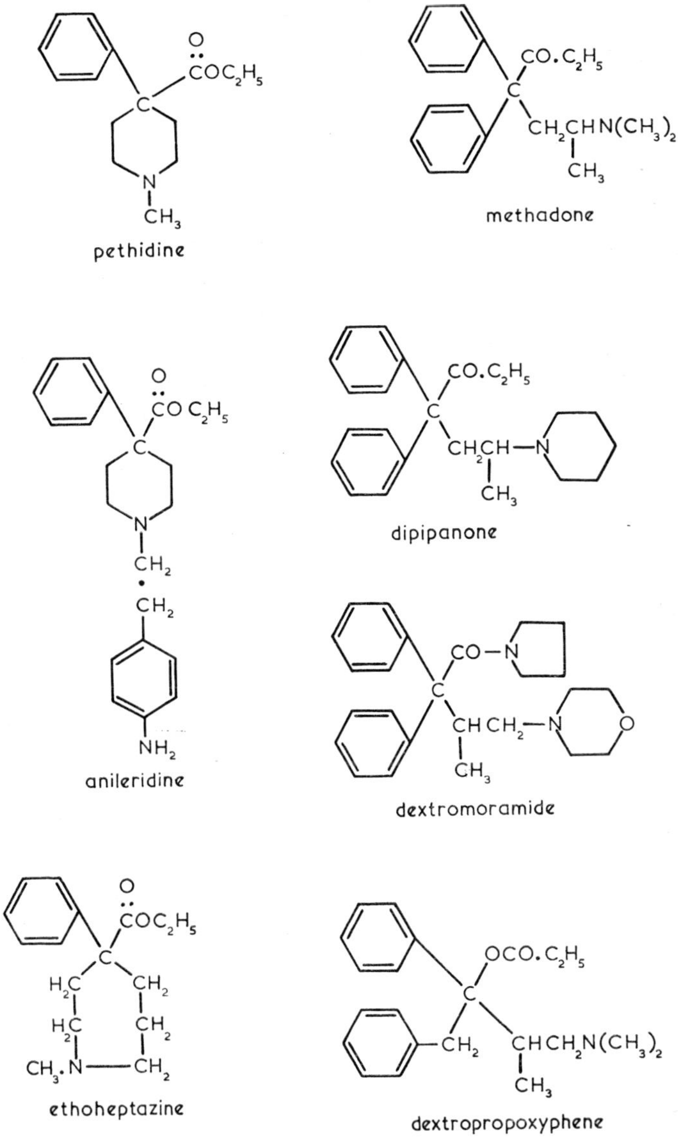

FIG. 67. Analgesics.

In equi-analgesic doses depression of respiration and circulation is similar. Addiction occurs and it has weak antihistamine and atropine-like actions. It has little sedative or constipating action and nausea is uncommon in patients confined to bed. It is eliminated by the liver and kidney and its duration of action is probably somewhat shorter than that of pethidine. It is reported (Wizenberg *et al.*, 1959) to be a satisfactory analgesic in labour and to cause less depression of foetal respiration than pethidine. It is not at present available in the U.K.

Ethoheptazine (Zactane) is structurally similar to pethidine but has a seven membered ring instead of a piperidine ring. It is considerably weaker as an analgesic and is only suitable for the relief of mild pain. It appears to be non-addicting though a longer experience is needed before this can be accepted without reserve (Eddy *et al.*, 1957). Compounded with aspirin (Zactirin) it has similar uses to other compound aspirin tablets.

Dipipanone (Pipadone) is related to methadone and has been used as a post-operative analgesic and found to compare favourably with papaveretum both in effectiveness and in freedom from unwanted effects (Cope and Jones, 1959). As an adjunct to anaesthesia it is liable to cause respiratory depression and hypotension.

Dextromoramide (Palfium), has been used for similar purposes but from the results of Cope and Jones (1959) appears to be less satisfactory for the relief of post-operative pain and to cause more side effects.

Dextropropoxyphene (Doloxene, Darvon) has an analgesic action similar to codeine and is of use only for the relief of mild pain but it appears to be non-addicting and to cause few side effects.

ANALGESICS WITH ANTIPYRETIC AND ANTI-INFLAMMATORY
    The studies of Brodie and his colleagues (see Burns *et al.*, 1960) have revealed a number of interesting facts about the fate of phenylbutazone in the body and have resulted in the introduction of two new compounds.
    After the oral administration of a single dose of phenylbutazone, absorption is rapid and complete and a peak blood concentration is reached in about 2 hours. After intramuscular injection, absorption is slower and peak blood concentrations are reached only after 6 hours, probably because of precipitation at the site of injection. In the blood it is almost entirely reversibly bound to plasma protein and in the bound state is protected from metabolism and thus forms a depot. This accounts for its very slow elimination which extends over a week or more after discontinuing administration.
    Two metabolites have been found (Fig. 68), a phenol formed by the introduction of a hydroxyl group into one of the rings and an alcohol by its introduction into the side chain. The phenolic compound is eliminated even more slowly than phenylbutazone and has been found in animal tests to be at least as potent in its anti-inflammatory and antipyretic actions but to have less analgesic action. Under the name of

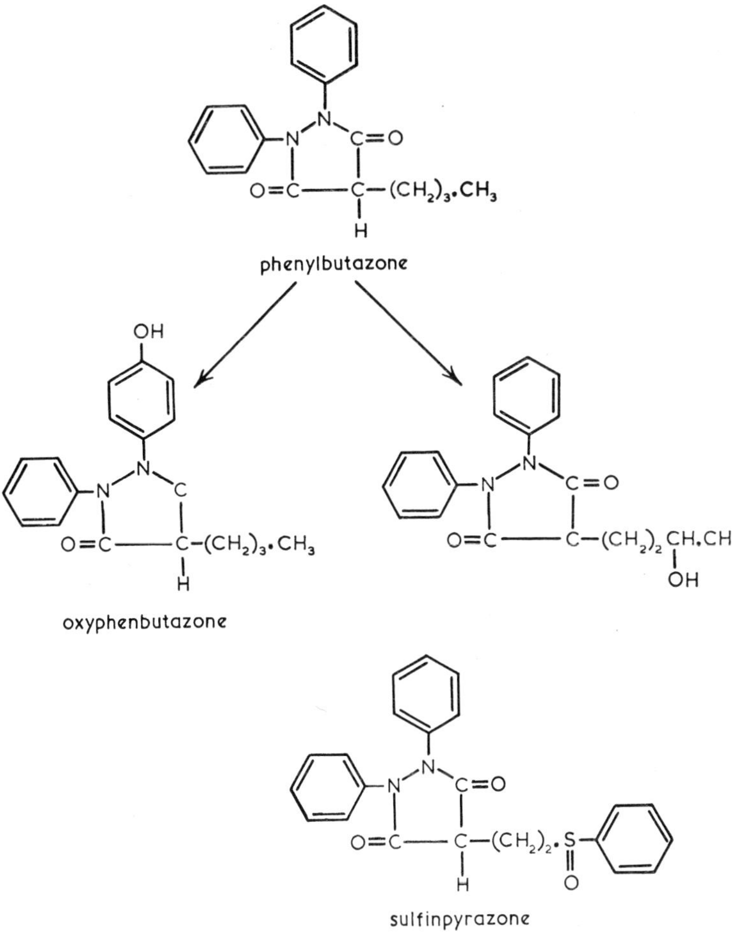

Fig. 68. Metabolism of phenylbutazone.

oxyphenbutazone (Tanderil) it has been used therapeutically and appears to cause less gastric irritation than phenylbutazone and has been reported to be of value in relieving the symptoms of rheumatic conditions (Hart and Burley, 1959). It is at present too soon to assess its value and in using it the likelihood of the development of toxic effects similar to those of phenylbutazone must be born in mind.

While investigating a number of phenylbutazone analogues, Brodie and his colleagues found that uricosuric activity was greatest in the most acidic compounds and selected *sulfinpyrazone* (Anturen), a sulphoxide of phenylbutazone, for testing in the treatment of chronic gout. Seegmiller and Grayzel (1960) have reported favourably on its clinical value. It has no anti-rheumatic or sodium retaining activity.

Chlorthenoxazin is reported to compare favourably in animal experiments with phenacetin and acetylsalicylic acid in antipyretic, analgesic and anti-inflammatory action. There is no evidence yet that in man it is superior to the well tried antipyretic analgesics.

In *summary* it may be said that none of the newer analgesics, to whichever category they belong, appears to be likely to supersede the established analgesics though there may, very occasionally, be circumstances where an individual patient might benefit by a change to one of them.

THE TESTING OF ANTI-TUSSIVE DRUGS

A large number of preparations are used widely in the treatment of cough. Thus, for example, an American investigator (Townsend, 1958) made a survey of local drug stores and found that 50 to 60 anti-tussive preparations are stocked by the average pharmacy, consisting of various expectorants, emollients, herbs, sedatives and narcotics. These preparations enjoy variable popularity, depending upon flavour more than anti-tussive properties! Anti-tussives can really be classified as (1) drugs which decrease the cough reflex, (2) spasmolytics and anticongestives, (3) local anaesthetics, and (4) inhalations of which steam is by far the most important (see review of cough mixtures, Oswald, 1959). Of these, only the first class will be discussed here. These are used extensively for many different types of cough and sometimes in mixtures, or in combination with expectorants.

New substances are being introduced for the control of cough, though in some cases little evidence is available about their therapeutic value and pharmacological actions. It seems, therefore, desirable to review the methods which can be used for assessing anti-tussive substances and briefly to consider a few of the recently introduced drugs. Pharmacological and pathological aspects of cough are reviewed by Bucher (1958) who also briefly discussed the evaluation of anti-tussive drugs, as do Bickerman and Itkin (1960). This can be done in experimentally induced cough (in animals or man) and clinically in patients suffering from various types of cough. The thoughtful discussion of Beecher (1959) will repay study.

The most common way of inducing experimental coughs is by stimulation or irritation of the respiratory passages. This has been done by many methods, e.g. mechanical, chemical and allergic, both in animals and man. Thus Kase (quoted by Bucher, 1958) used mechanical stimulation of the trachea of the unanaesthetized dog, while Mulinos (1960) produced mechanical tickling of the tracheal mucosa in the anaesthetized cat (and also used chemical stimulation with ammonia). Chemical irritation has also been used in the unanaesthetized guinea pig using ammonia and in the unanaesthetized dog exposed to a fine spray of dilute sulphuric acid. Dose response curves, for anti-tussive activity, were obtained in both species with a number of substances, including codeine (Winter and Plataker, 1954). Ammonia has also been used in unanaesthetized dogs in which it elicits 'realistic, vibrant coughs or paroxysms of coughing' (Rosiere et al., 1956). These authors include a review (in the form of a table) of the literature on the experimental production of cough. A number of investigators have used aerosolized antigen in sensitized animals for the production of cough. Winter and Plataker (1955) found that such cough was not inhibited by codeine.

Similar experimental methods have been used in man to produce coughing and to investigate the effect of drugs. An early investigation of this type was performed by Höglund and Michaëlson (1950) who introduced small amounts of ammonia into the airways of subjects during inspiration and were able to demonstrate the inhibitory effect of codeine on coughs so elicited. Citric acid aerosols were used by Bickerman and Barach (1954) both in normal subjects and in patients suffering from asthma. Tiffeneau (1957) has induced cough by the administration of acetylcholine, which can be inhaled as an aerosol. Coughing has also been induced in man by the intravenous injection of various drugs; for example intravenous administration of lobeline and of paraldehyde produces uncontrollable and explosive coughs lasting for a few seconds. Such cough, however, is not prevented by the common anti-tussive agents and thus does not seem very suitable for such investigations (Hillis and Kelly, 1951). It should be added here that Beecher (1959) investigated the action of some anti-tussive agents in cough produced in man by inhalation of ammonia or citric acid or by the intravenous injection of paraldehyde and did not observe any consistent reduction in the frequency of coughs so produced.

Stimulation of the central nervous system and of various peripheral nerves has also been used to produce experimental coughs in animals, in an attempt to get more information about the site of action of anti-tussive agents. Borison (1948) located an area in the medulla of the cat, electrical stimulation of which evokes a series of sharp coughs; by this method drugs which have a central action or an effect on the efferent pathways will be recognized. Using this method Chakravarty et al. (1956) obtained results suggesting that codeine and other drugs produce their anti-tussive effects by a central action. Schroeder (1951) has produced cough in unanaesthetized dogs by electrical stimulation of the vagus nerve; while stimulation of the superior laryngeal nerve of anaesthetized cats and unanaesthetized dogs has also been used (Domenjoz, 1952; Kase, 1958).

The final test of anti-tussive drugs is for the control of cough in human disease and a number of such investigations have been performed. Two main criteria have been used, namely (1) the effect on cough, as objectively measured (this may be a truly objective quantitative measurement, or the opinion of a third person, for example, a parent with a child suffering from cough, particularly nocturnal), and (2) the patient's subjective assessment of the drug in relieving his cough. It is interesting in this connection that a drug may not produce any objective measurable effect on coughing, yet a patient may say that it has relieved him and that he feels better for it, thus emphasizing the importance of subjective factors (Beecher, 1959).

There is no doubt that when the criterion of effectiveness is the patients subjective impression, various anti-tussive agents can be highly effective. For example, Snell and Armitage (1957) used the method of sequential analysis in comparing heroin and pholcodine with a placebo in patients with chronic cough due to various conditions and found that both drugs were about equally active and better than the placebo. Cass and Frederik (1956) observed, in a double blind trial, that dextromethorphan was as effective as codeine sulphate; both these were more effective than caramiphen ethanedisulphonate ('Toryn') and all three drugs were more effective than a placebo. Following experiments in dogs exposed to sulphuric acid aerosol, in which it was found that dihydrocodeinone in an ion exchange resin produced a more prolonged effect than the same drug in aqueous solution, Chan and Hays (1957) obtained evidence that the same applied to man, though the human experiments could be more convincing. These and other similar findings are supported by the careful experiments of Beecher (1959) in which he observed that patients with cough of pathological origin stated that they derived benefit from the use of codeine and heroin and believed that these drugs reduced the frequency of cough; in fact objective measurement showed that the cough frequency had not been significantly reduced. The difficulty of assessing the value of cough remedies is further emphasized by the following fact. There appears to be good evidence in the literature that carbetapentane citrate (Toclase) is valuable in treating cough in man (see for example Carter and Maley, 1957) yet the preparation has now been discontinued in Britain, though it is still available in the United States.

Conclusion: It is doubtful at present whether any experimental method in animals or in man, will reliably indicate whether a substance will be of value in treating cough clinically, though such methods can be used in a preliminary screening. There is great need for a careful assessment of anti-tussive remedies to determine (1) to what extent they affect cough, objectively, and (2) to what extent they modify the patient's response to cough, i.e. whether they decrease the disturbance caused by the cough. Pending such further investigation, the conclusion of Wade (1961) seems reasonable, that it is best to prescribe the simplest and cheapest remedies, like those in the British National Formulary.

REFERENCES

* Denotes review.

ANNOTATION. (1962). *Lancet*, **1**, 307

BEECHER, H. K. (1959). 'Measurement of Subjective Responses.' Oxford University Press

BEIN, H. J. and TRIPOD, J. (1958). *Schweiz. med. Wschr.* **88**, 1160

BIANCHI, C. and DAVID, A. (1960). *J. Pharm. Pharmacol.* **12**, 501

BICKERMAN, H. A. and BARACH, A. L. (1954). *Amer. J. med. Sci.* **228**, 156

BICKERMAN, H. A. and ITKIN, S. E. (1960). *Clin. Pharmacol. Ther.* **1**, 180

BORISON, H. L. (1948). *Amer. J. Physiol.* **154**, 55

*BUCHER, K. (1958). *Pharmacol. Rev.* **10**, 43

BURNS, J. J., YÜ, T. F., DAYTON, P. G., GUTMAN, A. B. and BRODIE, B. B. (1960). *Ann. N.Y. Acad. Sci.* **86**, 253

CARTER, C. H. (1960). *Dis. nerv. Syst.* **21**, 50

CARTER, P. H. and MALEY, M. C. (1957). *Amer. J. med. Sci.* **233**, 77

CASS, L. J. and FREDERIK, W. S. (1956). *J. Lab. clin. Med.* **48**, 879

CHAKRAVARTY, N. K., METALLANA, A., JENSEN, R. and BORISON, H. L. (1956). *J. Pharmacol. exp. Ther.* **117**, 127

CHAN, Y. T. and HAYS, E. E. (1957). *Amer. J. med. Sci.* **234**, 207

COHEN, H. (1960). *N.Y. med. J.* **60**, 280

COPE, E. and JONES, P. O. (1959). *Brit. med. J.* **1**, 211

DOBKIN, A. B. (1960). *Anaesthesiology*, **21**, 292

DOMENJOZ, R. (1952). *Arch. exp. Path. Pharmak.* **215**, 19

DOMINO, E. F., FOX, K. E. and BRODY, T. M. (1955). *J. Pharmacol. exp. Ther.* **114**, 473

EDDY, N. B., HALBACH, H. and BRAENDEN, O. J. (1957). *Bull. Wld. Hlth. Org.* **17**, 583, 709

ENGELMEIER, M. P. (1960). *Dtsch. med. Wschr.* **85**, 2207

FABISCH, W. (1959). *J. ment. Sci.* **105**, 448

FASTIER, F. W. (1958). *N.Z. med. J.* **57**, 171

FRIEBEL, H. and SOMMERS, S. (1960). *Dtsch. med. Wschr.* **85**, 2192

GRUBER, C. M., KOHLSTAEDT, K. G., MOORE, R. B. and PECK, F. B. (1954). *J. Pharmacol. exp. Ther.* **112**, 480

*HAHN, F. (1960). *Pharmacol. Rev.* **12**, 447

HART, F. D. and BURLEY, D. (1959). *Brit. med. J.* **1**, 1087

HILLIS, B. R. and KELLY, J. C. C. (1951). *Glasg. med. J.* **32**, 72

HOFFMANN, K. and KEBRLE, J. (1955). III int. Congress of Biochemistry

HÖGLUND, N. J. and MICHAËLSON, M. (1950). *Acta physiol. scand.* **21**, 168

HUGHES, W., KEEVIL, J. H. and GIBBS, I. E. (1958). *Brit. med. J.* **1**, 928

JOLLY, E. R. and DOMINO, E. F. (1956). *Fed. Proc.* **15**, 443

KASE, Y. Quoted by Bucher, 1958

LANGECKER, H., SCHÜMANN, H. J. and JUNKMANN, K. (1953). *Arch. exp. Path. Pharmak.* **219**, 130

LASAGNA, L. (1960). *J. chron. Dis.* **11**, 627

LAVECK, G. D. (1960). *Dis. nerv. Syst.* **21**, 230

McBAY, A. J. and KATSAS, G. G. (1957). *New Engl. J. Med.* **257**, 97

MULINOS, G. M. (1960). *Toxicol. appl. Pharmacol.* **2**, 635

OSWALD, N. C. (1959). *Brit. med. J.* **1**, 292

P'AN, S. Y., MARKARIAN, L., McLAMORE, W. M. and BAVLEY, A. (1953). *J. Pharmacol. exp. Ther.* **109**, 268

PARSONS, T. W. and THOMSON, T. J. (1961). *Brit. med. J.* **1**, 171

PEREMANS, J. (1958). *Gastroenterologia*, **90**, 29

ROSIERE, C. E., WINDER, C. V. and WAX, J. (1956). *J. Pharmacol. exp. Ther.* **116**, 296

ROWELL, N. R. (1957). *Lancet*, **1**, 407

SANDOVE, M. S., REUBEN, C. B., BRANION, J. M. and KOBAK, A. J. (1960). *Obstet. and Gynec.* **16**, 448

SCHREINER, G. E., BERMAN, L. B., KOVACH, R. and BLOOMET, H. A. (1958). *Arch. intern. Med.* **101**, 899

SCHROEDER, H. (1951). *Arch. exp. Path. Pharmak.* **212**, 433
SEEGMILLER, J. E. and GRAYZEL, A. I. (1960). *J. Amer. med. Ass.* **173**, 1076
SNELL, E. S. and ARMITAGE, P. (1957). *Lancet*, **1**, 860
SOMERS, G. F. (1960). *Brit. J. Pharmacol.* **15**, 111
TIFFENEAU, R. (1957). *Dis. Chest*, **31**, 404
TOWNSEND, E. H. (1958). *New Engl. J. Med.* **258**, 63
WADE, O. L. (1961). *Prescriber's Journal*, **1**, 40
WINTER, C. A. and PLATAKER, L. (1954). *J. Pharmacol. exp. Ther.* **112**, 99
WINTER, C. A. and PLATAKER, L. (1955). *J. exp. Med.* **101**, 17
WINTERS, W. and GRACE, W. J. (1961). *Clin. Pharmacol. Ther.* **2**, 40
WIZENBERG, M. J., SIEGEL, I. A., KORMAN, W. and ROSENTHAL, H. N. (1959). *Amer. J. Obstet. Gynec.* **78**, 405
WYANT, G. M. and HALEY, F. C. (1959). *Anaesthesiology*, **20**, 581
ZIMMERMAN, F. T. and BURGEMEISTER, B. B. (1958). *N.Y. St. J. Med.* **58**, 2054

INDEX

A 19120, 58, *see* pargyline
Acepromazine, 44, 69, 70
Acetazolamide, 241–244
  action as diuretic, 242, 243
  clinical use, 243, 244
  side effects, 244
Acetohexamide, 204, 205
Acetylcholine, 150
  biosynthesis, 4
  bretylium and, 110
  distribution in CNS, 4
  effect of injection, 9
    of intraventricular injection, 10
  in CNS, 4–9
  release, 7
    by catechol amines, 113
Acetyl-coenzyme A, 4
Acetylpromazine, 44, 69, 70
Acetylurea, 385
Acid–base balance, 217–219, 234, 235
  effect on bicarbonate reabsorption, 228
  metabolic change in, 257
  respiratory change in, 258
Acid, definition, 255
Acidosis, definition, 255, 256
Adenosine triphosphate (ATP), 12, 102
  amine storage by, 149
  estimation, 36
  in adrenal medulla, 101
  in CNS, 36
  in intestine, 149
  in platelets, 124
  liberation from sensory nerves, 36
Adrenal medulla, 125
  effect of insulin on, 101
    of reserpine on, 101
  release of amines, 100, 113
  staining, 100
  storage of amines, 101
Adrenaline, 95 *et seq.*, 150
  actions, 109
    on cell membrane, 108
    on CNS, 14–17
    on phosphorylase, 108
  antagonists, 107
  biosynthesis, 11, 98
  distribution, 96
  estimation, 97
  inactivation, 103
  infusion in man, 109
  potentiation, 105, 113
  release, 100, 114
    from adrenal medulla, 113
  storage, 100, 102
Adrenergic nerves, drugs blocking, 310
Albamycin, 338, *see* Novobiocin
Aldactone, 254, *see* spironolactone
Aldomet, 317, *see* α-methyldopa
Aldosterone, 268–270
  antagonists, 254
  control of secretion, 270, 271
  effect on body electrolytes, 230, 231, 270
    on renal secretion, 230, 231
  in familial paralysis, 273, 274

Aldosterone—*continued*
  inhibition of secretion, 253, 254
  relation to oedema, 272, 273
Aldosteronism, 230, 231, 271
Alkalosis, definition, 256
Allylmercaptopenicillin (Penicillin 'O'), 327
Amine binding, 124, 125
  by ATP, 36
  effect of drugs on, 106
    of reserpine on, 148, 149
  non-specific, 106
Amine oxidase (mono-amine oxidase, MAO),
  catechol amines and, 103
  distribution in brain, 2
  5-hydroxytryptamine and, 126
  in CNS, 13
  α-methyldopa and, 145
Amine oxidase inhibitors,
  assessment, 60
  biochemical actions, 61
  clinical use, 18, 57–68, 73–75, 129, 145
  effect on brain amines, 19–24, 65
  formulae, 59
  in hypertension, 318
  in mental disease, 73
  pharmacological actions, 65 *et seq.*
  toxic effects, 67
Aminoacids, use with mercurials, 238, 239
Amino-glutethimide, 381
  formula, 382
6-Aminopenicillanic acid, 326, 327
Aminophylline,
  effect on mercurial diuretics, 236, 237
Aminopterin,
  effect on blood cholesterol, 304
  on fertility, 285
4-Aminoquinoline derivatives, 359
  amodiaquine, 359
  chloroquine, 359
  combination with primaquine, 365, 366
8-Aminoquinoline derivatives, 362–365
  pamaquin, 362
  primaquine, 362–365
p-Aminobenzylpenicillin (penicillin T), 333
Amitriptyline, 56, 57, 75
Ammonium chloride,
  use with mercurials, 237, 238
p-Aminosalicylic acid,
  effect on blood cholesterol, 297, 298
Amodiaquine, 359
  combination with primaquine, 365, 366
Amphenone B, 253
Amphetamine, 20, 33, 73, 143
  formula, 59
Amphotericin B, 343
Ampicillin, 326, 331–333
  antibacterial activity, 331
  clinical use, 333
  fate in body, 332
  resistance to, 332
  toxicity, 333
Anabolex, 289, *see* stanolone
Anabolic steroids, 288, 289
Analgesics, 386–390

Spermine oxidase, inhibition, 61
Spindle poisons, effect on fertility, 285
Spiramycin, 336
Spironolactone, 254, 269, 274
Sporonticides, 358
Stanolone (Anabolex), 289
Stelazine, 45, *see* trifluoperazine
Stemetil, 45, *see* prochlorperazine
Steroids, 261–293
  aldosterone, 268–274
  anabolic and androgenic steroids, 288–290
  corticosteroids, 261–267
  metabolism, 274–276
  progestogens, 276–280, 282–284
Storage of amines, 148
  of catechol amines, 100, 102
  of 5-hydroxytryptamine, 124
Storage of oxytocin and vasopressin, 172
SU 4885, 435, 454
SU 5171, 23
Suavitil, 56, *see* benactyzine
Substantia nigra, 33
Substance P, 29, 133, 167–169
  action on CNS, 34
  anticonvulsant action, 34
  chemistry, 169
  distribution, 168
    in brain, 33
  effect of drugs on brain concentration, 33
  estimation, 33, 167
  inactivation, 167
  in CNS, 33–35
  pharmacological actions, 168
Succinic dehydrogenase, inhibition, 61
Sucrose gradient, 6
Sulfinpyrazone, 389
Sulphadimethoxine, 322, 324
Sulphafurazole (Gantrisin), 322
Sulphamethoxypyridazine, 322, 323
Sulphaphenazole, 322, 323, 324
Sulphonamides anti-malarial action, 361
  potentiation of pyrimethamine, 361
Sulphonamides, with prolonged action, 322–324
Sulphones, 361
  potentiation of pyrimethamine, 361
Sulphonylureas, 204–208
  chemistry, 204, 205
  clinical use, 207–208
  fate in body, 205
  mode of action, 205–207
  toxic effects, 208
Sultam derivatives, 386
Sweat, kinin formation by, 161
Sympathetic nerves, amines in, 101, 102
Sympathectomy, effect on amine stores, 105
Sympathin, 95
Sympathomimetic amines, mode of action, 114, 116
Synaptic vesicles, 7
Synnematin B, 334
Synthetic hypoglycaemic agents, 203–211
  biguanides, 208–211
  history, 203
  sulphonylureas, 204–208

Tachyphylaxis, 142
Tanderil, 389, *see* oxyphenbutazone
Tapeworms,
  treatment with dichlorophen, 378
    with extract of male fern, 377
    with organic tin compounds, 377
    with Yomesan, 378
Taractan, 57, *see* chlorprothixene
Temaril, 44

Tentone, 44
Tersavid, 58, *see* pivazide
Tetrabenazine, 50
  effect on brain amines, 24
Tetrachlorethylene, in hookworm infection, 372, 373
β-Tetrahydronaphthylamine, 33
  effect on brain amines, 25
Tetra-iodothyroformic acid, effect on blood cholesterol, 302, 303
Tetra-iodi-D-thyronine, effect on blood cholesterol, 302
Thalidomide, 383
  congenital abnormalities, 383
  formula, 382
  peripheral neuritis, 383
Thioperazine, 45, 69
Thiopropazate, 45
Thioridazine, 45, 48, 69, 70
Thorazine, 44
Thrombocytosis, 67
Thyroxine analogues, effect on blood cholesterol, 302–304
D-Thyroxine, effect on blood cholesterol, 303
Threadworms,
  treatment with dithiazanine, 374
    with gentian violet, 373
    with piperazine, 369, 370
    with pyrvinium, 373
Thyroid hormones, effect on blood cholesterol, 302–304
TM6, *see* choline *p*-tolyl ether
TM10, *see* xylocholine
Toad skin, 45
Toclase, 392, *see* carbetapentane
Tofranil, 56, *see* imipramine
Tolbutamide, 204–208
Toryn, 392, *see* caramiphen
Tranquillizers, 42, *see* psychotropic drugs
Transmission at sympathetic nerve endings, 110
  in CNS, 37
Transortin, 275
Tranylcypromine, 58, 74
  action, 64
  in hypertension, 319
Trematodes, 374–377
  life cycle, 374, 375
  treatment with lucanthone, 375, 376
    with organic antimonials, 375
    with phenoxyalkanes, 376, 377
Triacetyloleandomycin, 336
Trifluoperazine, 45, 47, 70
Trifluopromazine, *see* fluopromazine
  activity, 48, 70
  formula, 44
Triiodothyroacetic acid, effect on blood cholesterol, 303
Tri-iodo-D-thyronine, effect on blood cholesterol, 302
Triiodothyropropionic acid, effect on blood cholesterol, 304
Trilafon, 45, *see* perphenazine
Trimeprazine, 44
Trimetaphan, 307
Trimethidinium, 306, 307
Triton A20, 349
Trophenium, 307, *see* phenactropinium
Trophotropic division of the subcortical system, 43
Trypsin, formation of bradykinin by, 157
Tryptamine, 142–144
  formula, 144
  5-HT antagonism, 124
  infusion, 144
  in urine, 26

RECENT ADVANCES
IN
PHARMACOLOGY